Systemic Disorders in Pregnancy

Richa Sharma • Arvind Kumar
Editors

Systemic Disorders in Pregnancy

Management Principles

Springer

Editors
Richa Sharma
Director Professor, Department of
Obstetrics and Gynecology
UCMS–GTB Hospital
New Delhi, Delhi, India

Arvind Kumar
Professor, Department of Medicine
Lala Lajpat Rai Memorial Medical College
Meerut, Uttar Pradesh, India

ISBN 978-981-96-4875-7 ISBN 978-981-96-4876-4 (eBook)
https://doi.org/10.1007/978-981-96-4876-4

This Springer imprint is published by the registered company Springer Nature Singapore Pte Ltd.
The registered company address is: 152 Beach Road, #21-01/04 Gateway East, Singapore 189721, Singapore

Preface

Systemic disorders in Pregnancy: Insight and Management Algorithms is a comprehensive book that is designed to provide A to Z information about systemic disorders in pregnancy. There are always dilemmas and challenges in diagnosis and treatment; this book aims to guide the management, along with an easy understanding of complex issues associated with systemic problems during pregnancy. Recent advances and relevant guidelines have been incorporated. This book also deals with management algorithms and exact standard operating procedures. It also describes periconceptional management, differential diagnosis, prevention, and latest guidelines and recommendations regarding medical disorders during pregnancy. The contribution from various eminent authors has turned this book into an excellent piece of knowledge and information to the readers. This is the recommended textbook, for all family healthcare providers, gynecologists, and obstetricians.

Delhi, India
Meerut, UP, India

Richa Sharma
Arvind Kumar

Acknowledgments

We express our deepest gratitude to all the eminent authors, for sparing their time and contributing the chapters; their valuable contribution of knowledge has resulted this book into a signature piece of its own kind. The latest guidelines, illustrations, flowcharts, and key points are beautifully described and will be useful in everyone's routine practice. The best part of acknowledgments is that we get to thank all the people who have supported us in writing the book, since it is a combined effort of all people who have come together in many different ways. Foremost we want to offer this endeavor to Almighty for the wisdom he bestowed upon us, the strength, peace of mind, and good health in order to finish his book. Our heartfelt thanks to the Springer publication to convert our dream into reality. Their support has been indispensable in bringing this book to life. We are greatly thankful to our editorial team for perfect coordination of work, support, and encouragement. We cannot express enough thanks to our loving family for providing immense support and motivation to accomplish this endeavor.

Delhi, India
Meerut, UP, India

Richa Sharma
Arvind Kumar

Contents

About the Editors

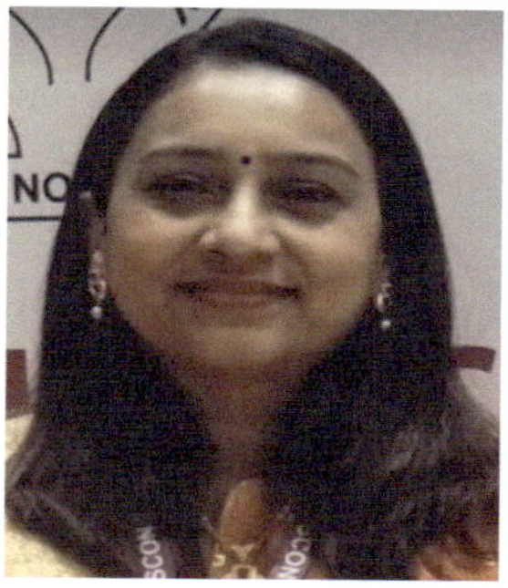

Richa Sharma (MS, MNAMS, FICOG, FICMCH, FMAS, FRM) is Director Professor in the Department of Obstetrics and Gynecology, University College of Medical Sciences & Guru Tegh Bahadur Hospital (UCMS & GTB Hospital), Delhi. Her area of interest is high risk pregnancy, Gyn Endoscopy. She is Gyn endoscopic & Robotic Surgeon and infertility and IVF specialist. Dr. Sharma has many publications in international and national journals and had presented various research papers and posters in international and national conferences. She has received several prestigious awards and prizes.

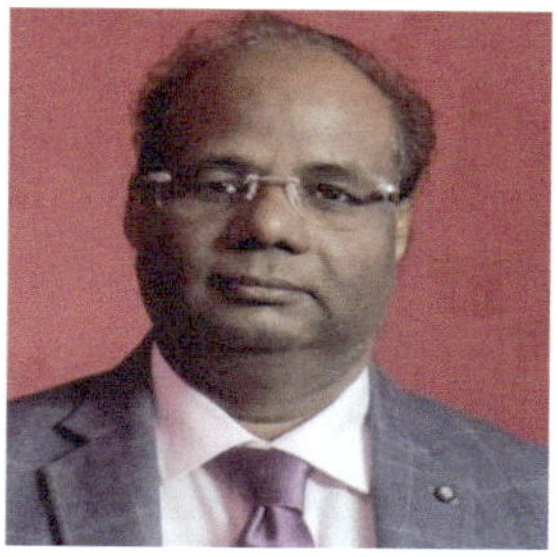

Arvind Kumar (MD FICP, FIACM) is Professor in the Department of Medicine and head of cardiology unit, LLRM Medical College, Meerut, Uttar Pradesh, India. Dr. Kumar achieved Fellowship in Cardiology from GB Pant Hospital, Delhi, India. He is an active governing body member of Indian Association of Clinical Medicine and UP Diabetes Association. He has authored various chapters in medicine and cardiology books and has many publications in national and international journals.

Physiological Changes in Pregnancy 1

Kanchan Rani and Divya Suman

A pregnant woman undergoes many anatomical and physiological changes in order to nurture the growing fetus. These changes are essential to fulfill the sudden increased metabolic demands and to prepare the woman for childbirth. The changes start to occur just after conception and restore prepregnancy status few weeks after birth with few residuals.

It is important to understand these physiological changes to differentiate a pathological condition from normal physiology or unmasking a preexisting condition that can aggravate during pregnancy. A thorough knowledge of these adaptions is required for better management of pregnancy.

1.1 Cardiovascular System

Pregnancy is affiliated with massive physiological and cardiovascular changes as increased heart rate, cardiac output, stroke volume, and decreased peripheral vascular resistance [1].

The vasodilatation caused by progesterone, NO, and prostaglandins results in peripheral vasodilatation. This phenomena causes 20% increase in cardiac output by 8 weeks of gestation [2]. This increase in cardiac output almost stabilizes between 28 and 32 weeks [+40–50%], but there is significant rise of almost additional 40% at delivery and up to 75% immediate postpartum (Fig. 1.1).

K. Rani (✉)
Obstetrics and Gynaecology, TMMC and RC, Moradabad, Uttar Pradesh, India

D. Suman
Consultant Department of Obstetrics and Gynaecology, Vaidyam Superspeciality Hospital, Patna, Bihar, India

R. Sharma, A. Kumar (eds.), *Systemic Disorders in Pregnancy*,
https://doi.org/10.1007/978-981-96-4876-4_1

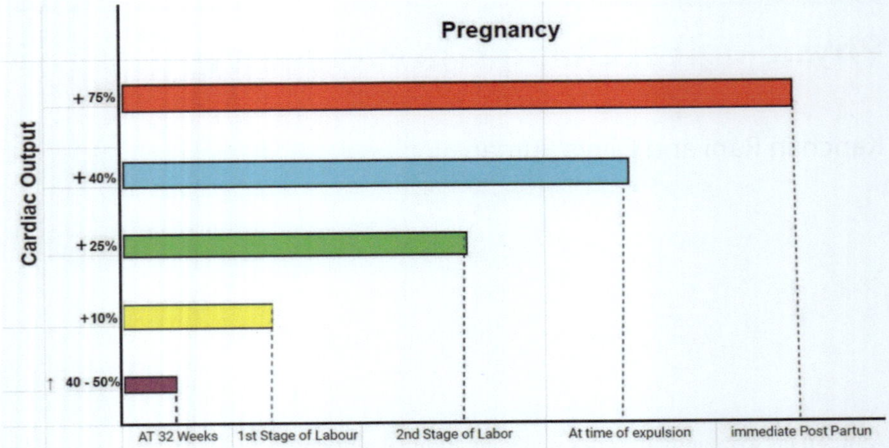

Fig. 1.1 Cardiac output changes during pregnancy

This increased cardiac output is mainly observed due to raised stroke volume and the increased heart rate [3]. This physiological change results in increased blood flow to uterus, placenta, skin, and extremities and helps in maintaining maternal thermal regulation. In the third trimester, the increased heart rate is responsible for maintaining the rise in cardiac output. This is particularly helpful to meet the tenfold increase in uterine blood flow and 50% increase in renal blood flow. There is also an autotransfusion of almost 500 ml of blood back to the maternal circulation due to uterine contraction in active labor.

The decreased peripheral vascular resistance causes a fall in blood pressure of mother in early pregnancy. This fall in blood pressure reaches its minimum by 20–24 weeks resulting in physiological hypotension of pregnancy. There is secondary rise in blood pressure, which results in prepregnancy level of blood pressure by term [4].

These cardiovascular changes will result in many clinical findings as majority of pregnant mothers can develop a systolic murmur, few can develop a diastolic murmur. Almost 80% of mothers can have a third heart sound and approximately 16% can have a fourth heart sound [5]. Small Q waves and inverted T waves in lead III, ST-segment depression and T-wave inversion in the lateral and inferior leads, and left-axis shift of the QRS complex are considered normal in pregnancy [3]. Maternal venous pressure is also markedly raised due to pressure effect of enlarged uterus on the common iliac veins. This physiological change explains the development of edema, varicose veins, and piles (Table 1.1).

Table 1.1 Cardiovascular changes during pregnancy

Cardiovascular physiology	Changes observed in pregnancy
Cardiac output	Increased up to 40–50% of prepregnancy value at 28–32 weeks. Increased up to 40% of pre-labor value at labor Increased up to 75% of pre-labor value at immediate postpartum
Stroke volume	Increased up to 20–30% of prepregnancy value.
Heart rate	Increased up to 15–20% of prepregnancy value
Venous pressure	Increased up to 100% of prepregnancy value
Systemic vascular resistance	Decreased up to 20% of prepregnancy value
Pulmonary vascular resistance	Decreased up to 30% of prepregnancy value

1.2 Hematological System

There is systemic vasodilatation and increased vascular capacitance in pregnancy, which can lead to undefiled vascular system [6]. As a result, to compensate for this physiology and blood loss during pregnancy, the maternal blood volume is raised by 40–50% [7]. Other than this there is also an increase in red blood mass of 20–30% due to increased erythropoiesis. This disproportionate rise in blood volume and RBC results in physiological anemia of pregnancy and lower blood viscosity [8]. The lower blood viscosity results in a decrease in the blood flow viscosity of utero-placental unit and hence helps in optimized oxygen flow to growing fetus and prevents red blood mass loss during childbirth. But this increase in red blood mass needs increased iron supplement throughout pregnancy. A pregnant mother requires 1gm of additional iron supplement till term, one-third of this value is needed for feta-placental unit and two-third for the mother herself. However, this requirement is more in third trimester (3.0–7.5 mg/day) than in first trimester (0.8 mg/day) [9]. Other than this the requirement of folate increased by 10–20 folds and a twofold increase in the requirement for vitamin B12 is seen during pregnancy (Tables 1.2 and 1.3).

Pregnancy is a physiological hypercoagulable state; this helps in early homeostasis in postpartum period [10]. There is a marked rise in fibrinogen level along with certain clotting factors as factor VIII, IX, and X. The concentration of protein s and antithrombin falls in pregnancy. There is shortened aPTT due to increase in the level of factor VIII; however, the prothrombin time and thrombin time is not changed [8]. The cumulative effect of these changes results in increased risk of venous thromboembolism in a pregnant women.

Although there is increased production of platelets, due to hemodilution and raised platelet destruction, pregnancy is associated with physiological thrombocytopenia, which restores its normal value in postpartum period [11].

A gradual increase in leucocytes count is also seen (around 15,000/mm) [12], as result the severity of infection rises during pregnancy.

Table 1.2 Coagulation system alteration during pregnancy

Coagulation system	Changes in pregnancy
Fibrinogen level	Significant rise
Clotting factor VIII, IX, X LEVEL	Increased
Protein S	Decreased
Antithrombin	Decreased
Platelet count	Static or decreased

Table 1.3 Hematological changes during pregnancy

Hematological parameters	Changes observed in pregnancy
Plasma volume	Additional rise up to 40–50%
Blood volume	Additional rise up to 30–40%
Red cell mass	Additional rise up to 20–30%
Hemoglobin concentration	Additional rise up to 18–20%
Hematocrit value	Decreased

1.3 Renal System

As a result of effects of progesterone and relaxin on smooth muscles, there is dilatation of urinary collecting system. This leads to urinary stasis in a pregnant mother and makes the woman more prone to UTI and pyelonephritis with asymptomatic bacteriuria [13].

There is increase in GFR (glomerular filtration rate) by almost 50% and approximately 80% enhancement in renal plasma flow due to the raised blood flow to the kidneys. This increased GFR causes decreased concentration of creatinine, urea, and uric acid. This is particularly important to diagnose an altered kidney function in pregnancy, as a slightest rise (above 0.8 mg/dL) is indicative of major dysfunction [4] (Fig. 1.2 and Table 1.4).

The increased production of aldosterone during pregnancy along with the estrogen produced by placenta leads to significant water and sodium retention in pregnancy. The cumulative effect can be seen as the rise of almost 1.5 L of water [13].

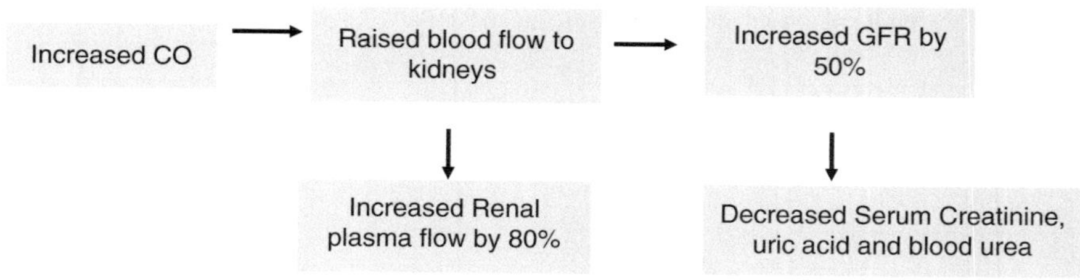

Fig. 1.2 Renal system alteration during pregnancy

Table 1.4 Renal system changes during pregnancy

Renal system	Physiological effects
Blood flow to kidneys	Increased
GFR	Increased by 50%
Renal plasma flow	Increased by 80%
Serum creatinine, uric acid, blood urea	Decreased
Aldosterone	Increased

1.4 Respiratory System

Pregnancy is associated with 15% increase in metabolic rate and 20% enhanced consumption of oxygen; this causes a large increase in oxygen demand. The gradual rise in progesterone level from the first trimester results in an increased tidal volume by approximately 30–50% [14]. As a result of this significant increase in tidal volume, the minute ventilation, which is a product of tidal volume and respiratory rate, rises by 30–50%. This is to note that respiratory rate of a pregnant woman remains almost unaffected during pregnancy.

This increase in minute ventilation causes the state of hyperventilation, resulting in the rise in arterial pO2 and fall in arterial pCO2 [15]. As a result of this, pregnancy is associated with slight respiratory alkalosis, which is metabolically compensated by fall in serum bicarbonate to18–22 mmol/L [16]. This physiological adaption of pregnancy causes a right shift of oxyhemoglobin dissociation curve, which finally results in better oxygen transfer to the fetus.

There is up to 200% rise in minute ventilation in labor, depending on the stage of labor, which causes more pronounced fall of PaCO2. During labor and delivery, oxygen consumption rises due to exaggerated maternal effects to deliver the baby and finally oxygen demand outpaces the supply and anaerobic metabolism sets resulting in lactic acid production [17, 18].

Other than progesterone, the increase in estrogen causes increased vascularity and edema of the upper respiratory tract [19]. This increase in vascularity and edema worsens the Mallampati scoring and makes the intubation difficult and also, causes increased risk of bleeding while putting a nasotracheal tube [20] (Table 1.5).

Table 1.5 Respiratory system alteration during pregnancy

Investigations	Results in pregnancy
pH	7.35–7.45
pCO2 mmHg	35–40
pO2 mmHg	90–100
Base excess	+2 to −2
Bicarbonates (mmol/L)	20–28

The intra-abdominal pressure is raised during pregnancy due the enlarging uterus and this causes the diaphragm to shift upward up to 5 cm. As a result of this, there is bibasilar alveolar collapse and basilar atelectasis, leading to decrease in the functional residual capacity and expiratory reserve volume [20]. Although, the vital capacity remains unaffected as the decrease in expiratory reserve volume is accompanied by increased inspiratory reserve volumes, this decreased functional residual capacity may result in hypoxemia to a pregnant woman during induction of general anesthesia [4].

1.5 Gastrointestinal System

In early weeks of pregnancy, nausea and vomiting is very common. The exact mechanism responsible for this is not known but pregnancy related hormones like human chorionic gonadotropin (hCG), estrogen, and progesterone could be involved in the etiology. This results in decreased drug absorption and lower plasma concentration of drugs.

The enlarged uterus and increased level of progesterone leads to delayed gastric emptying, reduced muscle tone of the lower esophageal sphincter, and prolonged small bowel transit time. The cumulative effect of all these results in pregnancy-associated gastroesophageal reflux disease (GERD) [21]. There is an increase in gastric pH leading to ionization of weak acids, reducing absorption. Also, drug interaction of antacid and iron causing chelation of co-administered drug is also important to take in account while prescribing medicines [22].

1.6 Endocrine System

1.6.1 Thyroid

In a nonpregnant woman, the anterior pituitary releases thyroid-stimulating hormone (TSH) and prolactin (PRL): this is mediated by thyrotrophin-releasing hormone (TRH),which is produced in the hypothalamus. In pregnancy, the level of TSH and prolactin increases due to additional release of placental TRH. There is increased level of thyroxine (T4) and tri-iodothyronine (T3). The production of thyroxine-binding globulin also increases, so, there is only slight alteration in the levels of serum-free T4 (fT4) and T3 (fT3) levels [23]. The concentrations of serum TSH are slightly decreased in the first trimester due to the thyrotropic effects of increased levels of hCG. Therefore, free T4 (fT4) and T3 (fT3) levels are the clinical determinants to rule out any thyroid condition in pregnancy. This approximate 50% enhancement of thyroid production helps in brain development and thyroid function of ingrowing fetus [24]. There is relative iodine deficiency in pregnancy due to increased demand by fetes and increased iodine excretion in urine. Therefore, WHO recommends an increased uptake of iodine (150–200 mg/day) to pregnant individuals [25].

1.6.2 Pituitary Gland

The lactotroph hyperplasia of pregnancy results in enlarged pituitary, which further leads to almost tenfold increase in prolactin levels. This physiological adaption is required for breast preparation for future lactation [24]. This increased level of prolactin is mainly due to increased serum estradiol during pregnancy. The enhanced level of estrogen, progesterone, and inhibin puts the negative feedback on pituitary and so the levels of LH and FSH are reduced. Production of oxytocin from posterior pituitary keeps increasing throughout pregnancy and peaks at term.

1.6.3 Adrenal Gland

Pregnancy is a state of physiological hypercortisolism [26]. This hypercortisolism is responsible for clinical manifestations like raised BP, impaired glucose metabolism, and few skin changes. Although, a balanced rise of cortisol is essential for the brain development of fetus, an excess rise can lead to impaired neural development [27].

The levels of endorphins and enkephalin is also raised in pregnancy; this causes increased pain threshold and helps to combat labor pain [28].

1.7 Metabolic Changes

1.7.1 Glucose Metabolism

Pregnancy is associated with major changes in glucose metabolism to deviate glucose to the growing fetus, while keeping maternal nutrition intact. So, there is development of a diabetogenic state during pregnancy [29].

Although there is increased insulin secretion and sensitivity in early pregnancy, insulin resistance develops progressively from second trimester and reaches its peak in the third trimester [30]. This insulin resistance along with relative hypoglycemia results in lipolysis, allowing the pregnant mother to preferentially use fat for fuel and preserve available glucose and amino acids for the fetus, minimizing protein catabolism. This physiological adaption is the result of enhanced secretion of human placental lactogen, growth hormone, progesterone, cortisol, and prolactin, which causes a decrease in insulin sensitivity [31]. Chances of gestational diabetes mellitus (GDM) increases in women whose pancreatic function is impaired as she is unable to overcome this physiological adaption of insulin resistance.

From a clinical point of view, fasting blood glucose should not be considered a parameter for glycemic assessment of a woman as fasting blood glucose can be decreased due to shunting of glucose to the fetus, decreased glucose production by liver, enhanced peripheral glucose use, and increased storage of tissue glycogen [32].

1.7.2 Iron Metabolism

There is an increase in iron demand during pregnancy, firstly due to the enhancement of red cell mass and secondly due to the placenta and fetus. This demand is mainly in the second half of the pregnancy when the daily requirement almost reach to 6–7 mg. To meet this increased demand, there is increased absorption from the gut, but dietary availability of iron is inadequate to meet the demands. Thus, iron supplementation is a must in pregnancy. The ferrous form of the iron is absorbed from duodenum and jejunum; this is only 10% of ingested iron. Now, this absorbed iron is released as transferrin to the maternal circulation and incorporates in hemoglobin and ferritin. The transportation of iron from placenta to fetus is not dependent on maternal iron deficiency. The active transportation continues even in severe maternal anemia.

1.7.3 Calcium Metabolism

There is increased intestinal absorption of calcium in a pregnant mother starting from the 12th week, which helps to meet the increased need of the growing fetus. Although, major calcium requirement to the fetus is needed in the last trimester, this early increased absorption helps in building a good store [33]. Hemodilution in pregnancy causes a decrease in serum albumin level, which further lowers the albumin bound fraction of calcium, resulting in decreased serum calcium levels. But the level of ionized calcium remains same; this helps in fulfilling the fatal demand of 30 gm of calcium [34].

1.7.4 Lipid Metabolism

There is an increase in the synthesis of triglyceride by liver and fall in the lipase activity of lipoprotein. This results in decreased catabolism of adipose tissues and rise in the level of triglycerides in maternal blood. This raised triglyceride is essential for the energy requirement of the pregnant woman. Total serum cholesterol also rises in pregnancy. At term pregnancy the level of high-density lipoprotein rises up to 15% along with up to 50% rise of the low-density lipoprotein (LDL) cholesterol. The increase in LDL cholesterol is important for placental steroidogenesis.

1.7.5 Protein Metabolism

The large demand of amino acids for developing fetus enhanced the requirement of protein for mother. As a results, maternal protein catabolism is decreased and fat stores are the primary source to provide energy to the mother.

Key Points

1. Pregnancy is associated with increased metabolic demands and physiological adaption in order to support the growing fetus. There are end numbers of anatomical and physiological changes that helps to prepare a mother to give birth.
2. Significant increase in cardiac output along with stroke volume and heart rate prepare the heart to fulfill the demand of increased blood flow during pregnancy and labor.
3. Pregnancy is a state of hypercoagulability due to significant rise in fibrinogen and some clotting factors along with decrease in the level of protein s and antithrombin.
4. Physiological anemia of pregnancy is the result of physiological hemodilution of pregnancy. For sufficient oxygen supply to fetus, slight respiratory alkalosis develops causing a rightward shift of oxyhemoglobin dissociation curve.
5. Endocrine system shows significant changes, especially in the thyroid, pituitary, and adrenal glands.
6. Increased demand of iron is met with changes in iron metabolism and iron supplementation and glucose metabolism is altered, making pregnancy a diabetogenic state.

References

1. Klein HH, Pich S. Cardiovascular changes during pregnancy. Herz. 2003;28(3):173–4.
2. Gaiser R. Physiologic changes of pregnancy. In: Chestnut DH, Wng CA, Tsen LC, Ngan Kee WD, Beilin Y, Mhyre JM, et al., editors. Chestnut's obstetric anesthesia: principles and practice. 5th ed. Philadelphia: Elsevier Saunders; 2014. p. 15–38.
3. Soma-Pillay P, Nelson-Piercy C, Tolppanen H, Mebazaa A. Physiological changes in pregnancy. Cardiovasc J Afr. 2016;27(2):89–94.
4. Pacheco L, Costantine MM, Hankins GDV. Physiologic changesduring pregnancy. In: Mattison DR, editor. Clincal pharmacology during pregnancy. San Diego: Academic Press; 2013. p. 5–14.
5. Breuer HW. Auscultation of the heart in pregnancy (author's transl). MMW Munch Med Wochenschr. 1981;123(45):1705–7.
6. Kepley JM, Bates K, Mohiuddin SS. Physiology, Maternal changes. [Updated 2023 Mar 12]. In: StatPearls [Internet]. Treasure Island (FL): StatPearls Publishing; 2024.

7. Rodger M, Sheppard D, Gandara E, Tinmouth A. Haematologicalproblems in obstetrics. Best Prac Res Clin Obstet Gynaecol. 2015;29(5):671–84.
8. Chandra S, Tripathi AK, Mishra S, Amzarul M, Vaish AK. Physiological changes in hematological parameters during pregnancy. Indian J Hematol Blood Transfus. 2012;28(3):144–6.
9. Brannon PM, Taylor CL. Iron supplementation during pregnancy and infancy: uncertainties and implications for research and policy. Nutrients. 2017;9(12)
10. Ramsay M. Normal hematological changes during pregnancy andthe puerperium. In: Pavord S, Hunt B, editors. The obstetric hematology manual. Cambridge: Cambridge University Press; 2010. p. 3–12.
11. Burrows RF, Kelton JG. Incidentally detected thrombocytopeniain healthy mothers and their infants. N Engl J Med. 1988;319:142–5.
12. Palmer SK, Zamudio S, Coffin C, Parker S, Stamm E, Moore LG, et al. Quantitative estimation of human uterine artery bloodflow and pelvic blood flow redistribution in pregnancy. Obstet Gynecol. 1992;80:1000–6.
13. Cheung KL, Lafayette RA. Renal physiology of pregnancy. Adv Chronic Kidney Dis. 2013;20(3):209–14.
14. McAuliffe F, Kametas N, Costello J, Rafferty GF, Greenough A, Nicolaides K. Respiratory function in singleton and twin pregnancy. BJOG. 2002;109:765–8. https://doi.org/10.1111/j.1471-0528.2002.01515.x.
15. Shankar KB, Moseley H, Vemula V, Ramasamy M, Kumar Y. Arterial to end-tidal carbon dioxide tension difference during anaesthesia in early pregnancy. Can J Anaesth. 1989;36(2):124–7.
16. Dayal P, Murata Y, Takamura H. Antepartum and postpartum acid-base changes in maternal blood in normal and complicated pregnancies. J Obstet Gynaecol Br Commonw. 1972;79(7):612–24.
17. Hägerdal M, Morgan CW, Sumner AE, Gutsche BB. Minute ventilation and oxygen consumption during labor with epidural analgesia. Anesthesiology. 1983;59(5):425–7.
18. Jouppila R, Hollmén A. The effect of segmental epidural analgesia on maternal and foetal acid-base balance, lactate, serum potassium and creatine phosphokinase during labour. Acta Anaesthesiol Scand. 1976;20(3):259–68.
19. Taylor M. An experimental study of the influence of the endocrine sys-tem on the nasal respiratory mucosa. J Laryngol Otol. 1961;75:972–7. https://doi.org/10.1017/S0022215100058746.
20. Baldwin GR, Moorthi DS, Whelton JA, MacDonnell KF. Newlung functions in pregnancy. Am J Obstet Gynecol. 1977;127:235–9.
21. Everson GT. Gastrointestinal motility in pregnancy. Gastroenterol Clin N Am. 1992;21(4):751–76.
22. Carter BL, Garnett WR, Pellock JM, Stratton MA, Howell JR. Effect of antacids on phenytoin bioavailability. Ther Drug Monit. 1981;3(333):340. https://doi.org/10.1097/00007691-198104000-00003.
23. Harada A, Hershman JM, Reed AW, Braunstein GD, Dignam WJ, Derzko C, Friedman S, Jewelewicz R, Pekary AE. Comparison of thyroid stimulators and thyroid hormone concentrations in the sera of pregnant women. J Clin Endocrinol Metab. 1979;48(5):793–7.
24. Napso T, Yong HEJ, Lopez-Tello J, Sferruzzi-Perri AN. The role of placental hormones in mediating maternal adaptations to support pregnancy and lactation. Front Physiol. 2018;9:1091.
25. Glinoer D. The regulation of thyroid function in pregnancy: pathwaysof endocrine adaptation from physiology to pathology. Endocr Rev. 1997;18:404.
26. Rosenthal HE, Slaunwhite WR, Sandberg AA. Transcortin: a corticosteroid-binding protein of plasma. X. Cortisol and progesterone interplay and unbound levels of these steroids in pregnancy. J Clin Endocrinol Metab. 1969;29(3):352–67.
27. Kapoor A, Dunn E, Kostaki A, Andrews MH, Matthews SG. Fetal programming of hypothalamo-pituitary-adrenal function: prenatal stress and glucocorticoids. J Physiol. 2006;572(Pt 1):31–44.
28. Abboud TK, Sarkis F, Hung TT, Khoo SS, Varakian L, Henriksen E, Noueihed R, Goebelsmann U. Effects of epidural anesthesia during labor on maternal plasma beta-endorphin levels. Anesthesiology. 1983;59(1):1–5.

29. Angueira AR, Ludvik AE, Reddy TE, Wicksteed B, et al. New insightsinto gestational glucose metabolism: lessons learned from 21st centuryapproaches. Diabetes. 2015;64:327–34.
30. Butte NF. Carbohydrate and lipid metabolism in pregnancy: normalcompared with gestational diabetes mellitus. Am J Clin Nutr. 2000;71:125S.
31. Newbern D, Freemark M. Placental hormones and the control of mater-nal metabolism and fetal growth. Curr Opin Endocrinol Diabetes Obes. 2011;18:409–16.
32. Brizzi P, Tonolo G, Esposito F, et al. Lipoprotein metabolism duringnormal pregnancy. Am J Obstet Gynecol. 1999;181:430.
33. Davison JM, Sheills EA, Barron WM, Robinson AG, Lindheimer MD. Changes in the metabolic clearance of vasopressin and in plasmavasopressinase throughout human pregnancy. J Clin Invest. 1989;83(4):1313–8.
34. Woodrow JP, Sharpe CJ, Fudge NJ, Hoff AO, Gagel RF, Kovacs CS. Calcitonin plays a critical role in regulating skeletal mineral metabolismduring lactation. Endocrinology. 2006;147:4010–21.

2 Anemia in Pregnancy

Indranil Dutta and Dilip Kumar Dutta

Anemia in pregnancy is defined as, hemoglobin value less than 11 g/dl (7.45 mmol/L) and hematocrit of less than 0.33 (33%) (WHO 1992; WHO 2001) (Table 2.1). The normal range of Hb in adult women is 12–14 gm%.

Iron deficiency is the main cause of anemia, which is the most prevalent nutritional deficiency worldwide, affecting 33% of nonpregnant women, 40% of pregnant women, and 42% of children worldwide (Table 2.2)

Table 2.1 Degree of anemia is graded according to hemoglobin level

Mild	Hb level	9.0–10.9 g/dL
Moderate		7.0–8.9 g/dL
Severe		4–6.9 g/dL
Very severe		<4 g/dL

Table 2.2 Classification of anemia in pregnancy

Acquired	Hereditary
1. Iron deficiency anemia 2. Anemia caused by blood loss 3. Acute 4. Chronic (Hook worm infestation, bleeding piles, etc.) 5. Megaloblastic anemia (vitamin B12/folic acid deficiency) 6. Acquired hemolytic anemia 7. Aplastic or hypoplastic anemia	1. Thalassemias 2. Sickle cell hemoglobinopathies 3. Other hemoglobinopathies 4. Hereditary hemolytic anemia (RBC membrane defects, spherocytosis)

I. Dutta (✉)
Department of OBG, IQ City Medical College, Durgapur, West Bengal, India

D. K. Dutta
GICE Hospital, Kalyani, West Bengal, India

R. Sharma, A. Kumar (eds.), *Systemic Disorders in Pregnancy*, https://doi.org/10.1007/978-981-96-4876-4_2

2.1 Physiological Changes in Pregnancy

Iron demand during pregnancy is nearly 900–1000 mg (Table 2.3) and the average daily requirement is 4–6 mg/day (Table 2.4). The red blood cell (RBC) mass and plasma volume increases by 30% and 40–50%, respectively, causing fall in Hb by 2 g/dL due to erythrocyte dilution by 5–15%.The picture on peripheral smear remains normocytic and normochromic, this phenomenon is called *physiologic anemia of pregnancy*. The decrease in blood viscosity results in a reduced load on the heart during pregnancy and may also facilitate blood flow through the placenta. The increased blood volume also offers a protective buffer against blood loss in the third stage of labor. Circulatory overload can be dangerous in women having anemia and cardiac diseases.

Table 2.3 Iron demand in pregnancy

Iron demand in pregnancy: 900 mg	
Fetus and placenta	500–600 mg
Loss in average blood loss during delivery	150–200 mg
Consumed in increased hemoglobin mass	500 mg
Saved as a result of amenorrhea	225 mg
This leaves an iron deficit of 600–700 mg	

Table 2.4 Iron daily needs

Daily intake should be 4–6 mg/day approximately	
Below 20 weeks	2.5 mg/day
20–32 weeks	5.5 mg/day
32 weeks onward	6–8 mg/day

2.2 Incidence and Prevalence

According to the prevalence of anemia, different geographical regions are categorized as follows:

High prevalence	>40% (of Sub-Saharan Africa, Southeast Asia)
Medium prevalence	15–39%
Low prevalence	5–14.9%
Not a problem	<5%

Anemia is responsible for 40–60% of maternal deaths in developing countries. It also increases perinatal mortality and morbidity rates (W.H.O 1997).

2.3 Prevalence of Anemia in Pregnancy

Overall prevalence—Nearly 40% of women worldwide are anemic and the prevalence of anemia is 3–4 times more in developing countries. According to WHO, 56% of Southeast Asian women are anemic.

India accounts for 88% prevalence of anemia in pregnancy (WHO Global Database 1997).

2.4 Causes of Increased Prevalence of Iron Deficiency Anemia (IDA)

- Dietary habits: Consumption of low bioavailability diet
- Food Faddism
- Defective iron absorption due to intestinal infections, hook worm infestation, amebiasis, and giardiasis
- Increased iron loss: Frequent pregnancies, menorrhagia, hook worm infestation, chronic malaria, excessive sweating, piles
- Repeated and closely spaced pregnancies and prolonged period of lactation

2.5 Iron Deficiency Anemia

Iron deficiency anemia is the most common type of anemia in pregnancy. Nutritional iron consists of heme iron pool and non-heme iron pool.

Heme Iron Pool: Usually its absorption is 15–30%, but it rises up to 50% in iron deficiency anemia. Food rich in heme molecules are meat, mutton, eggs, etc., and their absorption is not altered by any inhibitors.

Non-Heme Iron Pool: Their absorption is increased and decreased by enhancers and inhibitors, respectively. Food rich in non-heme contents are cereals, vegetables, milk, and eggs.

Enhancers: Ascorbic acid, ferrous iron, gastric acidity, alcohol, decreased iron stores, raised erythropoietic activity.
Inhibitors: Phytates, calcium, tannins, tea, and coffee.

- *Iron Metabolism*
- Total quantity of iron in the body—4–5gms
- 65%—hemoglobin
- 4%—myoglobin
- 1%—various heme compounds
- 0.1%—combined with protein transferrin in the plasma
- 15–30%—stored in RE system and liver parenchyma in the form of ferritin

2.5.1 Transport and Storage of Iron

Iron is absorbed from the small intestine, combines in the blood plasma to a protein called apo-transferrin to form transferrin, which is then transported in the plasma. Excess iron is deposited in the liver hepatocytes and reticuloendothelial cells of the bone marrow. Transferrin binds to receptors on cell surface and enters the cell. Iron is released and binds to apoferritin (high mol. Wt. and can store large amounts of iron) to form ferritin, This iron stored as ferritin is called storage iron. When storage iron is in excess, it is stored as hemosiderin, an extremely insoluble form. This occurs when the total quantity of iron in the body is more than the apoferritin storage pool can accommodate; when plasma transferrin levels fall, iron is released from its storage molecule, ferritin. This iron is then transported again in the form of transferrin in the plasma to the portions of the body where it is needed. When there are inadequate stores and plasma transferrin levels fall, it presents as severe hypochromic anemia.

2.6 Approach to a Case of Anemia (Figs. 2.1 and 2.2)

Primary steps in the evaluation of anemia during pregnancy are as follows:

1. To assess the severity of anemia by clinical and laboratory parameters
2. Typing of anemia
3. Identify the etiology of anemia

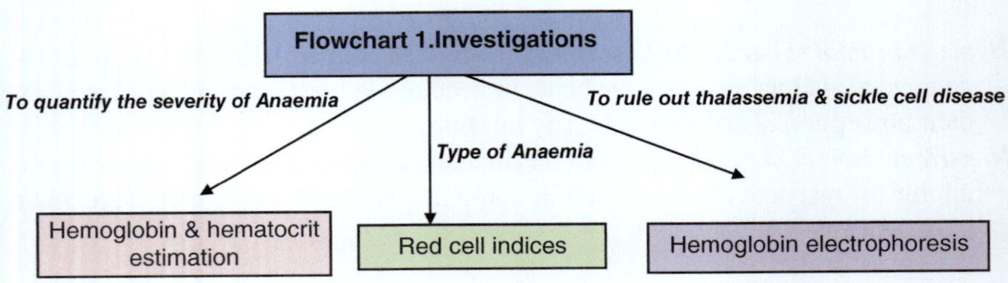

Fig. 2.1 Diagnosis and treatment

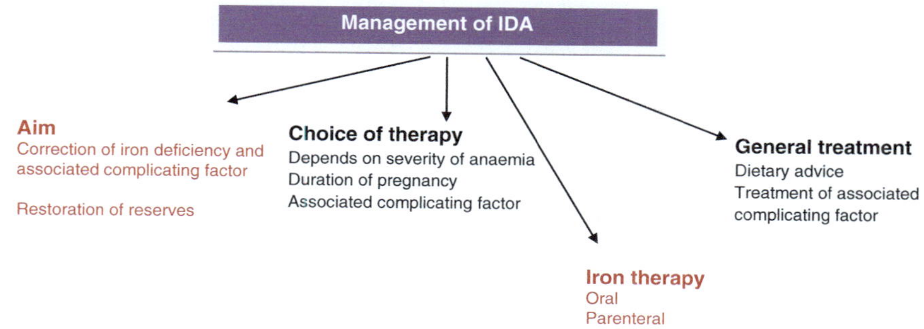

Fig. 2.2 Management of IDA

Table 2.5 Clinical features related to severity of anemia

Symptoms	Signs
1. Weakness	1. General physical examination
2. Light-headedness	2. Pallor of mucous membranes and nailbeds
3. Headache	3. Koilonychia or platonychia
4. Loss of appetite	4. Cheilosis
5. Dysphasia	5. Glossitis and stomatitis
6. Skin and nail changes	6. Features of cardiac decompensation: tachycardia, tachypnea, increased jugular venous pressure, heart murmurs, ankle edema, and postural hypotension
7. Ankle swelling	7. Specific features pointing toward the etiology
8. Dyspnea on exertion	8. Jaundice indicating hemolytic pathology
9. Palpitations	9. Leg ulcers in sickle cell anemia
10. Worsening of preexisting angina	10. Spotted nails and koilonychia suggesting iron deficiency
	11. Neurological deficit in megaloblastic anemia
	12. Hepatosplenomegaly in hemolytic anemias, malignancy, and parasitic infestations
	13. Frontal bossing in thalassemia
	14. Lymphadenopathy or sternal tenderness in blood dyscrasias and metastasis

4. Identify the predisposing and precipitating factors

History of passing worms in the stool, bleeding per rectum, hematuria, hyperemesis, Malabsorption. H/o chronic diseases like tuberculosis, malaria, bleeding diathesis, excessive menstrual blood loss, type of contraception practiced, obstetric hemorrhage & infections, H/o dietary intake of iron containing foods, hematinics & drugs causing bone marrow suppression or folate deficiency & h/o pica (Table 2.5)

Anemia during pregnancy has several devastating maternal and fetal effects (Tables 2.6 and 2.7)

Table 2.6 Effects of anemia on pregnancy

Antenatal	Intranatal	Postnatal
Poor weight gain	Dysfunctional labor	Puerperal sepsis
Preterm labor	Hemorrhage and shock	Subinvolution
Pre-eclampsia	Cardiac failure	Embolism
Abruptio placentae		
Premature rupture of membranes		
Intercurrent infections		

Table 2.7 Fetal effects. Poor perinatal outcome is seen in both, with excess or low maternal Hb levels

Excess levels of hemoglobin leads to hemoconcentration, blood clogging, and decreased placental flow	*Decreased hemoglobin* results in poor placental oxygenation
	2–four fold increased risk of preterm birth, FGR, LBW Low APGAR score
	Low iron store during neonatal and anemia during infancy
	Failure to thrive
	Hampered intellectual development

Table 2.8 RBC Indices (help in indicating the probable etiology of anemia)

↓MCV, ↓MCH, ↓MCHC. MCV is the most sensitive indicator *MCV:* average volume of a red cell [normal – 80–95 fl] *MCH:* average hemoglobin content in a red cell [normal – 27–32 pg] *MCHC:* average concentration of Hb in a RBC [t weight of Hb/vol in which it is contained] (normal – 34–37 g/d)
MCV is the most important of all the indices in distinguishing the type of anemia. *It increases by 3–4 fl during physiological macrocytosis of pregnancy, which makes it a poor indicator for iron deficiency.*
Since mixed nutritional deficiencies are common in pregnancy, MCV may be found normal with combined deficiency of iron and folic acid

- *Evaluation of peripheral blood smear stained with giemsa stain is the single most important tool in the diagnosis of anemia.*
  1. Different RBC morphologies provide clues to the diagnosis, like micro–/macrocytosis, hypo–/normochromia anisocytosis, poikilocytosis, Howell-Jolly and Heinz bodies, schistocytes, and target cells.
  2. Provides information on WBC count, differential count and morphology, platelets, presence of parasites and toxic granules.
- *The reduced size of RBCs in iron deficiency is masked by the macrocytosis caused by folic acid deficiency.*
  3. *RBC Indices* help in differentiating the different types of anemia (Tables 2.8 and 2.9).

Table 2.9 Sequence of abnormal test results

First abnormal laboratory test	Serum ferritin (normal-15–300 mcg/L)	↓ Serum ferritin – IDA – <12 mcg/L and in thalassemia is normal or increased
Second abnormal laboratory test	Transferrin saturation (20–45%)	↓ Transferrin saturation IDA < 15%
Third abnormal laboratory test	Free erythrocyte protoporphyrin FEP(<35)	Increased in IDA Normal in thalassemia

- *Serum transferring receptor*—by ELISA. In IDA—it is raised.
- *Red cell distribution width*—RDW (15%). It is an index of the presence of a heterogeneous red cell population with different cell diameters. IDA—>15% Thalassemia—normal.
- *Serum iron levels*—(60–120 mcg/dL) IDA < 60 mcg/dL. Levels vary during the day, falling during the latter part of the day and during infection.
- *Total iron binding capacity*—TIBC—(300–400 mcg/dL) IDA > 350 mcg/dL

2.7 Prevention or Preconception Precautions/Counseling

Iron prophylaxis to nonpregnant women—60 mg of elemental iron daily for 3 months.

Iron prophylaxis to *pregnant women*

Routine iron supplementation is debatable in the Western countries

It has to be given in nonindustrialized countries

2.7.1 Recommendations and Guidelines

2.7.1.1 WHO Recommendation

Universal oral iron supplementation for pregnant women (60 mg of elemental iron and 250 μg of folic acid) for 6 months in pregnancy and additional of 3 months postpartum where the prevalence is more than 40%.

Integrated Child Development Services (ICDS) Scheme of Ministry of Women and Child Development (MWCD), India, aims to provide supplementary nutrition of 600 Kcal and 18–20 gm of protein to the antenatal and lactating women at the rate of Rs.5/day/woman.

National Programs to Prevent and Treat Anemia [Ministry Of Health & Family welfare Government of India] (Table 2.10)

Table 2.10 Salient feature of national programs by GOI

1. Testing and treatment of anemia using digital methods (Digital Invasive Hemoglobinometer) in field settings, Sub Health Centers, Health and Wellness Centers; and Semi-auto analyzer in health facilities PHC and above; and point-of-care treatment.
2. Anemia management protocols to be followed are mentioned in Anemia Mukt Bharat.
3. Mandatory iron and folic acid fortified foods in government-funded health programs.
4. Intensifying awareness, screening and treatment of nonnutritional causes of anemia in endemic pockets, with special focus on malaria, hemoglobinopathies, and fluorosis.

2.8 National Iron Plus ± Initiative

This initiative recommends weekly supplementation for adolescents (10–19 years) and women in reproductive age groups and daily supplementation to pregnant and lactating mothers.

Anemia Mukt Bharat program was initiated to reduce anemia in following target groups

(i) Children (6–59 months)
(ii) Children (5–9 years)
(iii) Adolescents (10–19 years)
(iv) Pregnant and lactating women
(v) Women of reproductive age group (15–49 years)

2.8.1 Interventions

Pregnant women and lactating mothers up to 6 months

Must take **daily** one iron and folic acid tablet (*each tablet containing 60 mg elemental Iron + 500 mcg Folic Acid, sugar-coated, red color]* starting from second trimester or fourth month of pregnancy and to be continued throughout pregnancy (minimum 180 days during pregnancy) and for180 days postpartum

Women of reproductive age (nonpregnant, non-lactating) 20–49 years— Must take *weekly,* one tablet of iron and folic acid [*Each tablet containing 60 mg elemental Iron + 500 mcg folic acid, sugar-coated, blue color]*

Preconceptional period and up to the first trimester of the pregnancy—Must take 400 mcg of folic acid tablet daily

2.9 National Deworming Day (NDD) Program

Children and adolescents (10–19 years) receive mass deworming twice a year (tenth February and tenth August) and every year.

Pregnant women are provided services under the strategy through antenatal care contacts (ANC clinics/VHND) for deworming (in the second trimester).

Federation of Gynecological and Obstetrical Societies of India [FOGSI] Recommendations

- Universal screening for iron deficiency anemia with hemoglobin is recommended for all pregnant women at the first antenatal visit. A complete blood count is preferable wherever feasible (Grade A, level 4).
- With a presumptive diagnosis of mild iron deficiency anemia, a trial of oral iron (100 mg/twice a day) for 1 month is recommended. In pregnant women with established mild to moderate anemia, with a period of gestation less than 30–32 weeks, and those who respond to a trial of oral iron, the treatment should continue with 100 mg elemental iron twice daily and 500 μg of folic acid with an assessment for the rise in hemoglobin. A repeat hemoglobin test is recommended after 4 weeks of oral iron.(Grade A, level 3).
- After achieving the normalization of hemoglobin a prophylactic daily iron supplementation (60–100 mg of iron and 500 μg of folic acid) is recommended for at least 6 months during pregnancy and should be continued in postpartum for another 6 months.
- Pregnant women on oral iron supplements should be counseled to consume the tablets before meal or at least 1 h after the meal along with supplements like vitamin C to enhance absorption (Grade A, level 3).

"Nari Swasthya Janandolan Yatra—Anemia National Ride—Na Na Anaemia" an intiative by *The Federation of Obstetrics and Gynecological Societies of India (FOGSI)* under "Badlaav Campaign" aimed to bring holistic health awareness in Indian women, especially anemia prevention. The yatra was started from Rishikesh, Uttarakhand on November 28, 2022, and covered 5 states and over 20 cities, culminating at Kolkata in the first week of January 2023.

Treatment of iron deficiency anemia depends upon the gestational age. If a minimum of 10 weeks is available and the anemia is not severe, a satisfactory result can be obtained with oral therapy.

Oral preparations available are:

- Ferrous sulfate
- Ferrous fumarate
- Ferrous gluconate
- Ferrous succinate

Ferrous sulfate is the cheapest and is suitable for most patients, but the other expensive preparations may produce less gastric discomfort, nausea, vomiting, and constipation.

Iron preparations should preferably be taken on an empty stomach to prevent dietary factors from interfering with its absorption.

- If GI intolerance occurs, advice
- Ingestion of iron supplementation with meals, although absorption may be reduced.

Starting with a small dose and gradually increasing improves compliance

Newer Preparations:
1. Carbonyl iron
2. Iron sucrose (iv dose)
3. Iron polymaltose complex (iv dose)

Carbonyl iron is an effective nontoxic form of elemental iron and is more slowly absorbed and has a higher bioavailability than ferrous sulfate, and less risk of toxicity with overdose.

It has an additional advantage, it eliminates the risk of iron poisoning in children, if taken in lethal doses (LD). *LD of ferrous sulfate-200 mg/kg, LD of carbonyl iron-50,000 mg/kg*

Intravenous iron preparations for anemia in pregnancy are iron sucrose (IS) and ferric carboxymaltose (FCM).

2.10 Parenteral Iron Sucrose

It is non-dextran, complex of iron (III)-hydroxide in sucrose for iv use. Iron sucrose is available as 2.5 and 5 mL single dose ampoules. One ampoule of 2.5 mL contains 50 mg and one ampoule of 5 mL contains 100 mg of elemental iron. It leads to rapid erythropoiesis and quick rise in Hb levels within 5–7 days, due to its short half-life of 5–6 h

IV Iron sucrose is administered by intravenous Infusion

Total dose in mg = Body Wt. × (Target Hb – Actual Hb) × 2.4

This is followed by 10 mg/Kg body weight to replenish the iron stores

After 3 weeks of iron sucrose injection, the expected increase in Hb in pregnant women with severe anemia is approx. 2.5 gm/dL and in moderate anemia is 1.6 gm/dL.

Dose Max of 200 mg of elemental iron dissolved in 100 mL NS, infusion over 1/2 h on alternate days. A total dose of 1.0 gm can be given in 4–10 sittings (over a period of 1 month).

Prerequisites for IV Iron Sucrose Therapy
- Supervision and close monitoring
- Emergency tray to manage anaphylactic reactions, must contain Inj. adrenaline, inj. Hydrocortisone and oxygen
- Facilities for cardiopulmonary resuscitation

Contraindications
- Anemia other than IDA
- Hypersensitivity to iron sucrose

Patient Selection IV iron sucrose can be considered in IDA, Hb >7 gm % and blood transfusion must be considered If Hb <7 gm %

FCM (Ferric Carboxymaltose) Macromolecular ferric hydroxide carbohydrate complex with a ferric hydroxide core stabilized by a carbohydrate shell. In the bloodstream the iron from the iron-carbohydrate complex is released and is either taken by ferritin or serum transferrin. This iron-transferrin complex binds to receptors on erythroblasts situated in the bone marrow providing essential iron for hemoglobin synthesis. Thus, FCM is rapidly cleared from plasma and largely distributed to bone marrow. Infusion of FCM can correct iron deficiency anemia in the second and third trimester of pregnancy.

Evidence from National and International studies have shown that FCM is safe and effective for treatment of anemia in pregnancy and postpartum period. Common adverse drug reactions are nausea, vomiting, dizziness, headache, hypertension, and hypophosphatemia; the latter most is asymptomatic and self-limiting in most patients.

Hypersensitivity reactions are uncommon.

FCM is available in 10 mL (contain 500 mg of FCM, which is equivalent to elemental iron) and 20 mL vials (contain 1000 mg of FCM, which is equivalent to elemental iron)

Administration
1. Test dose is not required.
2. Calculated dose must be dissolved in 100 mL of 0.9% of normal saline and given as infusion over 15 min.
3. Check for the patency of the cannula, because extravasation will cause permanent discoloration of skin.

4. Maximum dose per sitting is 1000 mg (do not give more than 1500 mg in one pregnancy).
5. Never use leftover drug, or one opened and kept in refrigerator.
6. Do not give iron folic acid tablets after infusion for 3 months.
7. Additional doses must be given at weekly interval, i.e., 0, 7, 14 days gap.
8. Monitor BP, pulse, HR, temperature, fetal heart rate during the infusion and for next 30 min.
9. Always keep available all life-saving equipment and drugs.

Advantages of FCM over Iron Sucrose
FCM is more stable, short administration time (15 min versus 30 min), maximum dose is given in single infusion and greater Hb rise.

2.11 Refractory Cases

Cases are labeled as refractory if the hemoglobin level does not improve (Hb < 1 gm %/dL rise) despite 4 weeks of treatment.

Blood transfusion must be considered for non-iron deficiency anemia and refractory iron deficiency anemia.

Indications for Intravenous Iron Sucrose Therapy

(a) Gastrointestinal intolerance (GI) to oral iron
(b) Noncompliance
(c) Poor absorption due to GI disorders
(d) Severe iron deficiency anemia presenting late in pregnancy
(e) Moderate to severe IDA in second and third trimesters of pregnancy
(f) Postpartum anemia

Indications of Response to Therapy

- Sense of well-being
- Improved outlook of patient
- Increased appetite
- ↑Hemoglobin, hematocrit, and reticulocytosis within 5–10 days
- If no significant clinical or hematological improvement within 3 weeks, diagnostic re-evaluation is needed.

Causes of Failure of Oral Therapy

(a) Improper diagnosis
(b) Malabsorption syndrome
(c) chronic infection
(d) Continuous loss of iron
(e) Noncompliance
(f) Concomitant folate deficiency

Key Points

1. Anemia in pregnancy is defined as a hemoglobin value below 11 g/dL (7.45 mmol/L) and hematocrit of less than 0.33 (33%).
2. Iron demand during pregnancy is approximately 900 mg and average daily requirement is 4–6 mg/day.
3. IDA is the commonest type of anemia in pregnancy.
4. Poor perinatal outcome is seen both with too high and too low maternal hemoglobin levels.
5. First abnormal laboratory test in IDA is decreased levels of serum ferritin.
6. Evaluation of peripheral blood smear, stained with Giemsa stain, is the single most important tool in the diagnosis of anemia.
7. 100 mg of elemental iron with 500 μg of folic acid in second half of pregnancy for at least 100 days is recommended by GOI as prophylaxis.

Bibliography

1. IAN DONALDS Practical obstetric problems 6th edition
2. Arias F, Daftary SN, Bhide AG. Practical guide to high risk pregnancy & delivery, 3rd ed; 2008
3. Textbook of obstetrics – D.C.Dutta
4. Textbook of physiology – Guyton
5. Tandon R, Jain A, Malhotra P. Management of iron deficiency anemia in pregnancy in India. Indian J Hematol Blood Transfus. 2018;34(2):204–15. https://doi.org/10.1007/s12288-018-0949-6.
6. Kriplani A, Sharma A, Radhika AG, et al. FOGSI general recommendations for clinical practice; 2016.
7. Kriplani A, Mahey R, Dash BB, Kulshreshta V, Agarwal N, Bhatla N. Intravenous iron sucrose therapy for moderate to severe anaemia in pregnancy. Indian J Med Res. 2013;138(1):78–82.
8. Bayoumeu F, Subiran-Buisset C, Baka NE, Legagneur H, Monnier-Barbarino P, Laxenaire MC. Iron therapy in iron deficiency anemia in pregnancy: intravenous route versus oral route. Am J Obstet Gynecol. 2002;186(3):518–22. https://doi.org/10.1067/mob.2002.121894.
9. Mishra A, Dave N, Viradiya K. Fatal anaphylactic reaction to iron sucrose in pregnancy. Indian J Pharmacology. 2013;45(1):93–4.

3 Thrombocytopenia in Pregnancy

Upma Saxena and Sumedha Gupta

The normal platelet count in pregnancy is 150–400 × 10^9/L, and thrombocytopenia is defined as platelet count below 150 × 10^9/L. Platelets are responsible for primary hemostasis, plugging sites of endothelial damage and acting as a surface for secondary hemostasis via the coagulation pathway. According to the National Health and Nutrition Examination Survey (NHANES) the platelet count in the first trimester were significantly lower than platelet count in nonpregnant women.

Platelet count was studied in 7351 participants during pregnancy and delivery, at the Oklahoma University Medical Center from 2011 to 2014. Authors found that there was a mild decrease in platelet count during all uncomplicated pregnancies, and in twins it was slightly further lower than in singleton pregnancies [1].

Pregnant women have significant lower mean platelet count due to various causes, i.e., sequestration of platelets in placenta and spleen, dilutional effects, or rarely due to decreased production of platelets. Hence, there is a general downward trend leading to 10% decrease in platelet count, compared to the prepregnancy level. Most cases are mild having no effect on mother or fetus, but when it is part of a complex clinical disorder, it can have profound and even life-threatening effects. So, management of thrombocytopenia during pregnancy is challenging as it can occur due to causes specific and nonspecific to pregnancy (Table 3.1).

3.1 Incidence of Thrombocytopenia in Pregnancy

Thrombocytopenia occurs in 8–10% of pregnancies [1–6]. Spurious thrombocytopenia should always be excluded by doing peripheral smear, manual platelet count, or by sampling in citrate vial to rule out pseudo decrease due to clumping.

U. Saxena (✉) · S. Gupta
Department of Obstetrics and Gynecology, VMMC & Safdarjung Hospital, New Delhi, Delhi, India

R. Sharma, A. Kumar (eds.), *Systemic Disorders in Pregnancy*, https://doi.org/10.1007/978-981-96-4876-4_3

Table 3.1 Causes of thrombocytopenia in pregnancy

Pregnancy specific	Nonpregnancy specific
A. *Isolated—Gestational Thrombocytopenia (70%–80%)*	A. Spurious/pseudo—Due to platelet clumping or macrothrombocytes
B. *Associated with systemic disorders* 1. Preeclampsia (15%–20%) 2. HELLP (<1%) 3. Acute fatty liver of pregnancy (<1%) 4. Disseminated intravascular coagulation DIC 5. Sepsis	B. Immune thrombocytopenic purpura (ITP) (1%–4%)
	C. Drug induced (<1%)
	D. *Associated with systemic disorders* 1. Thrombotic Microangiopathies (TMA)-TTP/HUS (<1%) 2. SLE (<1%) 3. Antiphospholipid antibody syndrome (<1%)
	E. Infections—malaria, typhoid, dengue, HIV, HCV, Covid-19 (1–2%)
	F. Nutritional (<1%)—FA, B12, Cu deficiency
	G. Bone marrow disorders (<1%)—Hematological malignancy

3.1.1 Gestational Thrombocytopenia (GT)/ Incidental Thrombocytopenia

Gestational thrombocytopenia is the commonest cause (75%) of thrombocytopenia in pregnancy, occurring in 8–10% of all uncomplicated pregnancies. It is a benign and self- limited condition, incidental finding in second half of pregnancy and pathogenesis is still unclear. But it occurs most likely due to combination of dilutional effect and accelerated destruction of platelet across the placenta. A recent study observed that platelets were present at perivillous fibrinoid spaces throughout placenta demonstrating that GT occurs due to this sequestration and consumption of platelet [7, 8].

There is no other specific associated finding on complete blood count (CBC), physical examination, diagnostic test, and it is considered as diagnosis of exclusion with platelet counts typically 100–150 × 10^9/L, and in only 1% < 100 × 10^9/L [1]. So, platelet counts between 100 × 10^9/L and 150 × 10^9/L at any time during pregnancy is most likely GT unless other factors are present and only <100 × 10^9/L person should be investigated for an etiology other than gestational thrombocytopenia.

GT is not associated with maternal or fetal risks if counts are >100 × 10^9/L, and require no further investigations, except for a periodic monitoring of the platelet count [9].

If platelet count falls to 50–80 × 10^9/L, then the possibility of immune thrombocytopenic purpura cannot be ruled out.

Management: No treatment is required. Prenatal care and management of delivery also remain same. It spontaneously resolves after delivery and may recur in subsequent pregnancies.

3.1.2 Immune (Idiopathic) Thrombocytopenic Purpura (ITP)

ITP is a chronic condition, usually occurs in young women. It affects in approximately 1–3 in 10,000 pregnancies but platelet count is rarely $<50 \times 10^9$/L [11].

The incidence is estimated at 0.1–1/1000 pregnancies [10], accounting for 3% of cases of thrombocytopenia in pregnancy [11]. It is a diagnosis of exclusion, although in approximately two-thirds of cases the diagnosis is already established before pregnancy, allowing the opportunity for prepregnancy counseling [12].

3.2 Etiology

The thrombocytopenia in ITP is due to autoantibodies, resulting in immune-mediated platelet destruction especially in spleen. Platelet antibodies tests lack sensitivity and specificity and, therefore their absence also does not exclude the diagnosis of ITP [13]. Hence, careful history, examination, and laboratory test should be done to exclude other causes of thrombocytopenia. Difficulty to differentiate ITP from GT is not a clinical problem, because treatment is not required for either condition when the platelet count is $>50 \times 10^9$/L. ITP is commonly diagnosed during pregnancy, due to more frequent CBC testing done, while occurrence of GT leads to decreased platelet counts and increased incidence of autoimmune disorders in females [1].

Effects

Effect of Pregnancy on ITP

In ITP, platelet counts decrease at the same rate as healthy pregnancy, and there is 15 to 20 percent decrease in platelet count at delivery which is similar to as seen in uncomplicated pregnancies. Therefore, there is no correlation between decreased platelet count and severity of the ITP during pregnancy [1]

Pregnancy does not affect course of ITP but vigilance is needed at the time of delivery as optimal platelet count for vaginal delivery is >50x109 /L and for operative delivery and neuroaxial analgesia is > 80x109 /L. Recently in 2021, consensus from the Society for Obstetric Anesthesia in concordance further affirmed that the risk of spinal epidural hematoma is very low when platelet count >70x109 /L [14]

Effect of ITP on Pregnancy

Recent study found no increased risk of bleeding in the pregnant versus the nonpregnant group with ITP [15]

Bleeding and purpura is unlikely in mother if platelet count remains above 30x109 /L. IgG antibodies can cross the placenta and cause fetal thrombocytopenia in 0-1.5%. However only 5-10% neonate have platelet count below 50x109 /L which increases to 10-15% in women with diagnosed ITP who are symptomatic before index pregnancy [16]

Best predictor of decreased fetal count is history of severe fetal thrombocytopenia in previous pregnancy.

3.2.1 Prepregnancy Counseling in ITP

Women should be counseled on the following:

1. Relapses or worsening may occur during pregnancy.
2. Treatment is required in one-third of women, around the time of delivery, which carry both maternal and fetal risks.
3. Risk of hemorrhage during delivery, if platelet count is low and epidural anesthesia should be avoided.
4. Maternal counts cannot predict neonatal platelets but risk is higher if mother had undergone splenectomy or prior sibling had thrombocytopenia.
5. The risk of maternal death and intracranial hemorrhage in fetus/neonate is very low.

3.3 Management

3.3.1 Maternal

Multidisciplinary approach involves obstetricians, physicians, and hematologists. The aim of the management is to maintain an adequate platelet count by close monitoring, which will minimize the risk of bleeding during pregnancy, delivery, and postpartum. Majority of women do not require treatment in the antenatal period; unless the platelet count falls below 20×10^9/L before 36 weeks [17]. If platelet count is below 50×10^9/L prior to delivery then steroids or IVIG are the first-line therapy and cesarean delivery is carried out only for obstetrical indications.

Lower dose of prednisolone orally, 1 mg/kg, is advised, which is much less than those recommended for nonpregnant women (20–30 mg/d vs. 60–80 mg/d) to minimize the risk of adverse effects on the mother, such as gestational diabetes, postpartum psychoses, osteoporosis, and weight gain. Response to oral prednisolone is evident after 5–7 days and then its dose is tapered. If the counts are very low and the woman is experiencing hemorrhage, or there is an inadequate response to steroids, intravenous immunoglobulin (IVIG) should be considered, as it acts more quickly than steroids. IVIG at a dose of 1 g/kg for 2 days has a relatively rapid therapeutic response, evident within 1–3 days.

Anti-D immunoglobulin given as IV bolus appears to have efficacy equal to that of IVIG for non-splenectomized women who are Rhesus positive [18]. In unresponsive cases Azathioprine and Cyclosporine can also be given. TPO receptor agonist (TPO-RAs) such as Romiplostim and Eltrombopag are still under trial during pregnancy and evidence suggests they do not cause a high rate of adverse events. In a review of 92 pregnancies managed with Romiplostim, the adverse pregnancy outcomes were comparable to the general population [19].

In China recombinant human thrombopoietin (rhTPO) was administered to 31 pregnant individuals with platelet counts $<30 \times 10^9$/L, not responding to glucocorticoids, IVIG, or platelet transfusions and it was well tolerated with overall response rate of 74% [20].

Due to the risk of consumptive mechanism, platelet transfusion is not recommended. However, splenectomy, if indicated can safely be done in second trimester of pregnancy.

Platelet transfusions (if platelet count <50 × 10^9/L) along with IVIG is recommended, if an emergency cesarean is undertaken.

Unlike GT, the platelet count in ITP does not improve spontaneously postpartum and the therapeutic response to steroids or IVIG reconfirms the diagnosis.

3.3.2 Neonatal

Intracranial hemorrhage (ICH) is rare but devastating complication of ITP. Fetal scalp and percutaneous umbilical blood sampling should not be undertaken as the procedure carries a risk of fetal hemorrhage and death of approximately 2%, which is higher than <1% risk of ICH.

A cord sample should be taken to assess the neonatal platelet count and if the count is mildly reduced, it should be repeated on day 1 and 4 but if the initial result is normal, no further sampling is required [21]. Platelets should be administered in addition to IVIG if there is life-threatening hemorrhage.

3.3.2.1 Other Differential Diagnosis of Thrombocytopenia (Table 3.2)

The most common causes of thrombocytopenia in pregnancy are gestational thrombocytopenia and ITP. The other causes can be HELLP syndrome characterized by hemolysis, elevated liver enzyme levels and low platelet counts, Acute fatty liver of pregnancy (AFLP),Thrombotic thrombocytopenic purpura (TTP) /Hemolytic uremic syndrome (HUS), Severe Preeclampsia (PE) as summarized in Table 3.2.

3.3.2.2 Preeclampsia

Preeclampsia affects 5–10% of all pregnancies and is associated with endothelial dysfunction leading to the activation of platelets and the coagulation cascade. Preeclampsia with severe features affects 1% of individuals with preeclampsia and includes more severe hypertension, severe headache and/or visual symptoms, liver function abnormalities and epigastric pain, and thrombocytopenia (platelet count <100 × 10^9/L [22].

Preeclampsia is associated with a platelet count <100 × 10^9/L in only 7% of women, and with severe thrombocytopenia at platelet count <60 × 10^9/L in 3% [23].

Women with preeclampsia have 15% lower platelet counts than normal pregnancy and the condition resolves quickly after delivery [22]. Severe thrombocytopenia can be associated with disseminate intravascular hemolysis (DIC) requiring delivery after correction of the coagulopathy.

Table 3.2 Differential diagnosis of causes of thrombocytopenia in pregnancy

Characteristic	HELLP	AFLP	TTP	HUS	Severe PE
Incidence	0.5%	Rare	Rare	Rare	5–10%
Pathogenesis/genetic cause	–	LCHAD gene defect	ADAMTS 13 gene deficiency	–	–
Hypertension	+/–	–	–	–	++
Thrombocytopenia	++	+/–	+++	++	+
DIC	+	+++	–	+/–	+/–
Liver disease	Transaminases++	Bilirubin++	+/–	+/–	+/–
Renal disease	+ (With abruption)	–/+	+/–	+++	+
CNS disease	–	+	+++	+/–	+/–
Diagnostic criteria	Tennessee/Mississippi classification	Swansea criteria	Pentad of TTP	AKI postpartum	–
Male fetus	50%	70%	–	–	–
MAHA	++	+/–	+++	++	+
Cornerstone of management	Delivery	Delivery	Plasmapheresis	Plasmapheresis with dialysis	Delivery

3.3.3 HELLP Syndrome

This is characterized by hemolysis, elevated liver enzyme levels, and low platelet counts, which can complicate severe preeclampsia in about 10% of cases [5]. It occurs most frequently in the third trimester, but can develop and worsen in the postpartum period. Sometimes it can occur without hypertension or proteinuria and so there should be a high level of suspicion, needing confirmation with CBC showing thrombocytopenia, with microangiopathic hemolytic anemia (MAHA) and liver function tests showing a raised lactate dehydrogenase (LDH), increased bilirubin, and abnormal liver enzymes. DIC and abruption may be present in 20% and 16% cases, respectively.

Neonatal outcome depends on the duration of gestation at delivery:10–20% are preterm, as delivery is the mainstay of treatment. HELLP syndrome improves by sixth day postdelivery, although it may worsen during the first 24–48 h postpartum.

Acute Fatty Liver of Pregnancy (AFLP) It is a form of liver injury that typically occurs in the third trimester and women presents with nausea, vomiting, and abdominal pain. There is thrombocytopenia with severely deranged LFT with bilirubin levels much more elevated than transaminases, hypoglycemia, leukocytosis, and DIC. Delivery is cure as it prevents further progression of the pathology.

3.3.3.1 Thrombotic Microangiopathies (TMA)

It is characterized by microthrombi formation in small vessels leading to organ damage and includes thrombotic thrombocytopenic purpura (TTP), and complement-mediated TMA (C-TMA). TTP, both hereditary or acquired, is associated with increased risk to women during pregnancy [17, 24]. Almost all patients with hereditary TTP have worsening with pregnancy leading to an acute, severe episode of TTP [25].

Women with TMA worsens commonly during late pregnancy or postpartum, presenting with MAHA, thrombocytopenia, and end-organ injury, which persist for more than 3 days after delivery distinguishing it from preeclampsia with severe features, which almost always begins to recover before this time. TMAs are life-threatening, however majority women deliver healthy term infants, but intrauterine fetal death may occur from placental infarction caused by thrombosis of the decidual arterioles.

3.3.3.2 Thrombotic Thrombocytopenic Purpura (TTP)/Hemolytic Uremic Syndrome (HUS)

They both are continuum due to microvascular platelet aggregation leading to thrombocytopenia and MAHA [26, 27]. If this is systemic and extensive with central nervous system involvement then it is TTP [27] and if with predominant renal involvement then it is HUS. Both HUS and TTP are rare during pregnancy and puerperium.

Classic clinical features of TTP (pentad) are:

- Microangiopathic hemolytic anemia (MAHA)
- Thrombocytopenia
- Fever
- Neurological manifestation: headache, irritability, drowsiness, seizure, coma
- Acute kidney injury (AKI)

Pathogenesis

TTP has been shown to be due to a severe deficiency of von Willebrand's factor-cleaving protein (ADAMTS 13). The diagnosis of TTP is made on a thorough clinical assessment combined with a finding of ADAMTS13 activity most of time <10% [28].

The association with pregnancy may be due to the formation of endothelial cell autoantibodies associated with immune dysregulation during pregnancy.

Diagnosis

MAHA is diagnosed with fragments RBC (schistocytes) seen on the peripheral blood film along with severe thrombocytopenia, increased reticulocytes, unconjugated bilirubin, and LDH. Clotting time and fibrinogen concentrations are normal and consumptive DIC is rare. In HUS, there is severe AKI but hypertension is not seen in TTP/HUS. Both are severe conditions, associated with morbidity and mortality.

Effect of TTP/HUS on Pregnancy

The fetus is not affected by HUS/TTP and prognosis is related to gestational age at delivery.

Management

There is no evidence that delivery affects the course of HUS/TTP. Aggressive treatment with therapeutic plasma exchange (TPE) with fresh frozen plasma (FFP) and plasmapheresis may limit vascular injury and improve prognosis. TPE and anti-complement therapy can cause potentially serious adverse effects and are costly. So are reserved for individuals with strong supporting evidence for TTP [29].

Corticosteroids may be beneficial but platelet transfusion is contraindicated. Supportive therapy for AKI may necessitate dialysis, and supportive therapy for cerebral involvement involves investigation to exclude other causes of seizure [30].

3.4 Other Causes of Thrombocytopenia

Disseminated intravascular coagulation (DIC) It is a systemic process in which both coagulation and fibrinolysis become activated, leading to consumption of clotting factors and platelets, with severe bleeding and/or diffuse oozing. It is associated with an underlying cause, i.e., abruption, retained dead fetus, amniotic fluid embolism, septic abortion, and others. There may be MAHA, prolonged prothrombin time and activated partial thromboplastin time, low fibrinogen, and the elevated D-dimer and FDP.

Management It involves identifying and treating the underlying cause; in some cases, this may require delivery (e.g., retained dead fetus, abruption), and others (e.g., sepsis from a non-obstetric infection) require antibiotics therapy, along with supportive treatment.

Antiphospholipid Syndrome (APLA) It is associated with thrombocytopenia and is treated with aspirin and enoxaparin sodium during pregnancy, as this has been shown to improve outcome.

Viral Infection Almost any virus can cause thrombocytopenia but it is usually transient, and HIV and cytomegalovirus infections should be excluded.

Drug Induced Medication is an important cause of thrombocytopenia: it is a frequent adverse effect of commonly used drugs, i.e., unfractionated heparin.

Key Learning Points
1. Thrombocytopenia defined as platelet count below 150×10^9/L is the second most common hematological abnormality seen in pregnancy after anemia.
2. Gestational thrombocytopenia is the commonest cause.
3. A good history, physical examination, BP and lab test, i.e., CBC with peripheral smear, LDH, Antinuclear Antibody (ANA), LFT, KFT, HIV, and coagulation profile helps in differentiating among various causes.
4. Delivery in GT and ITP, only for obstetrical indications.

References

1. Reese JA, Peck JD, Deschamps DR, et al. Platelet count during pregnancy. N Engl J Med. 2018;379:32–43.
2. Verdy E, Bessous V, Dreyfus M, et al. Longitudinal analysis of platelet count and volume in normal pregnancy. Thromb Haemost. 1997;77:806–7.
3. Myers B. Diagnosis and management of maternal thrombocytopenia in pregnancy. Br J Haematol. 2012;158:3.
4. Boehlen F, Hohlfeld P, Extermann P, et al. Platelet count at term pregnancy: a reappraisal of the threshold. Obstet Gynecol. 2000;95:29–33.
5. Burrows RF, Kelton JG. Thrombocytopenia at delivery: a prospective survey of 6715 deliveries. Am J Obstet Gynecol. 1990;162:732–4.
6. Gernsheimer T, James AH, Stasi R. How I treat thrombocytopenia in pregnancy. Blood. 2013;121(1):38–47.
7. Aster RH. "Gestational" thrombocytopenia: a plea for conservative management. N Engl J Med. 1990;323:264.
8. Reese JA, Peck JD, Yu Z, et al. Platelet sequestration and consumption in the placental intervillous space contribute to lower platelet counts during pregnancy. Am J Hematol. 2019;94(1):E8–E11.
9. Burrows RF, Kelton JG. Fetal thrombocytopenia and its relation to maternal thrombocytopenia. N Engl J Med. 1993;329:1463–6.

10. Win N, Rowley M, Pollard C, et al. Severe gestational (incidental) thrombocytopenia: to treat or not to treat. Hematology. 2005;10:69–72.
11. Care A, Pavord S, Knight M, et al. Severe primary autoimmune thrombocytopenia in pregnancy: a national cohort study. BJOG. 2018;125:604.
12. Terrell DR, Beebe LA, Vesely SK, et al. The incidence of immune thrombocytopenic purpura in children and adults: a critical review of published reports. Am J Hematol. 2010;85:174.
13. Webert KE, Mittal R, Sigouin C, et al. A retrospective 11-year analysis of obstetric patients with idiopathic thrombocytopenic purpura. Blood. 2003;102:4306.
14. Bauer ME, Arendt K, Beilin Y, et al. The society for obstetric anesthesia and perinatology interdisciplinary consensus statement on neuraxial procedures in obstetric patients with thrombocytopenia. Anesth Analg. 2021;132:1531.
15. Guillet S, Loustau V, Boutin E, et al. Immune thrombocytopenia and pregnancy: an exposed/nonexposed cohort study. Blood. 2023;141:11.
16. Loustau V, Debouverie O, Canoui-Poitrine F, et al. Effect of pregnancy on the course of immune thrombocytopenia: a retrospective study of 118 pregnancies in 82 women. Br J Haematol. 2014;166:929.
17. Jiang Y, McIntosh JJ, Reese JA, et al. Pregnancy outcomes following recovery from acquired thrombotic thrombocytopenic purpura. Blood. 2014;123:1674.
18. Michel M, Bussel NMV, JB. Intravenous anti-D as a treatment for immune thrombocytopenic purpura (ITP) during pregnancy. Br J Haematol. 2003;123:142–6.
19. Bussel JB, Cooper N, Lawrence T, et al. Romiplostim use in pregnant women with immune thrombocytopenia. Am J Hematol. 2023;98:31.
20. Kong Z, Qin P, Xiao S, et al. A novel recombinant human thrombopoietin therapy for the management of immune thrombocytopenia in pregnancy. Blood. 2017;130:1097.
21. Burrows R, Kelton J. Pregnancy in patients with idiopathic thrombocytopenic purpura: assessing the risks forthe infant at delivery. Obstet Gynecol Surv. 1993;48:781–8.
22. Gestational Hypertension and Preeclampsia: ACOG Practice Bulletin, Number 222. Obstet Gynecol 2020; 135:e237. Reaffirmed 2023.
23. Perez Botero J, Reese JA, George JN, et al. Severe thrombocytopenia and microangiopathic hemolytic anemia in pregnancy: a guide for the consulting hematologist. Am J Hematol. 2021;96:1655.
24. Moatti-Cohen M, Garrec C, Wolf M, et al. Unexpected frequency of Upshaw-Schulman syndrome in pregnancy-onset thrombotic thrombocytopenic purpura. Blood. 2012;119:5888.
25. Kasht R, Borogovac A, George JN. Frequency and severity of pregnancy complications in women with hereditary thrombotic thrombocytopenic purpura. Am J Hematol. 2020;95:E316.
26. Scully M, Thomas M, Underwood M, et al. Thrombotic thrombocytopenic purpura and pregnancy: presentation, management, and subsequent pregnancy outcomes. Blood. 2014;124:211.
27. Martin JN Jr, Bailey AP, Rehberg JF, et al. Thrombotic thrombocytopenic purpura in 166 pregnancies: 1955–2006. Am J Obstet Gynecol. 2008;199:98.
28. Ayanambakkam A, Kremer Hovinga JA, Vesely SK, et al. Diagnosis of thrombotic thrombocytopenic purpura among patients with ADAMTS13 Activity 10%–20. Am J Hematol. 2017;92:E644.
29. Zheng XL, Vesely SK, Cataland SR, et al. ISTH guidelines for treatment of thrombotic thrombocytopenic purpura. J Thromb Haemost. 2020;18:2496.
30. Gupta M, Govindappagari S, Burwick RM. Pregnancy-associated atypical hemolytic uremic syndrome: a systematic review. Obstet Gynecol. 2020;135:46.

Hemoglobinopathies in Pregnancy

4

Pinki Lakra

Hemoglobinopathies encompass all genetic diseases of hemoglobin. They fall into two main groups: thalassemias (α and β thalassemias) and structural hemoglobin variants like HbS, HbE, HbD, HbC, etc. Sometimes both coexist in combinations.

4.1 Thalassemia

In India, β thalassemia comprises of 80–90% of all cases of thalassemia. A recent study in India showed that the overall prevalence of β-thalassemia trait was 2.78% [2]. A varied prevalence of α-thalassemia ranging from 1% to 18% has been reported in the general Indian population [3]. The communities commonly affected are Gujaratis, Maharashtrians, Bengalis, Sindhis, Goaneses, and people from Northern states like Punjab, UP, Rajasthan, and Haryana.

Hemoglobin molecule is composed of four globin chains. Each globin chain has a heme moiety (a protoporphyrin ring and a central iron ion). More than 95% of an adult's hemoglobin is in the form of HbA with two α and two β chains whereas 2.2–3.5% is HbA2, composed of two α and two δ chains. Fetal hemoglobin (HbF) comprises two α chains and two γ chains. The alpha and beta globin genes are located on chromosome number 16 and 11, respectively.

4.1.1 Pathophysiology

- α-Thalassemia results from the partial (α^+) or total (α^0) **deletion** of one, two, three, or all four genes, with a variation in clinical severity. The deletion of all four genes is incompatible with life (Table 4.1). In spite of its varied prevalence,

P. Lakra (✉)
BPS GMC(W) Khapurkalan, Sonipat, Haryana, India

R. Sharma, A. Kumar (eds.), *Systemic Disorders in Pregnancy*,
https://doi.org/10.1007/978-981-96-4876-4_4

Table 4.1 Types of α thalassemia

Phenotype	Arrangement of genes
Normal findings	αα/αα
Thalassemia minima	−α/αα
Thalassemia minor	− −/αα, −α/−α
HbH disease	− −/−α
Hb Barts's	− −/− −

no case of Hb Bart's hydrops fetalis syndrome has been reported from India. There are fewer sporadic case reports of Hb H disease with variable clinical severity from different regions.

- β-Thalassemia is usually due to a single-gene **mutation** and results in insufficient (β^+) or absent (β^0) production of β-globin chains. The excess α-globin chains combine with the available β, δ, or γ chains, forming abnormal amounts of HbA2 and HbF. β-thalassemias is classified into thalassemia minor/carrier/trait, thalassemia intermedia, and thalassemia major/Cooley's anemia.
- Ineffective erythropoiesis due to the release of damaged red blood cells and erythroid precursor into the peripheral circulation leads to extravascular hemolysis.

4.1.2 Clinical Presentation

Anemia is mild in thalassemia minor and it increases in severity from intermedia to major forms. Children develop pallor, jaundice, feeding problems, growth retardation, and hepatosplenomegaly. Ineffective erythropoiesis and compensated erythroid hyperplasia produce bone marrow expansion. Maxillary marrow hyperplasia and frontal bossing lead to characteristic "chipmunk" facies. Skeletal deformities like genu valgum and pathological fractures of long bones and vertebrae may occur early due to cortical invasion by erythroid elements. Susceptibility to infection and improper transfusion of blood may lead to death in the first decade of life in severe cases.

Thalassemia major requires lifelong transfusions with chelation therapy and bone marrow transplantation is the only curative option available. Multiple transfusions cause iron overload resulting in hepatic, cardiac, and endocrine dysfunction. Most of the women with β thalassemia major and severe β thalassemia intermedia suffer from hypogonadotrophic hypogonadism and are infertile. Artificial reproductive techniques involving ovulation induction with gonadotrophins are helpful for conception.

4.1.3 Diagnosis of Thalassemia

1. Naked Eye Single Tube Red Cell Osmotic Fragility Test (NESTROFT) is the preliminary screening test for β-thalassemia carriers.

Table 4.2 Differentiation between iron deficiency anemia and thalassemia trait

Tests	Iron deficiency anemia	Thalassemia trait
Serum ferritin	Low	Normal or high
Red cell distribution width (RDW)	High	Low <15.5%
RBC count	Low	>five million/μL
Mentzer index (MCV/RBC count)	>13	<13

2. Thalassemics have reduced MCV (<77 fl) and MCH (<27 pg) and thalassemia trait needs to be differentiated from iron deficiency anemia since both are microcytic and hypochromic [1]. Normal or high serum ferritin, RDW <15.5%, RBC count >five million/μL, and Mentzer index <13 (MCV/RBC count) indicate thalassemia.
3. High-performance liquid chromatography (HPLC) is a technique for detection and quantitative estimation of Hb variants, identification of an abnormal hemoglobin or elevated levels of HbA2 (≥3.5%) for beta thalassemia carriers.
4. Unlike β-thalassemia trait and iron deficiency, no simple biochemical test can detect α-thalassemia. α + thalassemia is often a diagnosis of exclusion; patients are microcytic with no evidence of iron deficiency and no abnormal findings in HPLC. Multiplex ligase-dependent probe amplification (MLPA) and gap-PCR are useful for deletional types and for nondeletional α-thalassemia, (Sanger) DNA sequencing is required.
5. Reticulocyte preparations made from anticoagulated blood with 1% methylene blue shows HbH inclusion bodies in alpha thalassemia carriers (Table 4.2).

4.2 Care of Pregnancy in Thalassemia

4.2.1 Thalassemias Carrier

1. Couples who are heterozygous carriers have 25% chance of having a baby with thalassemia major, 50% of having a carrier baby, and another 25% of normal baby.
2. Pregnancy is well tolerated in women with thalassemia trait.
3. Folic acid supplementation is advised.
4. Iron supplementation is not given, but advised only if iron deficiency is documented.
5. Parenteral iron is contraindicated.
6. All the women must be screened during their antenatal period and if they are the carriers then their husbands are also screened. If husband is a carrier, then prenatal diagnosis (Chorionic Villus sampling or Amniocentesis) is offered, to decide regarding termination of pregnancy or continuation.

4.2.2 Thalassemia Major

Multidisciplinary team including an obstetrician and a hematologist is required for the management of Thalassemia major.

4.2.3 Preconception Care

1. Stop all chelation therapy and bisphosphonates and start folic acid 5 mg at least 3 months before conception.
2. Screen for diabetes and thyroid dysfunction. HbA1c is not a reliable marker of glycemic control, so serum fructosamine is preferred for monitoring.
3. Do echocardiogram, T2* cardiac MRI, and Ferriscan or liver T2* for baseline iron concentrations. Bone density scan is done to document preexisting osteoporosis.
4. ABO and full blood group genotype should be done for transfusion.
5. If the partner is a carrier of a hemoglobinopathy, then offer genetic counseling. IVF/ICSI with a PGD should be considered in the presence of hemoglobinopathies in both partners so that a homozygous or compound heterozygous pregnancy can be avoided.
6. Hepatitis B vaccination and Hepatitis C testing is required. Women with splenectomy need penicillin prophylaxis.

4.2.3.1 Antenatal Care

Feto-maternal risk is increased in thalassemia due to iron overload, particularly risk of cardiomyopathy, diabetes mellitus, hypothyroidism, and hypoparathyroidism in the mother increased the risk of fetal growth restriction.

1. Monthly ANC visits until 28 weeks and fortnightly thereafter.
2. Monthly serum fructosamine in diabetics and thyroid function tests.
3. Monthly growth scans from 24 weeks onward.
4. Blood transfusions aiming for a pretransfusion hemoglobin of 10 g/dL.
5. Start low-dose aspirin (75 mg/day) in those with splenectomy or platelet count $>600 \times 10^9$/L and LMWH during antenatal hospital admissions.
6. Cardiac evaluation at 28 weeks, and monitoring of signs of cardiac decompensation and ejection fraction regularly, especially in those with myocardial iron loading. If present then intervention with chelation therapy is required.

4.2.3.2 Intrapartum Care

1. In the presence of red cell antibodies, blood should be cross-matched for delivery to avoid delays.
2. Start intravenous desferrioxamine 2 g over 24 h during labor.
3. Thalassemia is not an indication for cesarean, but must be considered if there is feto-maternal indication.

4.2.3.3 Postnatal Care

1. Breast feeding is safe.
2. LMWH prophylaxis is recommended during hospital stay and continued for 1 week (normal delivery) after discharge from hospital or for 6 weeks after cesarean [4, 5].

4.3 Sickle Cell and Other Abnormal Structural Variants

Sickle cell disease (SCD) is a hemoglobin disorder, with significant morbidity and mortality during lifetime. Hemoglobinopathies are more common in tribal population in India.

In sickle cell disease, valine is substituted for glutamate at position 6 of β-globin chain due to a single-base mutation in the β-globin gene. In homozygous state, both β-globin genes are abnormal, which results in sickle cell anemia. Similarly other aminoacid substitutions result in other variants like HbD, HbE, HbC, etc. A high frequency of HbD has been reported from the North in the Punjabi population, HbE in the eastern region of India, and HbS from tribes in different parts of the country. HbE may combine with thalassemias resulting in a serious major form of hemoglobinopathies.

National Sickle Cell Anemia Elimination Mission 2023

- Guidelines for National Sickle Cell Anemia Elimination Mission by the Ministry of health and family welfare, government of India, have been developed to eliminate sickle cell disease by 2047.
- Aim is integrated comprehensive approach for the prevention, screening, and management of SCD.

4.3.1 Pathophysiology

Rigid and fragile sickle-shaped red cells are formed due to polymerization of the abnormal hemoglobin in low-oxygen conditions. This leads to vaso-occlusion, sickling-induced membrane fragmentation, and complement-mediated lysis causing intravascular hemolysis. Poorly deformable sickle cells get trapped extravascularly and phagocytosed by macrophages and monocytes resulting in extravascular hemolysis.

4.3.2 Clinical Presentation

Anemia (and reticulocytosis) generally presents in HbSS by 4 months of age and is not detected in the newborn. Baseline anemia is intensified with aplastic crises or splenic sequestration. Pain crises are experienced as deep, throbbing pains, usually without physical findings. Children younger than 5 years may experience pain in the form of the "hand-foot syndrome," with swelling and tenderness of hands or feet. Other complications of SCD include stroke, pulmonary hypertension, renal dysfunction, retinal disease, leg ulcers, cholelithiasis, and avascular necrosis (mostly femoral head and may necessitate hip replacement). SCD was previously associated with a high early mortality rate, but now majority live to reproductive age and average life expectancy is at least the mid-50 s [6, 7].

SCD in pregnancy is associated with both maternal and fetal complications like hemolytic crises, acute painful crises, miscarriages, thromboembolism, antepartum hemorrhage, preeclampsia, cesarean section, postpartum sepsis maternal mortality, FGR, IUFD, prematurity, and perinatal mortality (Tables 4.3 and 4.4 and Fig 4.1).

Table 4.3 Diagnostic criteria and cardinal symptoms of sickle cell disease and trait

Diagnosis	Gene type	RBC count	Hemoglobin pattern on HPLC	Cardinal symptoms
Sickle cell disease	HbSS	Hb 6–9 g/dL Normochromic sickle cells Positive hemolysis parameters	HbS = 55–90% HbA2 > 3.5% HbF = 20%	Sickle cell crises/pain crises acute organ syndromes, chronic hemolytic anemia
Sickle cell trait	HbAS	Normal	HbS = 35–40% HbA2 ≥ 3.5%	No apparent illness

Table 4.4 Prenatal diagnosis

Prenatal diagnosis required	Prenatal diagnosis NOT required
If a sickle cell diseased and sickle cell trait marry 50% risk for the disease and 50% risk for the carriers in babies	If both having sickle cell disease marry, then 100% risk for SCD in babies
If both having sickle cell trait marry 25% risk for disease, 25% normal, and 50% risk for carriers in babies	If one has sickle cell disease and the other is normal 100% risk for trait in babies
	If one has sickle cell trait and the other is normal 50% will be normal and 50% risk of being carriers

Option 1 GoI-approved -One step approach -Point of Care test (Confirmatory test)

Option 2 Two-step approach
Mass screening / Initial screening-using Solubility test (Tube based)

↓ If + for Solubility test

Confirmation test - using GoI-approved Point of Care confirmatory test or Hb- HPLC/Capillary zone electrophoresis/Agarose gel/Cellulose Acetate Hb Electrophoresis testing

Fig. 4.1 Screening and diagnosis

4.4 Newborn Screening

Aim is to detect SCD in neonatal period, dried blood spot card is used for sickle screening and the routine Hb-HPLC equipment with the Hb variant program is used. *Informed consent* must be taken.

4.4.1 Sickle Cell Disease in Pregnancy

Pregnancy must be managed by a multidisciplinary team including an obstetrician and hematologist [8].

4.4.2 Preconception Care

1. Stop hydroxyurea, angiotensin-converting enzyme inhibitors, and angiotensin receptor blockers at least 3 months before conception. Start folic acid 5 mg preconceptually and continue throughout pregnancy.
2. Do echocardiography to rule out pulmonary hypertension, blood pressure, and urinalysis to identify hypertension and/or proteinuria, and retinal screening to rule out proliferative retinopathy.
3. Check hemoglobinopathy status of husband.
4. Give penicillin prophylaxis and check vaccination status of meningococcal, pneumococcal, Hib, and Hepatitis B vaccines. Give influenza and swine flu vaccine annually.
5. Tab. folic acid is 5 mg daily.

4.4.3 Antenatal care

1. Tab. folic acid is 5 mg daily and vitamin D supplementation.
2. Precipitating factors like exposure to extreme temperatures, dehydration, and overexertion will precipitate sickle cell crises. Aspirin 75 mg daily, starting from 12 weeks pregnancy to be considered. LMWH prophylaxis is given on hospital admissions. NSAIDs for analgesia can be given between 12 and 28 weeks pregnancy. Do urine culture monthly.
3. From 24 weeks onward monitor fetal growth with growth scans.
4. Routine prophylactic transfusion is not recommended during the antenatal period. If acute exchange transfusion is done to treat sickle cell crisis, then transfusion regimen must be continued for the remaining half of the pregnancy. Extended phenotype cross-match including full Rhesus typing (C, D and E) as well as Kell typing must be done.
5. Painful crisis is the most frequent complication of SCD during pregnancy and it is the most frequent cause of hospital admission. Fluids, oxygen, analgesics, and

thromboprophylaxis should be administered. Assess for infection and give therapeutic antibiotics.

6. SCD is associated with other acute complications including Acute Chest Syndrome (ACS), stroke, and acute anemia. ACS is reported in 7–20% of pregnancies. Tachypnea, chest pain, cough and shortness of breath, and the presence of a new infiltrate on the chest X-ray, indicated ACS. The signs and symptoms of ACS are the same as those of pneumonia, so both should be treated simultaneously.
7. Sometimes acute anemia may be attributable to erythrovirus infection. It causes red cell maturation arrest and aplastic crisis characterized by a reticulocytopenia. Treatment is isolation of women and blood transfusion. Erythrovirus infection can cause risk of vertical transmission and hydrops fetalis.
8. Any woman with SCD presenting with acute neurological impairment indicates acute stroke. Urgent brain imaging and exchange transfusion is required.

4.4.4 Intrapartum Care

1. Offer elective birth through induction of labor, or by elective cesarean section if indicated, after 38 + 0 weeks.
2. Blood should be cross-matched for delivery if there are atypical antibodies present.

4.4.5 Postpartum Care

1. If the baby is at high risk of SCD (i.e., the partner is a carrier or affected), early testing for SCD should be offered.
2. Adequate hydration.
3. Keep maternal spo2 > 94%.
4. LMWH should be administered while in hospital and 7 days post-discharge following vaginal delivery or for a period of 6 weeks following cesarean section. Antithrombotic stockings are recommended in the puerperium.
5. Progestogen-containing contraceptives are safe and effective.

4.4.6 Follow-Up

Regular checkup at 3–6 monthly:

- Monitoring for fever, jaundice, pallor, spleen size.
- Monitoring Hb levels.
- Counseling on diet, stress management, etc.

Key Points

1. Hemoglobinopathies are autosomal recessive conditions affecting the quantity and quality of hemoglobin molecules in red blood cells.
2. Beta-thalassemias is clinically more significant in India, with higher incidence in certain communities.
3. Screening for thalassemia trait in pregnancy should be an essential part of routine antenatal care.
4. Preconceptional care and counseling is recommended to optimize the fetomaternal outcome in hemoglobinopathies.
5. Antenatal care should be provided by a multidisciplinary team.
6. Thalassemia major is associated with cardiomyopathy in the mother due to iron overload and increased risk of FGR.
7. ACS, sepsis, and pulmonary embolism are the major causes of maternal mortality in SCD.
8. LMWH should be administered while in hospital and for 1 week post-discharge (vaginal delivery) or for 6 weeks (cesarean section).

Bibliography

1. Guidelines for National programme for prevention & management of sickle cell disease. Ministry of Health & Family Welfare, Government of India 2023.
2. Shukla S, Singh D, Dewan K, Sharma S, Trivedi SS. Antenatal carrier screening for thalassemia and related hemoglobinopathies: a hospital-based study. J Med Soc. 2018;32:118–22.
3. Mohanty D, Colah RB, Gorakshakar AC, Patel RZ, Master DC, Mahanta J, et al. Prevalence of β-thalassemia and other haemoglobinopathies in six cities in India: a multicentre study. J Community Genet. 2013;4:33–42.
4. Nadkarni A, Phanasgaonkar S, Colah R, Mohanty D, Kanjaksha G. Prevalence and molecular characterization of α-thalassemia syndromes among Indians. Genet Test. 2008;12(2):177–80.
5. Rachmilewitz EA, et al. Prevalence of thromboembolic events among 8,860 patients with thalassaemia major and intermedia in the Mediterranean area and Iran. Thromb Haemost. 2006;96:488–91.
6. Royal College of Obstetricians and Gynaecologists. Reducing the risk of thrombosis and embolism during pregnancy and the puerperium. Green-top Guideline No. 37a. London: RCOG; 2009.
7. Telfer P, Coen P, Chakravorty S, Wilkey O, Evans J, Newell H, et al. Clinical outcomes in children with sickle cell disease living in England: a neonatal cohort in East London. Haematologica. 2007;92:905–12.
8. Wierenga KJ, Hambleton IR, Lewis NA. Survival estimates for patients with homozygous sickle-cell disease in Jamaica: a clinic based population study. Lancet. 2001;357:680–3.

Hypertensive Disorders of Pregnancy

5

Munjal Jayeshkumar Pandya, Janki Munjal Pandya,
and Kanan P. Kotdawala

5.1 Introduction

Hypertensive disorders of pregnancy (HDP) is a spectrum of disorders complicating pregnancy, adversely affecting the mother as well as the fetus. Various classification systems have been suggested over the period of time, and the term "pregnancy-induced hypertension" has been discarded. Due to lack of uniformity in the classification system, there had been difficulties in studying various aspects of this disease spectrum, their pathophysiology, maternal and fetal outcomes, prevention and management, and long-term sequelae.

Incidence of preeclampsia is around 2–4% in more-developed nations, India reporting incidence of 2% preeclampsia.

5.2 Classification of Hypertensive Disorders of Pregnancy

ISSHP (International Society for the Study of Hypertension in Pregnancy and the American Heart Association) suggested classification of HDP as follows [1]:

A. Hypertension known before pregnancy or present in the first 20 weeks:
   (a) Chronic Hypertension (Essential/Secondary): Associated with adverse fetal and maternal outcome, making it necessary to monitor fetal growth and proper maternal BP management.
   (b) White coat hypertension: Elevated BP (>140/90 mmHg) at clinic, but normal BP at home/work (<135/85 mmHg); and carries increased risk of preeclampsia.

M. J. Pandya (✉) · J. M. Pandya · K. P. Kotdawala
Narendra Modi Medical College, Ahmedabad, Gujarat, India

R. Sharma, A. Kumar (eds.), *Systemic Disorders in Pregnancy*,
https://doi.org/10.1007/978-981-96-4876-4_5

(c) Masked hypertension: BP is normal at clinic, but raised at other times, on Ambulatory BP Monitoring (ABPM). Diagnosis can be made on the basis of unexplained features of end organ damage like chronic kidney disease (CKD), left ventricular hypertrophy, or retinopathy early in pregnancy.

B. Hypertension arising de novo at or after 20 weeks:

New onset hypertension (BP $\geq$ 140 mmHg systolic or $\geq$90 mmHg diastolic) at or after 20 weeks gestation), with documented normal BP either prepregnancy or in early pregnancy.

(a) Transient gestational hypertension: Usually arising in the second or third trimester, detected in clinic, but settles down after repeated BP recordings over few hours in a day. Follow-up of such cases is important as 40% of them may develop true gestational hypertension or preeclampsia.

(b) Gestational hypertension: Hypertension arising de novo after 20 weeks of gestation, in absence of proteinuria and without biochemical or hematological abnormalities; usually not accompanied by fetal growth restriction. About 25% of these cases (especially those presenting at <34 weeks) will progress to preeclampsia, leading to poorer outcome.

(c) Preeclampsia de novo or superimposed on chronic hypertension: Presence of de novo hypertension after 20 weeks of gestation, accompanied by proteinuria and/or evidences of liver dysfunction, cerebral or visual abnormalities, hemolysis/thrombocytopenia, maternal acute kidney injury (AKI), maternal pulmonary edema, or fetal growth restriction. Proteinuria is NOT a mandatory feature. ACOG (American College of Obstetricians and Gynecologists) has recommended elimination of the term “severe” preeclampsia, as preeclampsia can be a potential threat at any stage; thus, the recommendation has been made for usage of the term preeclampsia with or without severe features.

5.3 Pathophysiology of Preeclampsia

This involves abnormal placental implantation, due to defects in trophoblasts and defective spiral arteriole invasion, leading to high resistance vasculature. Low level of placental growth factor has been thought to be one of the factors. Genetic factors and thrombophilia have been strongly associated with occurrence of preeclampsia. Microscopically, vascular endothelial damage leads to micro-coagulation and initiation of cascade leading to preeclampsia.

5.4 Prediction, Risk Factors, and Prevention of Preeclampsia

No test can reliably predict the development of all cases of preeclampsia, but risk factors can be identified. Presence of Antiphospholipid antibodies, preeclampsia in a previous pregnancy, preexisting diabetes mellitus, family history of preeclampsia, multifetal gestation, nulliparity, body mass index>30 kg/m^2, and maternal age more than 40 years are the risk factors known for the development of preeclampsia [2]. As per ISSHP, women with any of these strong risk factors should be treated with low dose aspirin; ideally before 16 weeks, but definitely before 20 weeks of gestation. 150 mg/day of aspirin may show benefit to prevent preterm preeclampsia, but NOT term preeclampsia in women with combination of maternal risk factors, placental growth factors (PlGF), and abnormal uterine artery doppler [1].

1.2–2.5 gm/day of calcium is suggested for women taking low calcium (<600 mg/day) in "at risk" women. Physical exercise during pregnancy helps in reducing the risk of developing hypertension.

According to recent NICE 2023 guidelines on Hypertension in pregnancy, diagnosis and management and placental growth factor (PlGF)-based tests are used to rule in or rule out preeclampsia in patients with suspected preterm preeclampsia (20 weeks to 36 weeks and 6 days of pregnancy). These are:

- DELFIA Xpress PlGF 1–2–3.
- DELFIA Xpress sFlt-1/PlGF 1–2–3 ratio.
- Elecsys immunoassay sFlt-1/PlGF ratio.
- Triage PlGF Test.

5.5 Diagnosis

Preeclampsia can be defined by systolic BP ≥ 140 mmHg or diastolic BP ≥ 90 mmHg, on at least two separate occasions, at least 4 h apart, plus new onset proteinuria, or one of the "severe" features. Hypertension with only one severe feature is sufficient to stamp the case as preeclampsia.

Proteinuria is defined as 300 mg of protein in 24-h urinary sample or urinary protein/creatinine (PCr) ratio of >0.3. Urine dipstick level of at least 1+ (30 mg/dL), on two separate occasions at least 6 h apart, suggests preeclampsia level proteinuria. Massive proteinuria (>5 gm in 24-h urinary sample) is associated with more severe neonatal outcome, and PCr > 9 is associated with worse maternal outcome [3].

"Severe" features of preeclampsia include systolic BP ≥ 160 mmHg, diastolic BP ≥ 110 mmHg, elevated creatinine level (> 1.1 mg/dL), hepatic dysfunction/right upper-quadrant-epigastric pain, new onset headache/visual disturbances, platelet count <1 lakh/cmm, and pulmonary edema (due to increased peripheral vascular resistance/cardiac dysfunction). Glomerular filtration rate (GFR) decreases, which may progress to oliguria and renal failure. Elevated liver enzymes, with subcapsular hemorrhage, and occasionally, capsular rupture leading to intra-abdominal bleeding, represent possible liver dysfunction. Preeclampsia may proceed onto coagulopathies; i.e., HELLP syndrome and Disseminated Intravascular coagulation (DIC).

Table 5.1 Diagnostic criteria for HELLP syndrome

Hemolysis	Serum bilirubin >1.2 mg/dL Damaged RBC in peripheral blood smear
Elevated liver enzymes	Alanine/aspartate transaminase more than double the upper limit of normal Lactate dehydrogenase >600 U/L
Low platelet count	< 1 lakh/microL

5.5.1 HELLP Syndrome

This occurs in around 20% of pregnancies having preeclampsia with severe features. HELLP syndrome occurs majorly at preterm stage (53%) and postpartum (30%), as compared to at term (18%) [4].Diagnostic criteria have been mentioned in Table 5.1. Eternal vigilance is of utmost value, as nearly 12–18% of women with HELLP syndrome can be normotensive, and nearly 13% women may not have proteinuria [5].

5.5.2 Eclampsia

This life-threatening emergency can occur antepartum (53%), intrapartum (19%), or postpartum (28%), and may be preceded by headache (80%) and visual changes (45%). Usually, these seizures are associated with hypertension; they may occur in the absence of severe features with normal BP [6].

Generalized tonic-clonic in nature, 60–90 s cycle, followed by post-ictal confusion/agitation, usually lead to fetal hypoxia-bradycardia.

If any of the following criteria (Eden's criteria) is present, CT scan needs to be done: temperature > 39^0 C, pulse >120/min, coma for more than 6 h, respiratory rate > 40/min, systolic BP > 200 mmHg, number of convulsions more than ten.

Major complications may arise, such as abruptio placentae, neurological deficits, aspiration pneumonia, pulmonary edema, cardiopulmonary arrest, acute renal failure, and maternal death.

5.6 Management

Earliest diagnosis and finding balance between continuation and termination of pregnancy with proper control of BP and vigilant monitoring need to be the aim.

5.6.1 Fetal Monitoring

Fetal biometry, amniotic fluid index, fetal doppler should be monitored regularly. In case of confirmed preeclampsia or stamped case of intrauterine fetal growth restriction (FGR/IUGR), monitoring should be done 24 weeks gestation onward until birth. In case of high resistance of umbilical artery doppler study (Pulsatility Index (PI) > 95th percentile) or absent or reduced end-diastolic flow, decision must be taken keeping in mind optimal fetal outcome, with more frequent vigilant monitoring. Fetal growth restriction is stamped on the basis of umbilical and uterine artery doppler changes along with placental morphology, as per the Society of Obstetricians and Gynecologists of Canada. Estimated fetal weight (EFW) less than tenth percentile suggests reflect IUGR. EFW less than third percentile with abnormal umbilical artery doppler suggest adverse perinatal outcome [1].

Antenatal corticosteroids are recommended between 24 and 34 completed weeks, and should be continued up to 38 completed weeks, in case of elective cesarean section.

$MgSO_4$ for fetal neuroprotection should be given to pregnancies less than 32 weeks of gestation.

Mode of delivery should be decided on basis of maternal and fetal condition, with cesarean section being necessary in majority of cases of absent or reversed end diastolic flow in umbilical artery doppler or in cases of very preterm labor.

Placental histopathological examination is recommended is cases of FGR.

5.6.1.1 Management of Maternal Hypertension

Target BP should be of systolic 110–140 mmHg, diastolic 80–85 mmHg.

Oral antihypertensives used are: Labetalol, as first-line agent, 100 mg twice a day to maximum dose of 400 mg twice a day. Oral methyldopa can be given in dose of 250 mg twice a day/thrice a day to maximum dose of 4 gm in 24 h. Oral nifedipine in dose of 20–60 mg a day to maximum dose of 120 mg/day.

Patients with *chronic hypertension* should be put on labetalol as first choice, followed by methyldopa and nifedipine as alternatives. Prazosin and hydralazine are recommended as the second- and third-line agents, respectively. Pregnancy can be continued up to 39 completed weeks of gestation, with proper BP control and stable fetal condition.

White Coat Hypertension needs to be managed conservatively, at least up to BP of 160/110 mmHg in hospital setting. Regular home-based BP monitoring is needed, as nearly half of these cases may develop gestational hypertension or preeclampsia.

Gestational Hypertension should be treated with antihypertensives and monitored regularly. Hospital admission is needed in cases where BP is recorded ≥160/110 mmHg, or when patient develops preeclampsia. In case of proper control of BP, reassuring fetal condition, and absence of preeclampsia, pregnancy can be continued at least up to 39 completed weeks of gestation.

5.6.1.2 Preeclampsia

Target systolic BP of <160 mmHg and diastolic BP of around 85 mmHg are preferred to avoid severe maternal hypertension and related maternal and fetal complications. Caution must be taken to avoid fall of diastolic BP to less than 80 mmHg. Once the patient gets stabilized, with absence of any severe features, she can be managed on outpatient basis; but if severe features develop, she needs to be given prophylactic $MgSO_4$. $MgSo_4$ has been found to be more effective at preventing recurrent seizures and decreasing maternal mortality as compared to phenytoin, diazepam, chlorpromazine, promethazine, and meperidine [7].

Table 5.2 describes injectable antihypertensives and Table 5.3 mentions continuous infusions.

In case of admitted patients, routine fetal monitoring, along with maternal monitoring in the form of assessment for proteinuria, twice weekly blood investigations (Complete blood count, liver enzymes, renal function test, uric acid, and blood sugar), fundus examination for retinopathy, ultrasonography of abdomen with fetal doppler should be performed.

Pregnancy with preeclampsia can be continued upto 37 completed weeks, but has to be terminated earlier if any of the severe features of preeclampsia develops. Proteinuria or uric acid should not be used for indication of delivery [1].

In low resource setting, convulsion prophylaxis should be given in the form of $MgSO_4$ in loading dose of 4 gm i.v. or 10 gm i.m., followed by 5 g i.m. every 4 h or an infusion of 1 g/h until delivery and for at least 24 h postpartum. In tertiary care centers, this prophylaxis is usually initiated in cases with severe hypertension and proteinuria or in the presence of premonitory signs [1]. As per ISSHP guidelines, timing of delivery can be offered as given below (Table 5.4).

In case of conservative management, delivery becomes necessary, when one or more of the following emerge:

- Maternal $SPO_2 < 90\%$.
- Persistently high BP with all three classes of antihypertensives in adequate doses.
- Intractable headache, visual disturbances, or eclampsia.
- Non-reassuring cardiotocograph, reversal of end diastolic flow in umbilical artery doppler, or intrauterine fetal death.
- Abruptio placentae.
- Worsening liver function tests, hemolysis, or thrombocytopenia.

Table 5.2 Antihypertensive for severe preeclampsia [8]

Antihypertensive	Dose
Hydralazine	5–10 mg i.v. over 2 min. If systolic BP > 160 mmHg or diastolic BP > 110 mmHg, after 20 min; additional 10 mg i.v. if still above desired level, switch to i.v. labetalol
Labetalol	20 mg i.v. initial dose, if target BP not achieved after 10 min, double the dose to 40 mg, and if target BP not reached after next 10 min, dose needs to be 80 mg. Maximum dose: 220–300 mg in 24 h (contraindicated in asthma, heart disease, congestive heart failure)
Nifedipine	10 mg initial dose. Additional 20 mg, if target BP not achieved after 30 min. If BP is still not controlled after next 30 min, can add 20 mg, followed by 10–20 mg every 4–6 h accordingly.

Table 5.3 Continuous i.v. infusions

Antihypertensive	Infusion dose
Labetalol	1 mg/min
Nicardipine	5–10 mg/h
Nitropruside	0.2 microgram/kg/min every 5 min, up to max. dose of 4 microgram/kg/min (only for few hours, as it will lead to fetal cyanide toxicity, and increased maternal intracranial pressure with worsening of cerebral edema)
Nitroglycerine	5 microgram/min, can be doubled every 5 min, up to maximum of 100 microgram/min

Table 5.4 Decision of delivery in relation to onset of preeclampsia

Onset of preeclampsia	Management
At ≥37 weeks of gestation	Delivery
Between 34 and 37 completed weeks of gestation	Expectant management
<34 weeks of gestation	Conservative approach with maternal and fetal monitoring
Before 24 weeks of gestation	Counseling and termination of pregnancy should be offered

Intrapartum: Antihypertensives should be given as scheduled, and in case of severe cases, injectable labetalol should be started. Fluid should be restricted to 60–80 mL/h to avoid pulmonary edema.

Postpartum: Treatment threshold for postpartum phase is systolic BP ≥ 150 mmHg and diastolic BP ≥ 100 mmHg, on two separate occasions at least 4 h apart. BP monitoring every 4–6 h, as preeclampsia or even eclampsia may occur de novo intra- or postpartum phase. Blood investigations, assessment for retained product should be done when any of the reports are abnormal before delivery, or in case of de novo preeclampsia. Lowering of dose of antihypertensive should be done gradually after third to sixth day postpartum, or if the patient goes into hypotension. NSAIDs should be avoided, mainly when the patient has developed acute kidney injury. Increase in urine output will be a sign of improvement.

5.7 Preferred Anesthesia for Cesarean Section (CS)

- Spinal anesthesia is preferred over epidural, as the former has quicker onset and better quality of sensory blockage.
- General anesthesia (G/A) is preferred in cases of coagulopathy and fetal bradycardia.
- Neuraxial anesthesia techniques are preferred over G/A for elective CS, as the former leads to decrease in serum catecholamines and improvement in uteroplacental blood flow. G/A may lead to pressor response, may result in dangerous rise in BP leading to intracranial hemorrhage [9].

- Neuraxial anesthesia can be given 10–12 h after prophylactic dose of LMWH (low molecular weight heparin), 24 h after therapeutic dose of LMWH, and 4 h after last dose of unfractionated heparin (UFH) with normal aPTT.

5.7.1 Eclampsia

Call for further assistance, place patient on her left side, insert mouth gauge for avoiding tongue bite. Usage of soft padding and side rails do prevent injuries from fall. $MgSO_4$ is the drug of choice for initial as well as recurrent convulsions. Multiple medications can lead to maternal and fetal adverse effects such as respiratory depression and aspiration. The following are the regimens for $MgSO_4$ usage:

Sibai regimen: 4–6 gm of loading dose i.v. over 15–20 min, followed by continuous infusion of 2 gm/h. In case of convulsion with ongoing continuous infusion, additional 2 gm can be given i.v.

Pritchard regimen: 5 gm i.m. doses on both buttocks each, along with 4 gm i.v. slowly, followed by 5 gm on alternate buttocks every 4 hourly till 24 h after delivery/from last convulsion; whichever is last.

Monitoring of Mg levels is required if there is renal dysfunction, increased creatinine, urine output <30 ml/h, or loss of deep tendon reflexes.

CT brain (with abdominal shield, if predelivery), MRI are helpful to diagnose PRES (posterior reversible encephalopathy syndrome), intracranial hemorrhage, or other neurological damages.

5.7.2 HELLP Syndrome

$MgSO_4$ should be administered from the time of admission 24–48 h postpartum. Platelet-rich plasma is indicated when women have abnormal bleeding, or platelets <20,000/microL before vaginal delivery or <50,000/microL before Cesarean section.

5.8 Differential Diagnosis

Acute fatty liver of pregnancy, thrombotic thrombocytopenic purpura, hemolytic uremic syndrome, sepsis, and vasculitis/other systemic rheumatic conditions may imitate preeclampsia.

5.8.1 Follow-Up

Patient should be followed up 1 week after discharge to assess requirement of antihypertensive medications. A follow-up at 3 months needs to be done for confirming normalized BP and blood investigations. Longer time hypertension persists postpartum, more will be the consequences of chronic vascular diseases.

Patients with HDP may suffer from stroke, cardiovascular disease, diabetes mellitus, chronic kidney disease, venous thromboembolic disorder, and death as compared to normotensive pregnancies. Counseling should be done that patients with preeclampsia can have 15% chances of developing preeclampsia and gestational hypertension in future pregnancies. Women with gestational hypertension can develop preeclampsia in 4% cases, and gestational hypertension in 25% cases [10].

Key Points

- HDP covers a wide spectrum, and uniform classification will help in properly documenting, understanding, and improving maternal and fetal outcomes.
- Aspirin should be started in patients with high risk factors. At least before 20 weeks of gestation.
- "Severe" features should be watched for, as hypertension with even a single such feature should be considered as preeclampsia
- Being watchful will help, as patients with HELLP syndrome and eclampsia, may occur even in normotensive patients.
- Umbilical artery doppler is a useful tool for fetal monitoring and guides timing and mode of delivery.
- MgSO4 has been proven to be effective in preventing recurrent convulsions as well as in reducing maternal mortality.
- Spinal anesthesia is preferred for Cesarean section, except in cases of coagulopathy and fetal bradycardia, where General Anesthesia is preferred.
- Patients with preeclampsia are more prone to chronic vascular diseases in the long run, and chances of developing preeclampsia is higher in the subsequent pregnancy.

References

1. Brown MA, Magee LA, Kenny LC, et al. Hypertensive disorders of pregnancy. AHA J. 2018;72:24–43.
2. Leeman L, Dresang LT, Fontaine P, et al. Hypertensive disorders of pregnancy. Am Fam Physician. 2016;93(2):121–7.
3. Chan P, Brown M, Simpson JM, Davis G. Proteinuria in pre-eclampsia: how much matters? BJOG. 2005;112:280–5. https://doi.org/10.1111/j.1471-0528.2004.00395.x.
4. Sibai BM, Ramadan MK, Usta I, et al. Maternal morbidity and mortality in 442 pregnancies with hemolysis, elevated liver enzymes, and low platelets (HELLP syndrome). Am J Obstet Gynecol. 1993;169(4):1000–6.
5. Sibai BM. Diagnosis, controversies, and management of the syndrome of hemolysis, elevated liver enzymes, and low platelet count. Obstet Gynecol. 2004;103(5 pt 1):981–91.
6. Mattar F, Sibai BM. Eclampsia. VIII. Risk factors for maternal morbidity. Am J Obstet Gynecol. 2000;182(2):307–12.
7. Duley L, Henderson-Smart DJ, Walker GJ, et al. Magnesium sulphate versus diazepam for eclampsia. Cochrane Database Syst Rev. 2010;(12):CD000127.

8. Committee on Obstetric Practice. Committee opinion no. 623: emergent therapy for acute onset, severe hypertension during pregnancy and the post-partum period. Obstet Gynecol. 2015;125(2):521–5.
9. Reynolds F. Labour analgesia and the baby: good news is no news. Int J Obstet Anesth. 2011;20:38–50.
10. Brown MA, Mackenzie C, Dunsmuir W, Roberts L, Ikin K, Matthews J, Mangos G, Davis G. Can we predict recurrence of pre-eclampsia or gestational hypertension? BJOG. 2007;114:984–93. https://doi.org/10.1111/j.1471-0528.2007.01376.x.

6 Hyperglycemia in Pregnancy

Bhanupriya

Hyperglycemia in pregnancy (HIP) is the most common medical disorder of pregnancy. HIP affects 16.9% of pregnancies worldwide in some or other forms. The prevalence is as high as 25.0% in the South-East Asia region, which is much higher than North America and Caribbean Region where it is 10.4%. The low- and middle-income countries encounter more than 90% of cases of HIP [1]. Hyperglycemia is one of the most common medical complications in pregnancy, affecting an estimated 15.8% of live births in 2019. Out of this, approximately 84% were affected by gestational diabetes mellitus (GDM) and 16% had preexisting diabetes, which preceded pregnancy or were first time diagnosed during antenatal period [2]. The occurrence of maternal and fetal complications is on the higher side in women with GDM, e.g., preeclampsia, fetal macrosomia (resulting in shoulder dystocia and birth injury), and neonatal hypoglycemia (Fig. 6.1) [3, 4].

Bhanupriya (✉)
Department of Obstetrics & Gynaecology, University College of Medical Sciences & Guru Teg Bahadur Hospital, New Delhi, Delhi, India

R. Sharma, A. Kumar (eds.), *Systemic Disorders in Pregnancy*,
https://doi.org/10.1007/978-981-96-4876-4_6

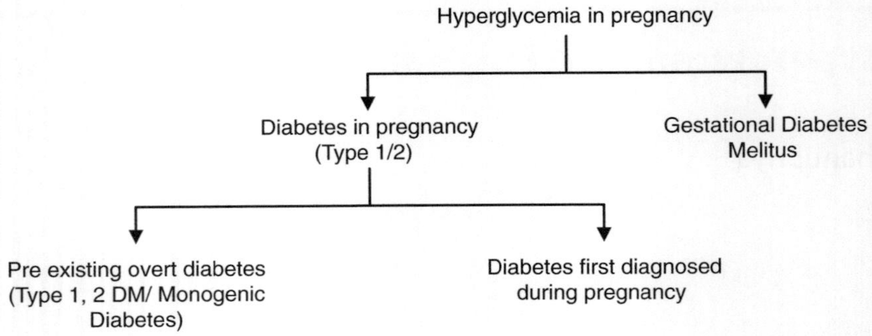

Fig. 6.1 Classification of hyperglycemia in pregnancy

6.1 Pathophysiology of Hip

Maternal metabolism changes in pregnancy to allow for the fetus growth and nourishment. Placental hormones mediated modified maternal carbohydrate, lipid, and amino acid metabolism. Maternal insulin secretion increases in response to rising insulin resistance in pregnancy for maintaining euglycemia. As the pregnancy advances, insulin resistance continues to rise and maximum insulin resistance is established by the 24th week. Hyperglycemia is prevented till maternal pancreas continues to increase insulin production and secretion. Maternal hyperglycemia ensues when this capacity is exhausted by rising insulin resistance [5].

6.2 Feto–Maternal Complications

Fetal Implications It has been hypothesized that the mother with diabetes mellitus have an abnormal metabolic environment, which affects the development of fetal tissues and eventually has permanent long-term functional implications in adult life. As per Frienkel's hypothesis, aberrant fuel mixture modifies the phenotypic expression in newly formed cells. The effect on fetus depends on the timing of (embryonic–fetal) exposure to the aberrant fuel mixture. Early in the first trimester, "fuel-mediated teratogenesis" may lead to intrauterine growth restriction and organ malformation. During the second trimester, brain development and differentiation may be affected leading to behavioral, intellectual, or psychological damage. During the third trimester, hyperplasia of pancreatic beta cells and abnormal proliferation of fetal adipocytes may be responsible for the development of obesity, hypertension, and T2DM later in life (Fig. 6.2) [6, 7].

Maternal Implications: Increased risk of maternal morbidity and mortality are found in such women. Also, there is a higher risk of vascular dysfunctions like retinopathy and nephropathy and long-term increased risk of diabetes and cardiovascular diseases (Fig. 6.3).

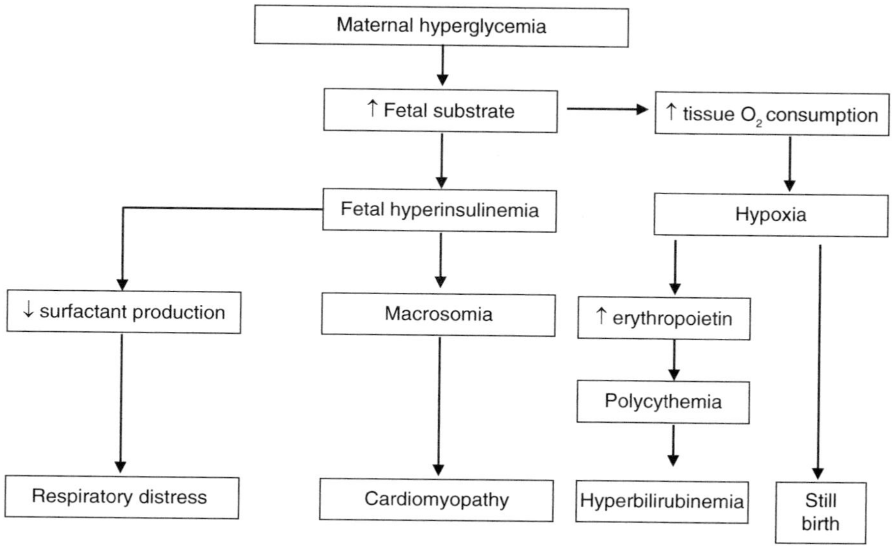

Fig. 6.2 Pathophysiology of maternal hyperglycemia on fetus

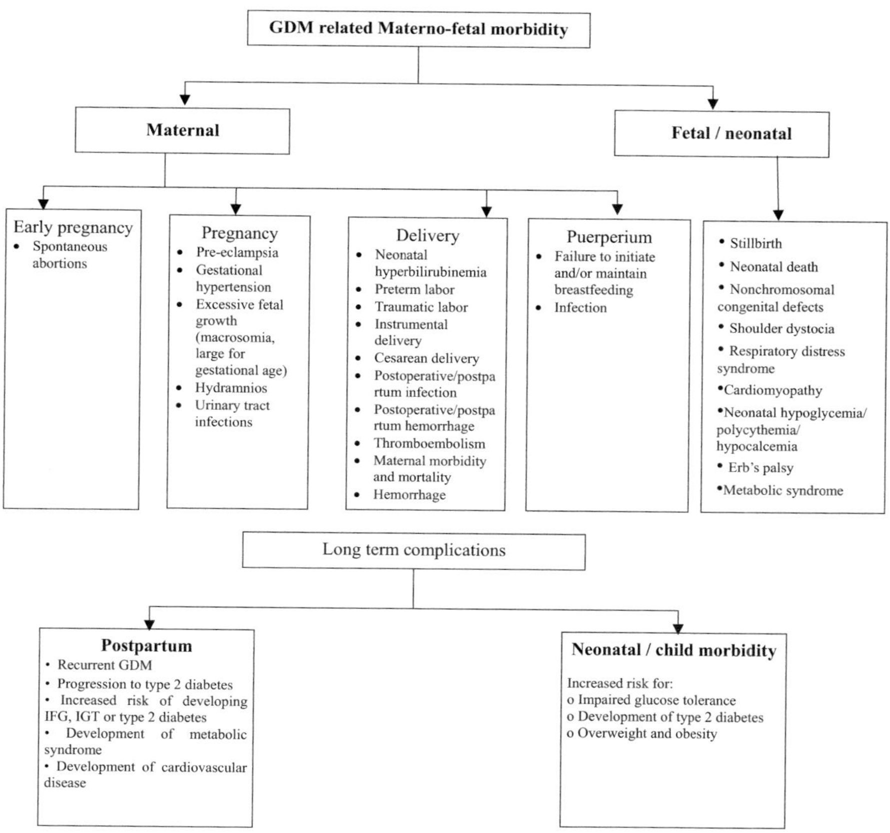

Fig. 6.3 GDM-associated maternal and fetal morbidity

6.3 Diagnosis of GDM

Glucose criteria are used to diagnose GDM. Most nations and societies have agreed on 75 g oral glucose tolerance test (OGTT) to be performed between 24 and 28 weeks of pregnancy for diagnosing GDM. Majority of societies recommend risk-based screening and do not suggest universal screening before 24 weeks (Table 6.1). FIGO recommends universal screening in low–middle income countries, where due to lack of awareness leads to nearly 90% of all cases of GDM [8].

Study comparing the WHO 2009 criteria IADPSG criteria concluded that a single WHO 2hPG of ≥140 mg/dL appears to be sufficient to diagnose GDM and appears to be suitable for large-scale screening for GDM in India and other developing countries [9]. Hence, India being a high-risk population, Diabetes in Pregnancy Study Group of India (DIPSI) criteria for diagnosing GDM is appropriate for screening. One Indian study by Saxena et al. in 2017 suggested that non-fasting DIPSI criteria has comparable diagnostic value than WHO oral GTT and is a practical alternative to OGTT [10]. The diagnostic criteria recommended by different societies have been described in Table 6.2.

6.3.1 How to Perform DIPSI Test

(a) *Procedure*

It is a single-step testing using 75 gm oral glucose, blood glucose is measured 2 h after ingestion (Table 6.3) 0.75 gm glucose is dissolved in 300 ml water irrespective of fasting status. The solution must be completed within 5–10 min. BG is detected after 2 h of oral glucose load by a plasma standardized glucometer. If vomiting occurs within 30 min of oral glucose intake, the test is repeated the next day.

Table 6.1 Risk factors warranting early screening to detect DIP

Testing advised in obese/overweight (BMI > 23 kg/m²) with one or more additional risk factors
Advanced maternal age
History of GDM, family history of diabetes
Racial/ethnic group that is at increased risk for developing type 2 diabetes (Hispanic, Native American, South or East Asian, or Pacific Islander descent)
Physical inactivity
Have previously given birth to an infant weighing 4000 g or more
Hypertension (>140/90 mm Hg or on therapy for hypertension)
High-density lipoprotein cholesterol level less than 35 mg/dL (0.90 mmol/L), a triglyceride level greater than 250 mg/dL (2.82 mmol/L)
Women with polycystic ovarian syndrome
HbA1C greater than or equal to 5.7%, impaired glucose tolerance, or impaired fasting glucose on previous testing
Other clinical conditions associated with insulin resistance (e.g., prepregnancy body mass index greater than 40 kg/m², acanthosis nigricans)
History of cardiovascular disease

Table 6.2 Screening guidelines of professional organizations

Organization	Screening (selective/ universal)	Testing methodology	Diagnostic value
American college of Obstetricians and Gynecologists [11] (ACOG) 2018	At 24 weeks or more Early pregnancy screening in high risk women	Two-step method 50 gm oral glucose challenge test (**If screen positive ≥ 130–140 mg/dL**)100 gm, 3 h 75 gm Oral Glucose Tolerance Test (OGTT)	Carpenter and Coustan or NDDG Fasting ≥ 95/ Fasting ≥ 10 5 1-h ≥ 180/ 1-h ≥ 190 2-h ≥ 155/2–h ≥ 165 3-h ≥ 140/ 3-h ≥ 145 wo abnormal values needed for diagnosis
US Preventive Services Task Force Recommendation Statement (2021) [12]	At 24 weeks or more Insufficient evidence for early screening	Two-step screening method (non-fasting 50 gm glucose challenge test (GCT) f/b OGTT with 75 gm glucose)	GCT- screen positive: ≥130–140 mg/dL OGTT: Carpenter and Coustan or NDDG (as above) Two abnormal values needed for diagnosis
American Diabetes Association (ADA) 2023 [13]	Test for undiagnosed prediabetes and diabetes at the first prenatal visit High risk	Two-step screening method (non-fasting 50 gm GCT f/b OGTT with 75 gm glucose)	Fasting ≥ 92 mg/dL 1-h ≥ 180 2-h ≥ 153 mg/dL One abnormal value needed for diagnosis
British National Institute for Health and Care Excellence (NICE) [14]	Targeted screening only in high risk	75-g 2-h oral glucose tolerance test (OGTT)	Fasting ≥ 100 mg/dL 2 h ≥ 140 One abnormal value needed for diagnosis
The Society of Obstetricians and Gynaecologists of Canada 2019 [15]	Universal screening between 24 and 28 weeks Women with risk factors to be screened earlier, repeat at 24–28 weeks if earlier negative	Preferred two-step approach (non-fasting GCT followed by OGTT) Acceptable (one step)—OGTT with 75 gm glucose (fasting and 1 h)	**2 Step** Screen positive GCT ≥ 140 mg/dL OGTT: Fasting: ≥ 95 1 h ≥ 190 2 h ≥ 162 **1 Step** Fasting: ≥ 90 1 h ≥ 180 2 h ≥ 153

(continued)

Table 6.2 (continued)

Organization	Screening (selective/ universal)	Testing methodology	Diagnostic value
IADPSG/WHO [16]	Universal screening	75-g 2-h oral glucose tolerance test (OGTT	Fasting ≥ 92 mg/dL 1-h ≥ 180 2-h ≥ 153 mg/dL One abnormal value needed for diagnosis
Indian guidelines (national health Mission) 2018 [17]	Universal screening, any time/repeat test at 24–28 weeks	75-g 2-h oral glucose tolerance test (OGTT) irrespective of fasting	2-h ≥ 140 mg/dL

Table 6.3 Diagnostic criteria for HIP

Blood glucose test	Plasma glucose level
Fasting	≥126 mg/dL
1 h	Not used
2 h	≥200 mg/dL
Random	≥200 mg/dL Confirm with additional standard test
HbA1C	6.5% in early pregnancy

The threshold blood sugar level of ≥140 mg/dL (more than or equal to 140) is taken as cut off for diagnosis of GDM.

(b) *Instrument for testing*

In low resource countries where laboratory facilities are not close by, FIGO 2015/National Health Mission (NHM) India 2018 recommends plasma-calibrated handheld glucometer. It is recommended to do the parallel testing of few samples from time to time. Generally, the glucometer performance is considered satisfactory and current glucometer recommendations (compared with laboratory methods) range widely from ±5% to ±20% [18].

6.3.2 Role of HbA1C in Diagnosis

This test reflects the average glucose level in the prior 3 months. It is correlated with the congenital malformations risk but not with any other adverse pregnancy outcomes.

It is best used for prenatal care in women with overt diabetes. HbA1c does not replace the OGTT for the diagnosis of GDM. However, HbA1c may be used to verify the results of self-monitored glucose reports in women with GDM [19].

HbA1c levels may be assessed in the second and third trimesters of pregnancy for women with overt diabetes, to assess the level of risk for the pregnancy (NICE 2020).

6.3.3 Management of Hyperglycemia

Good fetal and maternal outcomes are directly correlated with tight maternal glycemic control. The primary goal of treatment for pregnancies complicated by diabetes is to ensure a near normal feto–maternal outcome by controlling maternal hyperglycemia.

6.3.4 Preconceptional Counseling (ADA 2023)

- The importance of achieving glucose levels as close to normal as is safely possible should be emphasized in preconception counseling. If HbA1C <6.5%, then risk for congenital anomalies, macrosomia, preterm birth, preeclampsia, etc., is minimized [20].
- Effective contraception (long acting reversible contraception) should be discussed and advised to avoid unplanned pregnancy until a treatment plan and A1C are optimized for pregnancy.
- Greater emphasis on nutrition, diabetes education, and screening for diabetes comorbidities and complications.
- Women with preexisting diabetes should be counseled about the progression/development of retinopathy. Fundus examination before pregnancy or in the first trimester and then every trimester (Table 6.4).

Table 6.4 The checklist for preconceptional care

Individualized weight management recommendation and healthy prepregnancy weight
Folic acid 2.5–5 mg daily to be started ideally 3 months prior to conception and continued until 12 weeks gestation
Physical activity
Self-monitoring of blood sugars
Target HbA1c ≤6.5%
Contraception
Review and cease or replace medications not advised during pregnancy medications
Screen for comorbidities and complications and manage/refer as appropriate: blood pressure (BP)/coronary artery disease (CAD)/retinal disease/kidney disease/autonomic neuropathy/diabetic foot disease/thyroid disease
Arrange baseline investigations: HbA1c (repeat every 2–3 months)/lipid profile/thyroid-stimulating hormone (TSH) and thyroid peroxidase (TPO) autoantibodies (for type 1 diabetes)
healthy eating/glycemic index/carbohydrate content

6.3.4.1 Antenatal Care

Objectives for antenatal care of women diagnosed with GDM:

- Effectively manage of the diabetes
- Monitor for maternal complications
- Prevent fetal/neonatal complications
- Provide routine antenatal care (Table 6.5)

Table 6.5 Key point for antenatal visits in pregnancy with diabetes

Antenatal visit	Care of women during visit
First booking appointment Preferably by 10 weeks	Preconception checklist to complete if not yet performed Provide education: Healthy eating in pregnancy hysical activity and reduction in sedentary time in pregnancy ndividualized weight gain recommendation Optimal glycemic control for better maternal and neonatal outcomes Assessment: Retinal/renal assessment (if done more than 3 months ago) Glycemic monitoring: Measure HbA1C in pregestational diabetes women to know level of risk Offer self-monitoring of blood glucose (SMBG) Ultrasound (USG) to confirm viability and gestational age of pregnancy at 7–9 weeks. Monitoring of maternal weight gain/ proteinuria Medications: Review medications and replace with pregnancy safe drugs Review insulin doses every 1–2 weeks or as required Preeclampsia prevention: Commence aspirin 100–150 mg daily with evening meal (unless contraindicated) from 12 weeks gestation and cease at 36 weeks gestation (ADA 2023) Commence calcium supplementation (total 1.5 g daily including dietary calcium) from 12 weeks gestation
At 16 weeks	Repeat retinal examination Review SMBG/titrate insulin doses every 1–2 weeks
At 20 weeks	Targeted ultrasound scan to detect fetal structural abnormalities, including examination of the fetal heart (four chambers, outflow tracts and three vessels). 2D ECHO of fetal heart is advised, if any abnormality detected in targeted scan
At 28 weeks	Fetal growth and amniotic fluid volume monitoring scan. Repeat retinal assessment to all women with preexisting diabetes. Women diagnosed with gestational diabetes in routine antenatal testing enter the care pathway at 24–28 weeks

(continued)

Table 6.5 (continued)

Antenatal visit	Care of women during visit
At 32 weeks	Fetal growth and amniotic fluid volume monitoring scan. Fetal AC on USG ≥75th percentile for gestational age, at 29 + 0 to 33 + 6 weeks gestation, correlates with excess fetal growth/adiposity and an increased risk of an LGA baby. Weekly nonstress test (NST) from 34 weeks gestation
At 34 weeks	No differences in care for women with diabetes
At 36 weeks	Fetal growth and amniotic fluid volume monitoring scan Counseling about: Timing, mode, and management of birth Analgesia and anesthesia Changes in glucose lowering drugs after birth Care of the baby after birth Breastfeed initiation and the effect of breastfeeding on blood glucose control Contraception and follow-up.
At 37—38 + 6 weeks	Induction of labor or (if indicated) cesarean section is offered to women with pregestational diabetes. Await spontaneous labor for other women
At 39 weeks	Offer tests of fetal well-being. Advise women with uncomplicated gestational diabetes to give birth no later than 40 weeks plus 6 days

Table 6.6 Institute of Medicine recommendations for weight gain during pregnancy

Prepregnancy body mass index	Total weight gain, Kg	Mean (range) rates of weight gain at the second and third trimester, kg/weeks)
Underweight <18.5	12.5–18	0.51 (0.44–0.58)
Normal weight 18.5–24.9	11.5–16	0.42 (0.35–0.50)
Overweight 25.0–29.9	7–11.5	0.28 (0.23–0.33)
Obese ≥30.0	5–9	0.22 (0.17–0.27)

6.3.5 Weight Gain During Pregnancy

Overweight and obese women have increased risk of pregnancy-related complications like diabetes, hypertensive complications, stillbirth, and increased risk for cesarean delivery. Based on prepregnancy body mass index, the Institute of Medicine (IOM) has given recommendations for weight gain during pregnancy (Table 6.6) [21].

6.3.6 Blood Sugar Monitoring

Self-monitoring of blood glucose is recommended. The target BG values are: fasting plasma glucose <95 mg/dL, 1-h postprandial glucose <140 mg/dL, and 2-h postprandial glucose <120 mg/dL. The target HbA1C in pregnancy is <6% without significant hypoglycemia, but the target value may be relaxed to <7% if patient is experiencing hypoglycemia (ADA 2023).

Glycemic targets decide the frequency of monitoring of blood glucose. There are insufficient RCT to support the optimal frequency. ACHOIS trial group et al. recommended initially daily glucose monitoring four times a day, once after fasting and again after each meal then daily monitoring at rotating times [22]. If blood glucose level (BGL) is elevated on two occasions at the same test point within 1 week, review recent dietary modifications, physical activity interventions, and pharmacologic interventions. If average BGL over 1 week is elevated (BGL at the same time each day) consider pharmacological therapy [23].

6.3.7 Target During Labor and Delivery

Transplacental transfer of high maternal glucose leads to neonatal hypoglycemia as a result of reflex hyperinsulinemia. Maternal hyperglycemia during labor and delivery is associated with neonatal hypoglycemia, in both GDM [24] and T2DM [25]. Maternal hyperglycemia during labor is also related with birth asphyxia and non-reassuring fetal heart rate tracings [26]. A target glucose levels in the range of 72–126 mg/dL during labor is associated with a lower risk of maternal hypoglycemia as well as reduction in the incidence of neonatal hypoglycemia, birth asphyxia, and non-reassuring heart rate tracings (Table 6.7). [27]

6.3.8 Medical Nutrition Therapy

Medical nutritional therapy in pregnancy is a carbohydrate-controlled meal, planned in a manner to balance appropriate weight gain with adequate nutrition; normoglycemia is aimed in absence of ketosis. [28] The fundamental treating modality of HIP is nutritional intervention. The ADA 2023 recommends development of a personalized nutrition plan based on the individual's body mass index by a registered dietitian for all patients with GDM. A clinician may also provide recommendations regarding nutritional plan, if dietician is not available. The basic plan is based on three major nutritional components: (1) caloric allotment, (2) carbohydrate intake, and (3) caloric distribution.

Calories restriction is effective in controlling weight gain, maintaining euglycemia and prevents macrosomia in women with GDM. A restricted caloric intake varying from 1500 to 2800 calories per day is reported to have successful pregnancy outcomes [29]. The dietary plan of GDM has been suggested as carbohydrate intake of 33–40% of calories, with the remaining calories divided between protein (20%)

Table 6.7 Recommendations for glycemic targets for gestational diabetes mellitus

Targets for glucose control during pregnancy:	FBS <95 mg/dL 1-h PP <140 mg/dL 2-h PP <120 mg/dL
Target for glucose control during labor and delivery	72–126 mg/dL

Table 6.8 Recommendations for nutrition therapy and physical activity (FIGO 2015)

Appropriate dietary plan in terms of BMI, prepregnancy weight, physical activity, personal and cultural preferences.
Provide regular follow-up and dietary adjustments achieve treatment goals.
Offer training, and follow-up by a qualified dietician for issues like: weight optimization, food records, carbohydrate calculation, prevention of hypoglycemia, healthy food habits, and physical activity.
Caloric intake as per prepregnancy BMI and desirable weight gain is as follows:
35–40 kcal/kg desirable body weight for underweight women
30–35 kcal/kg desirable body weight for normal weight women
25–30 kcal/kg desirable body weight for overweight women
Carbohydrate intake restriction to 35%–45% of total calories count, with a minimum of 175 g carbohydrate per day, which should be divided into three small-to-moderate sized meals and 2–4 snacks.
Caloric intake may be cut by 30% in obese women, but not below 1600–1800 kcal/d
Protein may be restricted to 0.6–0.8 g/kg ideal body weight in women with diabetic nephropathy
Recommendations for Physical Activity
Moderate intensity planned physical activity- 30 min/day
Physical activity can include aerobic exercise (e.g., walking, stationary cycle, swimming, prenatal exercise classes) and light or moderate resistance exercises
Women physically active prior to pregnancy should be encouraged to continue like before
Advise women to:
Remain hydrated and avoid dehydration during and after physical activity
Wear loose light clothes to avoid over heating
Avoid exercise when hungry, unwell, or with an elevated temperature
Avoid exercising in high temperatures and humidity

and fat (40%). The complex carbohydrates digest more slowly and does not cause postprandial hyperglycemia, hence is recommended over simple carbohydrates [30].

Exercise is adjuvant to Medical nutrition therapy (MNT), especially in overweight or obese women with GDM and improves glycemic control. Therefore, a moderate exercise program is a recommended treatment plan in women with GDM (Table 6.8) [31].

6.3.9 Medical Therapy

Pharmacologic treatment is recommended when nutrition therapy and exercise are not able to achieve the target glucose levels consistently. However, a systematic review deciphered no conclusive evidence for a specific threshold value to start medical therapy. [32]

Insulin was considered the gold standard for GDM management after MNT. Insulin does not cross the placenta, provides a tighter metabolic control and traditionally added if fasting blood glucose ≥95 mg/dL, 1-h ≥ 140 mg/dL, or 2-h ≥ 120 mg/dL. These thresholds are mostly extrapolated from recommendations for managing pregnancy in women with preexisting diabetes. In women with pregestational diabetes where insulin is used throughout the day, a typical starting total

Table 6.9 Action profile of commonly used insulin agents [33]

Type	Onset of action	Peak action(h)	Duration of action(h)
Insulin lispro	23–27 min	~1	~5
Insulin aspart	21 min	1–3	4–5
Regular insulin	60 min	2–4	5–8
Isophane insulin (suspension) (NPH insulin)	1–4 h	4–10	>14 h
Insulin glargine	1.5 h	Flat	24
Insulin detemir	3–4 h	Minimal peak at 6–8	20–26

dosage is 0.7–1.0 units/kg daily as per the period of gestation (POG). This dosage is divided in multiple injections using long-acting or intermediate acting insulin in combination with short-acting insulin.

Traditionally, NPH insulin is the commonly used insulin, but more recently insulin glargine and insulin detemir have been added in the list for long-acting use. Insulin lispro and insulin aspart are short-acting insulins. These insulin analogues are safer than regular insulins as they do not cross the placenta; both have a more rapid onset of action. Hence allows the patient to administer her insulin immediately before meal rather than 10–15 min before the meal. This avoids hypoglycemic episodes and provides better glycemic control (Table 6.9).

Oral antidiabetic agents (OAD) Glyburide has been acknowledged in the Fifth International Workshop-Conference on Gestational Diabetes Mellitus [34] and both are considered in the NICE guidance [14] and ACOG practice bulletin [11].

Metformin belongs to biguanide group that inhibits hepatic gluconeogenesis and glucose absorption and stimulates peripheral glucose uptake. Despite limited evidence to suggest that such use decreases the risks of adverse pregnancy outcomes and first-trimester loss, metformin is often continued until the end of the first trimester, in women with polycystic ovary syndrome [35]. The long-term metabolic influence on the offspring is still under research as it crosses the placenta with levels that can be as high as maternal concentrations [36].

Glyburide is a sulfonylurea that binds to pancreatic beta-cell adenosine triphosphate potassium channel receptors to increase insulin secretion and insulin sensitivity of peripheral tissues. Langer et al. conducted an RCT and reported no differences in the maternal and neonatal adverse outcomes between the glyburide and insulin treated groups, as well as no detection of glyburide in cord blood [37].

In a recent meta-analysis compared the efficacy and safety of metformin, glyburide, and insulin in treating gestational diabetes mellitus (GDM). It included 41 studies. Compared with metformin, insulin had a significant increase in the risk of preeclampsia (RR, 0.57; 95% CI, 0.45 to 0.72; $P < 0.001$), NICU admission (RR, 0.75; 95% CI, 0.64 to 0.87; $P < 0.001$), neonatal hypoglycemia (RR, 0.57; 95% CI, 0.49 to 0.66; $P < 0.001$), and macrosomia (RR, 0.68; 95% CI, 0.55 to 0.86; $P < 0.05$).

Table 6.10 Recommendations for pharmacological treatment in women with GDM (FIGO 2015, ADA 2023)

Oral Antidiabetic drugs (OAD): Insulin, glyburide, and metformin are considered safe and effective in the second and third trimesters, and in failed MNT cases may be offered as the first-line treatment.
Metformin is considered a better OAD than glyburide [38]
Insulin may be considered as the preferred OAD in women with GDM who have more chances of failure on OAD therapy, which includes following indication [39]: Diabetes diagnosed <20 weeks gestation Pharmacological therapy required >30 weeks FBS >110 mg/dL 1-h PP >140

Regarding birth weight and gestational age at delivery, insulin caused a significant increase when compared with metformin. Of the two groups, glyburide treated and metformin treated, metformin had lower gestational weight gain compared with glyburide (MD, 1.67; 95% CI, 0.26 to 3.07; $P < 0.05$). Glyburide had a higher risk of neonatal hypoglycemia compared with insulin. Hence, in the short term, in women with GDM requiring drug treatment, glyburide seems inferior to both insulin and metformin, while metformin (plus insulin when required) performs slightly better than insulin (Table 6.10) [40].

6.3.10 Management of Hypoglycemia

Pregnancy tends to have lower fasting BGLs and levels of 63 mg/dL may be physiologically normal [41].

Women with GDM who are not on pharmacotherapy uncommonly have hypoglycemia. It is more commonly associated with insulin therapy. In the absence of symptoms of hypoglycemia, confirm the BGL before initiating the treatment for hypoglycemia. The management of hypoglycemia as per degree is described in Table 6.11.

6.3.11 Preterm labor in GDM

Use of antenatal corticosteroid prophylaxis for threatened preterm labor has become more prevalent in recent years. Diabetes is not considered a relative contraindication for antenatal corticosteroids. NICE guideline recommends that diabetic women receiving steroids should have additional insulin according to an institutional protocol [14]. The national Indian guidelines on indoor management of diabetes recommend more vigorous blood glucose monitoring and increase in the dose of insulin in persons with diabetes who receive steroid therapy [17]. Women on insulin therapy will warrant an increase in dosage or a change in insulin regime. If poor glycemic control is still there even after increasing the dose of insulin by 20–30%, it is

Table 6.11 Management of hypoglycemia [17, 41]

Definition	Hypoglycemia (BGL > 70 mg/dL)
Precipitating factors	Excessive physical activity Overdosing of insulin Missed, delayed, or inadequate carbohydrate with meal [42] Infections
Presenting features	*Early symptoms*: Hunger, tremor, sweating, shaking, weakness. Light headedness, headache, tingling around lips *Severe symptoms:* Blurred vision, confusion, irritability occasionally loss of consciousness
Treatment	Pregnant woman to take *one 15 g serve (three heaped tablespoons)* of glucose powder in a glass of water; if glucose not available, alternatives include: a glass of soft drink *or* Half a glass of fruit juice *or* Six tablespoons of sugar or honey dissolved in water Take rest after the episode/avoid physical exertion If repeat episode, then retake the same amount of glucose Check BGL If more than one episode in a day, report to clinician Avoid over treating of hypoglycemia
Hypoglycemia prevention	Eat at regular interval Carry snacks all the times Take intermediate/long-acting insulin at the same time of the day Carry Glucometer in case feeling symptoms of hypoglycemia Identify the causal factors for hypoglycemia

suggested to increase the number of injections per day. Better glycemic control may be achieved by adding rapid acting insulin and substituting premixed insulin with rapid acting insulin or by changing to basal insulin from premixed regimen [43].

6.3.12 Intrapartum Care

6.3.12.1 Timing of Birth (NICE 2020)

- Women with good glycemia control and on medical therapy—Do not deliver before 39 weeks of gestation.
- Type 1 or type 2 diabetes (no complications)—Elective birth by induction of labor or cesarean section (if indicated), between 37 weeks and 38 weeks plus 6 days of pregnancy.
- Type 1 or type 2 diabetes (metabolic/maternal or fetal complications)—Elective birth <37 weeks.
- Women with diabetes with ultrasound-diagnosed macrosomic fetus—The risks and benefits of vaginal birth, induction of labor, and cesarean section to be explained.
- Vaginal birth after a previous cesarean section in pregnant women with diabetes should not be considered a contraindication.

6.3.13 Mode of Birth

The relative risk of stillbirth in overt diabetes after 39 weeks is increased, 7.2 (95% CI 1.31–39.63), with an absolute risk increase of nearly 1% [44].

Therefore, termination of pregnancy should be planned by the end of 38 completed weeks gestation in women with preexisting diabetes. The induction of labor for a suspected large-for-gestational-age, in women without diabetes is associated with a reduced risk of shoulder dystocia and associated morbidity compared with expectant management, but sparse data exist for women with diabetes [45].

If fetal weight is estimated at:

- Less than 4000 g—Vaginal birth is usually appropriate (NHM 2018, Australian 2020)
- 4000–4500 g—Vaginal birth may be appropriate after considering other individual factors (e.g., maternal stature, obstetric and birth history, previous macrosomia with or without shoulder dystocia, limitations of estimating fetal weight)
- More than 4500 g—consider elective CS. If the estimated fetal weight (EFW) at the time of birth is
- >4500 g in women with preexisting diabetes, the risk of shoulder dystocia is >20% [46]
- The risk of instrumental extraction for shoulder dystocia is increased in women with GDM compared to spontaneous vaginal birth

6.3.14 Preparation for Labor

Preparation for Induction of labor (IOL) (Table 6.12) [41].

Elective cesarean section in women with preexisting diabetes must be done early in the morning to avoid the risk of maternal hypoglycemia (Table 6.13).

Table 6.12 Preparation for induction of labor

IOL	Metformin	Insulin
In the prior night before the induction of labor	Take usual dose of metformin	The usual dose of predinner rapid-acting insulin is taken The usual dose of pre-bed intermediate-acting insulin (e.g., isophane) is taken. The dose of pre-bed long-acting insulin (e.g., detemir, glargine) is reduced by 30–50%.
On the morning of induction of labor	Stop metformin when in established labor	Dose of rapid-acting insulin before breakfast (BBF) is decreased 50% decrease in dose of intermediate/long-acting insulin, BBF 1–2 hourly SMBG (target range of 72–126 mg/dL) is done
Spontaneous labor	Stop metformin when in established labor	Titrate BGL and start insulin accordingly

Table 6.13 Preparation for elective cesarean section

Elective cesarean section	Metformin	Insulin
In the prior night before the elective cesarean section	Omit the evening dose of metformin	Usual dose of rapid-acting insulin before dinner and intermediate-acting insulin at bed time must be taken Reduce the dose of pre-bed long-acting insulin (e.g., detemir, glargine) by 30–50%
On the morning of the elective LSCS		Omit rapid-acting insulin and decrease dose of intermediate/long-acting insulin by 50%, BBF Perform hourly SMBG target range of (72–126 mg/dL)

6.4 Glycemic Management During Labor

The aim of glycemic management during labor is to avoid neonatal hypoglycemia and optimize feto–maternal outcomes. One of the study observed neonatal hypoglycemia in all cases of type 1 diabetes, where maternal blood sugar levels were >180 mg/dL during labor [47].

The mother with preexisting diabetes is just not at the risk of hyperglycemia but the work during labor and increased whole-body glucose utilization also predisposes 56% of mother to hypoglycemia during labor and immediately after birth [48]. Hourly SMBG is advised during labor, with glycemic goal of 72–126 mg/dL [14]. Intravenous insulin or glucose infusions may be required (Table 6.14).

6.4.1 Intrapartum Fetal Monitoring

Continuous electronic fetal monitoring is advisable to detect fetal compromise during labor. [49] In case of high chances of shoulder dystocia, skilled senior obstetrician and staff are required for delivery to manage it.

6.4.2 Diabetic Ketoacidosis (DKA)

DKA is a life-threatening obstetric emergency for mother as well as fetus and warrants prompt diagnosis and management. Pregnant individuals with diabetes, especially with type 1 DM are at higher risk of developing DKA. It may occur due to increased glucagon to insulin ratio along with simultaneous rise in counter-regulatory hormones (cortisol, growth hormone), resulting in absolute or relative insulin deficiency. This process overall leads to abnormal metabolism of carbohydrate, protein, and fat and produces a state of hyperglycemia and subsequent ketoacidosis [50]. The precipitating factor of DKA includes protracted vomiting, infections, steroid treatment, insulin noncompliance or condition like gastroparesis [51]. The clinical signs and symptoms are shown in Table 6.15.

Table 6.14 Insulin infusion preparation/starting doses and BGL targets

Insulin infusion	Start by infusion pump Start glucose infusion @80 ml/h (5% glucose solution with 0.9% normal saline) in the main line Start insulin infusion ((Add 50 units (0.5 mL of 100 units per mL) neutral insulin to 49.5 mL of sodium chloride 0.9% to give a concentration of 1 unit/mL) in a side line
BGL (mg/dL)	Insulin infusion
≤72 mg/dL	Discontinue infusion Notify and review by medical officer
73–108 mg/dL	1 unit/hr. (1 ml/h)
109–144 mg/dL	2 unit/h (2 ml/h)
145–180 mmol/L	3 unit/h (3 ml/h)
≥180 mg/dL	Continue infusion Notify and review by medical officer

Table 6.15 Signs and symptoms of DKA

Fatigue
Nausea/vomiting
Abdominal pain
Polyuria/ polydipsia
Blurred vision
Drowsiness, altered mental status
Kussmaul breathing (hyperventilation with fruity odor)
Tachypnea, hypotension, tachycardia, coma, shock
Abnormal fetal heart tracing

The diagnostic criteria as per Joint British Diabetes Societies Inpatient Care Group guidelines are as follows [52]:

1. Blood ketone level more than or equal to 3.0 mmol/L or urine ketone level more than 2+
2. Blood glucose level > 198 mg/dL or known diabetes mellitus
3. Bicarbonate level less than 15.0 mmol/L and/or venous pH less than 7.3
4. Additionally, an anion gap (Na– [Cl + HCO3]) of >12 mmol/L indicates the presence of an increased anion gap metabolic acidosis

6.4.2.1 Management of DKA [53, 54]

The principles of management of DKA in pregnancy are broadly the same as non-pregnant women. It includes identification and treatment of precipitating factors, fluid replacement, insulin therapy, and electrolyte repletion (Fig. 6.2). In addition, fetal monitoring is warranted to identify any deleterious consequences of maternal acidosis on the fetus. All suspected or confirmed patients should be admitted to highly specialized units (preferably intensive care units), which can manage DKA as well as provide continuous fetal monitoring. The management includes a multidisciplinary approach.

1. Intravenous fluid management
2. Intravenous insulin therapy
3. Electrolyte correction
4. Identification and treatment of precipitating factors
5. Monitoring of maternal and fetal response

6.5 Post Natal Care

6.5.1 Blood Glucose Monitoring and Insulin Titration

In immediate postnatal period, insulin requirements drop rapidly [55] because the insulin resistance attributed by the placental hormone secretions are immediately ameliorated after the delivery of placenta [56]. Hence, the insulin/glucose infusion should be ceased postdelivery. Hourly measurement of BGL should continue.

A. The insulin requirement continues to persist in majority of type 1 diabetes women. The principles to restart insulin are:
   - Restart subcutaneous insulin at the 50% dose of prepregnancy requirement when the BGL reaches around 144–180 mg/dL.
   - Ketone testing should be done if fasting >6 h or BGL >180 mg/dL or any clinical complications.
   - Subcutaneous insulin should then be titrated according to blood glucose levels. Close monitoring and regular adjustment are required. In the first 24–48 h after birth, insulin requirements are usually dramatically less than during pregnancy [55].
B. Women with type 2 diabetes majority of the times do not require insulin/oral glucose-lowering agents as diet alone will suffice to achieve adequate glycemia after the birth. SMBG (fasting, 2-hour post-meal and overnight) is advisable in the early postpartum period, with a target range of 70–180 mg/dL, to assess the need of glucose-lowering treatment.

If maternal hyperglycemia persists after delivery, the treatment options include insulin, metformin, or glibenclamide [57, 58]. Lifestyle advice, including healthy eating, regular physical activity, social connection, and supporting good psychological health should be provided to women with type 2 diabetes in the early postpartum period. A biannual BGL should be done.

6.5.2 Risk of Infections

Mothers with diabetes are more prone to infections like genitourinary, uterine, or surgical site infections.

6.5.3 Breastfeeding

Breastfeeding should be encouraged in mothers with GDM and diabetes in pregnancy. Breastfeeding has been proven to be protective against the infant and maternal complications [59] including reduction in childhood obesity, T2/T1 DM [60, 61]. Moreover, breastfeeding promotes postpartum weight loss. Treatment with insulin or commonly used OADs, such as glyburide and metformin, is not contraindicated in breastfeeding as secretion of OAD in breast milk are negligible and do not cause hypoglycemia in the baby [57, 58].

6.5.4 Contraception

The World Health Organization has devised Medical Eligibility Criteria (MEC) to guide for choice of contraception. Women with diabetes without any complications has the advantage of choosing from the full range of contraceptive methods including hormonal contraception, as the benefits of usage outweigh the risk. Women with diabetic complications may require advice of specialist to assess the risk–benefit ratio, particularly for hormonal contraception. Copper intrauterine contraception device and oral emergency contraceptive is no restrictive usage (Tables 6.16 and 6.17).

6.5.5 Postpartum BG Surveillance

The glycemic status reevaluation should be done for all women diagnosed with HIP (GDM and diabetes in pregnancy) first time during pregnancy with a 75-g oral OGTT at 6–12 weeks after delivery [63] The diagnosis is made as per the recommendation by WHO criteria for diabetes [64], impaired fasting glucose (IFG), and impaired glucose tolerance (IGT) in the nonpregnant state. The risk of progression to diabetes and other cardiovascular problems persist even if the test does not show abnormal results (diabetes or prediabetes) and require ongoing surveillance (Fig. 6.4) [65].

Table 6.16 WHO MEC criteria for contraceptive eligibility for diabetic women [62]

Category	Clinical judgment
1	Unrestricted use
2	benefit outweighs theoretical or proven risk
3	Method not recommended; risk outweighs benefit
4	Method contraindicated

Table 6.17 Contraceptive methods for women with Diabetes [62]

Diabetic women	Complications	Copper intrauterine device	LNG IUD	Implanon	Depot Medroxy progesterone acetate	Progestin only pill	Combined hormonal contraceptives
	History of GDM	1	1	1	1	1	1
	Nonvascular disease						
	(a) Non-insulin dependent	1	2	2	2	2	2
	(b) Insulin dependent	1	2	2	2	2	2
	Nephropathy/neuropathy/retinopathy	1	2	2	3	2	3/4
	Other vascular disease/DM > 20 years duration	1	2	2	3	2	3/4

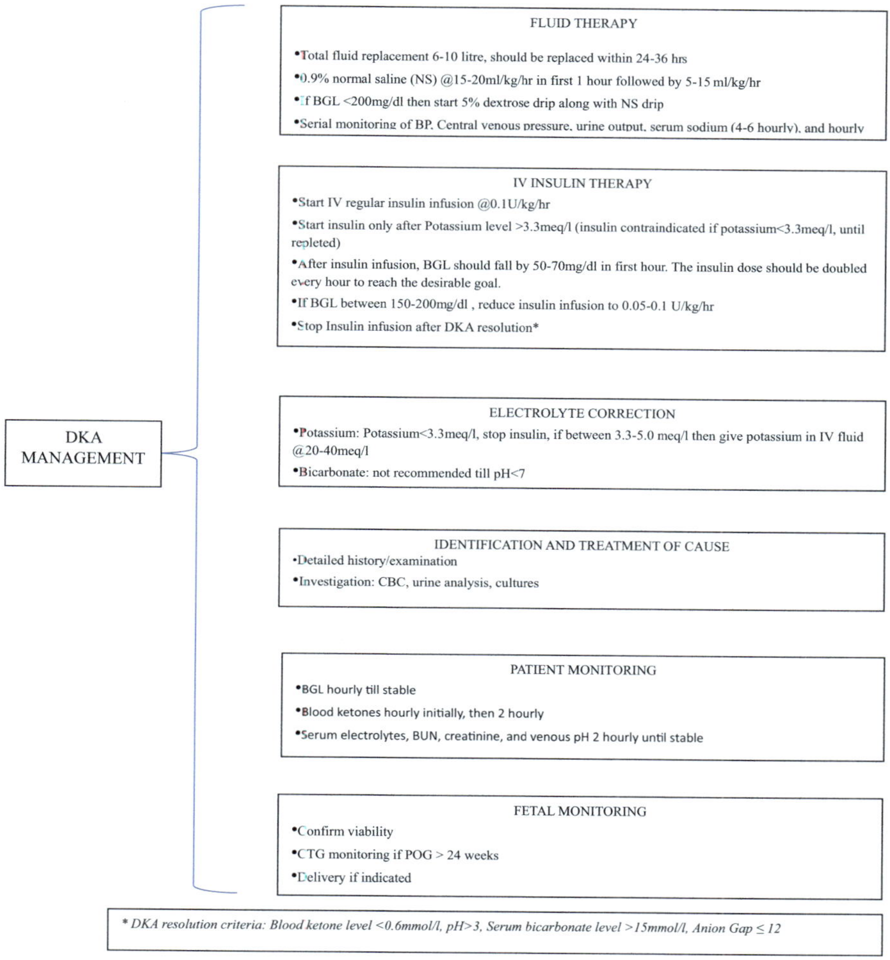

Fig. 6.4 Management of DKA in pregnancy

6.6 Long-Term Risk

The women with GDM have either the same or higher level of developing long-term risk of T2DM and cardiovascular disease irrespective of the glycemic status in the early postpartum period. Healthy lifestyle with regular exercise, nutritious diet, and maintenance of normal body weight should be advised. "Intensive lifestyle" and metformin are helpful highly in delaying or preventing diabetes in women with IGT and a history of GDM. [66] Data from the Diabetes Prevention Program Outcomes Study (DPPOS) reports beneficial effects of lifestyle intervention and metformin, over a longer period.

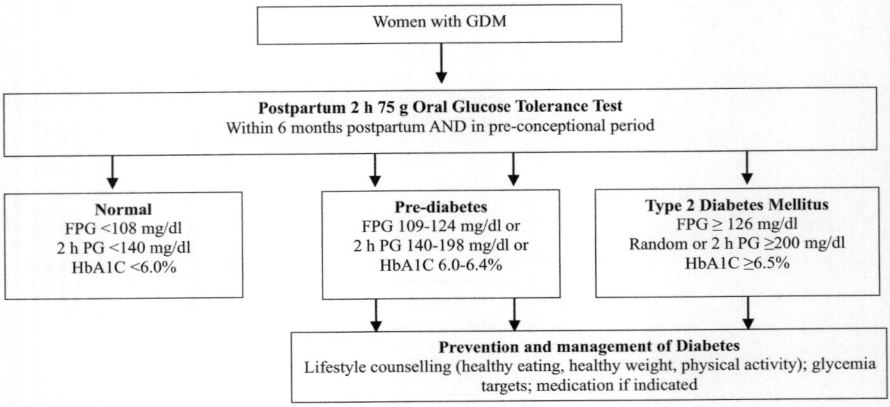

Fig. 6.5 Long-term follow-up of women with GDM

Aroda et al. [67] and show that the benefits of lifestyle intervention and metformin seen in the DPP study continue over a longer period (Fig. 6.5).

Key Points

1. Hyperglycemia in pregnancy has serious adverse outcomes to mother and fetus, so early detection and management is advisable.
2. There is lack of consensus on the methods of screening worldwide. The Ministry of Healthy and Family advocates for DIPSI criteria with 2-h BGL level > 140 mg/dL as the diagnostic criteria.
3. The blood glucose level targets in pregnancy are: fasting <90 mg/dL, 1 h and 2 h postprandial are <130–140 mg/dL and <120 mg/dL, respectively, which are the maintenance criteria.
4. Insulin and metformin are drug therapies used in hyperglycemia in pregnancy. Basal bolus regimen is the preferred regimen for insulin.
5. Careful timing and mode of delivery should be decided as the type of HIP.
6. Perioperative management of labor to maintain euglycemia in mother and prevent neonatal hypoglycemia.
7. Intrapartum fetal monitoring is like the other high-risk pregnancies.
8. Postpartum BGL monitoring and BG screening after 6–12 weeks are important components of postnatal surveillance.

References

1. Guariguata L, Linnenkamp I, Beagley J, et al. Global estimates of the prevalence of hyperglycemia in pregnancy. Diabetes Res Clin Pract. 2014;103:176–85.
2. International Diabetes Federation. IDF Diabetes Atlas. 9th ed. 2019. https://www.diabetesatlas.org.

3. Hartling L, Dryden DM, Guthrie A, et al. Screening and diagnosing gestational diabetes mellitus. Evid Rep Technol Assess (Full Rep). 2012;210:1–327.
4. Lowe WL Jr, Scholtens DM, Lowe LP, et al; HAPO Follow-up Study Cooperative Research Group. Association of gestational diabetes with maternal disorders of glucose metabolism and childhood adiposity. JAMA. 2018;320(10):1005–16.
5. Plows JF, Stanley JL, Baker PN, Reynolds CM, Vickers MH. The pathophysiology of gestational diabetes mellitus. Int J Mol Sci. 2018;19(11):3342.
6. Freinkel N. Banting Lecture 1980. Of pregnancy and progeny. Diabetes. 1980;29(12):1023–35.
7. Mitanchez D, Yzydorczyk C, Siddeek B, Boubred F, Benahmed M, Simeoni U. The offspring of the diabetic mother–short- and long-term implications. Best Pract ResClin Obstet Gynaecol. 2015;29(2):256–69.
8. Hod M, Kapur A, Sacks DA, Hadar E, Agarwal M, Di Renzo GC, Roura LC, McIntyre HD, Morris JL, Divakar H. The International Federation of Gynecology and Obstetrics (FIGO) Initiative on gestational diabetes mellitus: a pragmatic guide for diagnosis, management, and care. Int J Gynecol Obstet. 2015;131(Suppl. 3):S173.
9. Sagili H, Kamalanathan S, Sahoo J, Lakshminarayanan S, Rani R, Jayalakshmi D, Kumar KT. Comparison of different criteria for diagnosis of gestational diabetes mellitu. Indian J Endocrinol Metab. 2015;19(6):824–8.
10. Saxena P, Verma P, Goswami B. Comparison of diagnostic accuracy of non-fasting DIPSI and HbA1c with fasting WHO criteria for diagnosis of gestational diabetes mellitus. J Obstet Gynaecol India. 2017;67(5):337–42.
11. American College of Obstetricians and Gynecologists' Committee on Practice Bulletins—Obstetrics. ACOG Practice Bulletin No. 201: Pregestational Diabetes Mellitus. Obstet Gynecol. 2018;132(6):e228–48.
12. US Preventive Services Task Force, Davidson KW, Barry MJ, Mangione CM, Cabana M, Caughey AB, Davis EM, Donahue KE, Doubeni CA, Krist AH, Kubik M, Li L, Ogedegbe G, Owens DK, Pbert L, Silverstein M, Stevermer J, Tseng CW, Wong JB. Screening for prediabetes and type 2 diabetes: US Preventive Services Task Force Recommendation Statement. JAMA. 2021;326(8):736–43.
13. ElSayed NA, Aleppo G, Aroda VR, Bannuru RR, Brown FM, Bruemmer D et al; American Diabetes Association. Erratum 2. Classification and diagnosis of diabetes: Standards of Care in Diabetes-2023. Diabetes Care 2023;46(Suppl. 1):S19-S40. Diabetes Care. 2023;46(5):1106.
14. Tsakiridis I, Giouleka S, Mamopoulos A, Kourtis A, Athanasiadis A, Filopoulou D, Dagklis T. Diagnosis and management of festational diabetes mellitus: an overview of national and international guidelines. Obstet Gynecol Surv. 2021;76(6):367–81.
15. Berger H, Gagnon R, Sermer M. Guideline No. 393-Diabetes in Pregnancy. J Obstet Gynaecol Can. 2019;41(12):1814–1825.e1. Erratum in: J Obstet Gynaecol Can. 2020;42(10):1288
16. International Association of Diabetes and Pregnancy Study Groups Consensus Panel, Metzger BE, Gabbe SG, Persson B, Buchanan TA, Catalano PA, Damm P, Dyer AR, Leiva AD, Hod M, Kitzmiler JL, Lowe LP, McIntyre HD, Oats JJ, Omori Y, Schmidt MI. International association of diabetes and pregnancy study groups recommendations on the diagnosis and classification of hyperglycemia in pregnancy. Diabetes Care. 2010;33(3):676–82.
17. Government of India. Maternal and Health Division, Diagnosis and Management of Gestational Diabetes Mellitus: Technical and Operational Guidelines. New Delhi, India: Ministry of Health & Family Welfare, New Concept Information Systems; 2018.
18. Sacks DB, ed. Guidelines and recommendations for laboratory analysis in the diagnosis and management of diabetes mellitus. https://www.aacc.org/~/media/practice-guidelines/diabetes-mellitus/diabetesmellitusentirelmpg.pdf?la=en. Published 2011.
19. Jovanovic L, Savas H, Mehta M, Trujillo A, Pettitt DJ. Frequent monitoring of A1C during pregnancy as a treatment tool to guide therapy. Diabetes Care. 2011;34(1):53–4.
20. Charron-Prochownik D, Sereika SM, Becker D, et al. Long-term effects of the booster-enhanced READY-Girls preconception counseling program on intentions and behaviors for family planning in teens with diabetes. Diabetes Care. 2013;36:3870–4.

21. Institute of Medicine. Weight gain during pregnancy: reexamining the guidelines. Washington (DC): National Academies Press (US); 2009.
22. Crowther CA, Hiller JE, Moss JR, McPhee AJ, Jeffries WS, Robinson JS, et al. Effect of treatment of gestational diabetes mellitus on pregnancy outcomes. N Engl J Med. 2005;352(24):2477–86.
23. Hernandez TL, Anderson MA, Chartier-Logan C, Friedman JE, Barbour LA. Strategies in the nutritional management of gestational diabetes. Clin Obstet Gynecol. 2013;56(4):803–15.
24. Balsells M, Corcoy R, Adelantado JM, García-Patterson A, Altirriba O, de Leiva A. Gestational diabetes mellitus: metabolic control during labour. Diabetes Nutr Metab. 2000;13(5):257–62.
25. Curet LB, Izquierdo LA, Gilson GJ, Schneider JM, Perelman R, Converse J. Relative effects of antepartum and intrapartum maternal blood glucose levels on incidence of neonatal hypoglycemia. J Perinatol. 1997;17(2):113–5. Lean ME, Pearson DW, Sutherland HW. Insulin management during labour and delivery in mothers with diabetes. Diabet Med. 1990;7(2):162–4.
26. Mimouni F. Perinatal asphyxia in infants of diabetic mothers is associated with maternal vasculopathy and hyperglycemia in labour. Neonatal Epidemiol Follow-up. 1987:400A.
27. Carron Brown S, Kyne-Grzebalski D, Mwangi B, Taylor R. Effect of management policy upon 120 Type 1 diabetic pregnancies: policy decisions in practice. Diabet Med. 1999;16(7):573–8.
28. American Dietetic Association. Medical Nutrition Therapy Evidence-Based Guides for Practice: Nutrition Practice Guidelines for Gestational Diabetes Mellitus [CD ROM]. Chicago, IL: American Dietetic Association; 2001.
29. Rae A, Bond D, Evans S, North F, Roberman B, Walters B. A randomised controlled trial of dietary energy restriction in the management of obese women with gestational diabetes. Aust N Z J Obstet Gynaecol. 2000;40(4):416–22.
30. Moses RG, Barker M, Winter M, Petocz P, Brand-Miller JC. Can a low-glycemic index diet reduce the need for insulin in gestational diabetes mellitus? A randomized trial. Diabetes Care. 2009;32:996–1000.
31. Management of diabetes in pregnancy. American Diabetes Association. Diabetes Care. 2017;40:S114–9.
32. Agency for Healthcare Research and Quality. Therapeutic management, delivery, and postpartum risk assessment and screening in gestational diabetes. Rockville (MD): Evidence Report/ Technology Assessment No. 162, AHRQ; 2008.
33. Donnor T, Sarkar S. Insulin-pharmacology, therapeutic regimens and principles of intensive insulin therapy; 2023.
34. Metzger BE, Buchanan TA, Coustan DR, de Leiva A, Dunger DB, Hadden DR, et al. Summary and recommendations of the Fifth International Workshop-Conference on Gestational Diabetes Mellitus. Diabetes Care. 2007;30(Suppl2):S251–60.
35. De Leo V, Musacchio MC, Piomboni P, Di Sabatino A, Morgante G. The administration of metformin during pregnancy reduces polycystic ovary syndrome related gestational complications. Eur J Obstet Gynecol Reprod Biol. 2011;157:63–6.
36. Eyal S, Easterling TR, Carr D, Umans JG, Miodovnik M, Hankins GD, et al. Pharmacokinetics of metformin during pregnancy. Drug Metab Dispos. 2010;38:833–40.
37. Langer O, Conway DL, Berkus MD, Xenakis EM, Gonzales O. A comparison of glyburide and insulin in women with gestational diabetes mellitus. N Engl J Med. 2000;343(16):1134–8.
38. Balsells M, García-Patterson A, Solà I, Roqué M, Gich I, Corcoy R. Glibenclamide, metformin, and insulin for the treatment of gestational diabetes: a systematic review and meta-analysis. BMJ. 2015;350:h102.
39. Pertot T, Molyneaux L, Tan K, Ross GP, Yue DK, Wong J. Can common clinical parameters be used to identify patients who will need insulin treatment in gestational diabetes mellitus? Diabetes Care. 2011;34(10):2214–6.
40. Guo L, Ma J, Tang J, Hu D, Zhang W, Zhao X. Comparative efficacy and safety of metformin, glyburide, and insulin in treating gestational diabetes mellitus: a meta-analysis. J Diabetes Res. 2019;2019:9804708.
41. Queensland Clinical Guidelines. Gestational diabetes mellitus (GDM). Guideline No. MN21.33-V6-R26. Queensland Health; 2022.

42. Australian Medicines Handbook. Insulin. [Internet]. Adelaide: Australian Medicines Handbook Pty Ltd; 2020. [cited 2020 July 7]. Available from: http://www.amhonline.amh.net.au
43. Kalra S, Kalra B, Gupta Y. Glycemic management after antenatal corticosteroid therapy. N Am J Med Sci. 2014;6(2):71–6.
44. Holman NBR, Murphy H, Maresh M. Women with pre-gestational diabetes have a higher risk of stillbirth at all gestations after 32 weeks. Diabet Med. 2014;31(9):1129–13.
45. Boulvain MSM, Perrotin F, Winer N, et al. Induction of labour versus expectant management for large-for-date fetuses: a randomised controlled trial. Lancet. 2015;385:2600–5.
46. Bulletins—Obstetrics ACOG. Practice bulletin no. 173: fetal macrosomia. Obstet Gynecol. 2016;128(5):e195–209.
47. Effect of management policy upon 120 Type 1 diabetic pregnancies: policy decisions in practice. Diabet Med. 1999;16(7):573–8.
48. Kline GA, Edwards A. Antepartum and intra-partum insulin management of type 1 and type 2 diabetic women: Impact on clinically significant neonatal hypoglycemia. Diabetes Res Clin Pract. 2007;77(2):223–30.
49. The Royal Australian and New Zealand College of Obstetricians and Gynaecologists. Intrapartum Fetal Surveillance Clinical Guideline - fourth edition 2019.
50. Kitabchi AE, Umpierrez GE, Miles JM, Fisher JN. Hyperglycemic crises inadult patients with diabetes. Diabetes Care. 2009;32:1335–43.
51. Sibai BM, Viteri OA. Diabetic ketoacidosis in pregnancy. Obstet Gynecol. 2014;123:167–78.
52. Joint British Diabetes Societies Inpatient Care Group. The management of diabetic ketoacidosis in adults; 2013.
53. Dhanasekaran M, Mohan S, Egan AM. Diabetic ketoacidosis in pregnancy: an overview of pathophysiology, management, and pregnancy outcomes. EM J Diabet. 2022;
54. Mohan M, Baagar KAM, Lindow S. Management of diabetic ketoacidosis in pregnancy. Obstet Gynaecol. 2017;19:55–62.
55. Achong N, Duncan EL, McIntyre HD, Callaway L. Peripartum management of glycemia in women with type 1 diabetes. Diabetes Care. 2014;37(2):364–71.
56. Lain KY, Catalano PM. Metabolic changes in pregnancy. Clin Obstet Gynecol. 2007;50(4):938–48.
57. Simmons D. Safety considerations with pharmacological treatment of gestational diabetes mellitus. Drug Saf. 2015;38:65–78.
58. Feig DS, Briggs GG, Kraemer JM, et al. Transfer of glyburide and glipizide into breast milk. Diabetes Care. 2005;28(8):1851–5.
59. Mayer-Davis EJ, Rifas-Shiman SL, Zhou L, Hu FB, Colditz GA, Gillman MW. Breast-feeding and risk for childhood obesity: does maternal diabetes or obesity status matter? Diabetes Care. 2006;29(10):2231–7.
60. O'Reilly M, Avalos G, Dennedy MC, O'Sullivan EP, Dunne FP. Breast-feeding is associated with reduced postpartum maternal glucose intolerance after gestational diabetes. Ir Med J. 2012;105(5 Suppl):31–6.
61. Owen CG, Martin RM, Whincup PH, Smith GD, Cook DG. Does breastfeeding influence risk of type 2 diabetes in later life? A quantitative analysis of published evidence. Am J Clin Nutr. 2006;84(5):1043–54.
62. WHO Medical Eligibility Criteria for Contraceptive Use. Geneva: 2015. Accessed Jan 19, 2024.
63. Metzger BE, Buchanan TA, Coustan DR, de Leiva A, Dunger DB, Hadden DR, et al. Summary and recommendations of the Fifth International Workshop- Conference on Gestational Diabetes Mellitus. Diabetes Care. 2007;30(Suppl 2):S251–60. American Diabetes Association. Standards of medical care in diabetes–2011. Diabetes Care. 2011;34(Suppl 1):S11–61.
64. World Health Organization. Diagnostic Criteria and Classification of Hyperglycemia First Detected in Pregnancy. http://apps.who.int/iris/bitstream/10665/85975/1/WHO_NMH_MND_13.2_eng.pdf. Published 2013.
65. American Diabetes Association. Standards of medical care in diabetes–2011. Diabetes Care. 2011;34(Suppl 1):S11–61.

66. Ratner RE, Christophi CA, Metzger BE, Dabelea D, Bennett PH, Pi-Sunyer X, et al. Prevention of diabetes in women with a history of gestational diabetes: effects of metformin and lifestyle interventions. J Clin Endocrinol Metab. 2008;93(12):4774–9.
67. Aroda VR, Christophi CA, Edelstein SL, Zhang P, Herman WH, Barrett-Connor E, et al. The effect of lifestyle intervention and metformin on preventing or delaying diabetes among women with and without gestational diabetes: the diabetes prevention program outcomes study 10-year follow-up. J Clin Endocrinol Metab. 2015;100(4):1646–53.

Asthma in Pregnancy

7

Richa Sharma and Sushma V. Dev

Asthma is a syndrome characterized by airflow obstruction. Chronic airway inflammation causes airway hyperresponsiveness to a variety of triggers, leading to airflow obstruction and respiratory symptoms including dyspnea and wheezing [1]. Pregnancy represents a unique physiologic state that makes management of this chronic disease challenging. It is the most common chronic condition in pregnancy complicating 4–12% of pregnancies [2, 3]. This illness is a rising concern, as its prevalence has increased among all women over the recent decades. Studies have shown that pregnant asthmatic women have an increased risk of adverse maternal and perinatal outcomes, whereas controlled asthma is associated with reduced risks [4, 5]. Severe asthma tends to worsen during pregnancy than mild asthma [6, 7].

7.1 Pathophysiology

- The pathogenesis of asthma remission or aggravation during pregnancy is related to the physiological or pathological changes caused by pregnancy. Asthma has an unpredictable course during pregnancy due to alterations in maternal pulmonary physiology, immune function, and hormonal balance [7].

R. Sharma (✉)
Department of Obstetrics and Gynecology, UCMS–GTB Hospital, New Delhi, Delhi, India

S. V. Dev
Mysore Medical College and Research Institute, Mysore, Karnataka, India

R. Sharma, A. Kumar (eds.), *Systemic Disorders in Pregnancy*,
https://doi.org/10.1007/978-981-96-4876-4_7

- Asthma is a chronic inflammatory airway syndrome with a major hereditary component. This increased airway responsiveness and persistent subacute inflammation have been associated with genes on chromosomes 5, 11, and 12 that include cytokine gene clusters, beta-adrenergic and glucocorticoid receptor gene, and the T-cell antigen receptor gene [8].

7.2 Pulmonary Changes

- Decrease in lung functional residual capacity (FRC) by 10–25% occurs due to elevation of the diaphragm by 4–5 cms. But this does not typically result in significant changes to forced vital capacity, peak expiratory flow rate, or forced expiratory volume in 1 s (FEV1) (Fig. 7.1).
- Respiratory alkalosis occurs due to increase in VE, which is compensated by increased renal excretion of bicarbonate [7] (Tables 7.1 and 7.2).
- Dyspnea is common and presents with shortness of breath at rest or with mild exertion. The pulmonary changes are exaggerated in an asthmatic women.

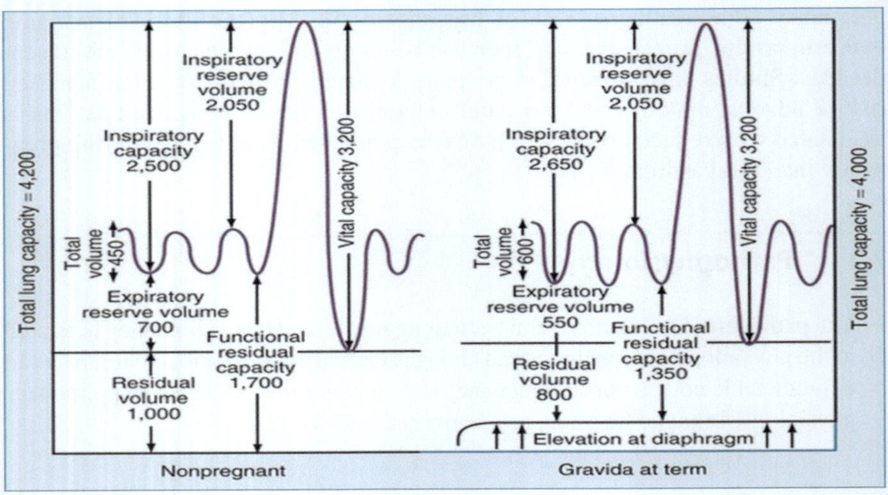

Fig. 7.1 Pulmonary volumes and capacities during pregnancy [9]

Table 7.1 Pulmonary function in pregnancy [8]

Parameter	Change
Oxygen consumption	Increases by 20–50%
Minute ventilation	Increases by 50%
Tidal volume	Increases by 40%
Respiratory rate	Unchanged/slightly increases
PaO_2	Increases by 10%
$PaCO_2$	Decreases by 15%
HCO_3	Decreases by 15%
FRC	Decreases by 20%

PaO_2 partial pressure of oxygen, *$PaCO_2$* partial pressure of carbon dioxide, *HCO_3* bicarbonate, *FRC* functional residual capacity

Table 7.2 Changes in lung function values during pregnancy [8]

Parameter	Change
Inspiratory capacity	Increased by 5–10%
Expiratory reserve volume	Decreased by 15–20%
Tidal volume	Increased by 40–50%
Minute ventilation	Increased by 30–50%
Residual volume	Decreased by 20–25%
Functional residual capacity	Decreased by 20–30%
Total lung capacity	Unchanged or decreased by less than 5%
FEV1	Unchanged
Peak expiratory flow rate	Unchanged
FEVl/FVC	Unchanged
Maximum mid-expiratory flow rate	Unchanged

FEV1 Forced expiratory volume in 1 s, *FVC* forced vital Capacity

7.3 Immunologic Changes

- Physiological immunosuppression occurs in pregnancy. Shift in the helper T cell (Th1)/Th2 ratio toward a Th2-predominant immune state and an increase in regulatory T cells (Tregs) that work to suppress activation of effector T cells and natural killer cells.
- Asthma is Th2-predominant disease state, with allergic Th2-type inflammation leading to airway hyperresponsiveness in patients. Pregnancy-associated Th2 immunological shift leads to worsening of the Th2-driven manifestations of asthma [7].
- No differences in Th1/Th2 ratio between healthy pregnant women and asthmatic pregnant women.

- Decrease in Treg cells can result in decreased suppression of the effects of pro-inflammatory Th17 cells and may contribute both to worsening of symptoms as well as increased likelihood of poor fetal outcomes in asthmatics.
- The pregnancy-associated decrease in cell-mediated immunity can make them prone to viral respiratory infections, which is a precipitating factor.

7.4 Hormonal Changes [7]

- Increase in serum-free cortisol during pregnancy can cause improvement in asthma. Increased progesterone levels relax the smooth muscle of the lungs and improve asthma symptoms, but relaxation of the smooth muscle controlling the esophageal sphincter may lead to exaggerated gastroesophageal reflux, which can worsen the symptoms of asthma.
- Increased estrogen during the third trimester can cause increased bronchial mucus production and airway edema, which can worsen the symptoms of asthma.
- Increasing progesterone levels can cause downregulation of β2-adrenoreceptors and thus failure of response endogenous catecholamines and exogenous beta-agonists [7].
- Increased secretion of prostaglandin E2 (PGE2) during pregnancy can have a protective effect on asthma [10].
- Maternal asthma is more likely to worsen in the presence of a female fetus [10].

7.5 Effect of Pregnancy on Asthma

- The natural course of asthma during pregnancy is extremely variable. Generally, asthma in pregnancy follows the "one-third rule" [11, 12]
- One-third will improve
- One-third will deteriorate
- One-third will remain unchanged

- In a large prospective study, pregnant patients with mild asthma had exacerbation rates of 12.6% and hospitalization rates of 2.3%, those with moderate asthma had exacerbation rates of 25.7% and hospitalization rates of 6.8%, and those with severe asthma had exacerbation rates of 51.9% and hospitalization rates of 26.9% [11] (Fig. 7.2).

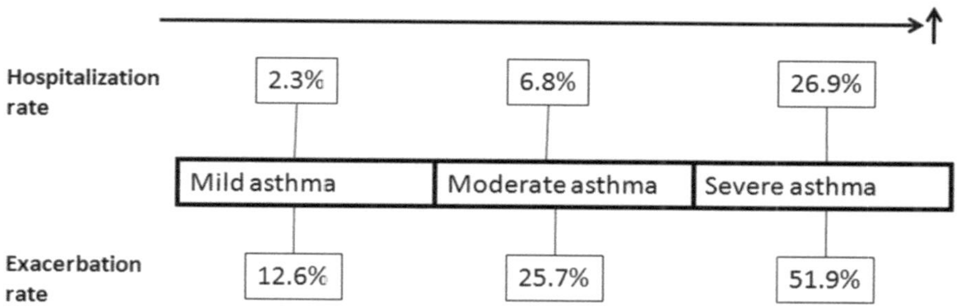

Fig. 7.2 Rate of exacerbation and hospitalization as per severity of asthma [11]

- Women with mild asthma have a favorable course.
- The most severe symptoms were experienced by patients between the 24th and 36th week of pregnancy. Thereafter symptoms decreased significantly in the last 4 weeks and 90% had no asthma symptoms during labor or delivery [12].
- In some women, asthma severity returns to the prepregnant state within 3 months of delivery; but in rare cases, it may worsen than before pregnancy.
- Deterioration in disease control is commonly caused by reduction or even complete cessation of medication due to fears about its safety.

7.6 Effects of Asthma on Pregnancy

- During pregnancy mild or moderate asthma can have excellent maternal and perinatal outcomes. Women with more severe asthma are at increased risk of asthma exacerbations in pregnancy and have been shown to have poorer maternal and perinatal outcomes [11, 13].
- There is evidence that exacerbations, oral steroid use, and severe asthma are associated with maternal complications, possibly due to maternal hypoxia, the effects of maternal inflammation, and/or changes in uterine smooth muscle function. The fetal response to maternal hypoxemia is decreased umbilical blood flow, increased systemic and pulmonary vascular resistance, and decreased cardiac output. The more severe the maternal asthma, the more is the fetal growth restriction.
- Maternal asthma is linked with small risk of fetal malformations than the healthy pregnant women [7, 11].

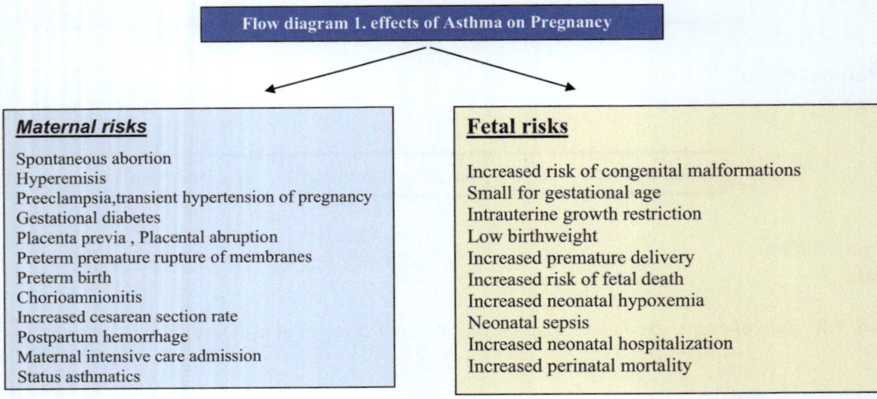

7.7 Clinical Features of Asthma

Diagnosis of asthma in a pregnant patient is the same as that for a nonpregnant patient. Typical clinical presentation in asthma includes:

Symptoms

Breathlessness, cough, wheeze, chest tightness, nocturnal waking due to cough

Signs

Raised respiratory rate, wheeze, use of accessory muscles, tachycardia

Triggering Factors (Table 7.3)

Allergens, cold, upper respiratory infections, emotions, medications (aspirin, beta blockers)

Table 7.3 Triggers of asthma

Atopy
Allergens, such as house dust mite, pollen, etc.
Smoking
Exercise
Occupational exposure
Pollution
Drugs, such as aspirin, β-blockers
Food and drinks such as dairy produce, alcohol, peanuts, and orange juice
Additives such as monosodium glutamate and tartrazine
Medical conditions, such as rhinitis and gastric reflux
Hormonal, such as premenstrual conditions and pregnancy

7.7.1 Diagnosis of Asthma

- History and examination consistent with the symptoms and signs of asthma as listed above; history of atopy (personal or family)
- Measurement of FEV1 (forced expiratory volume) and FVC (forced vital capacity) by spirometry. Ideally this will be supplemented by evidence of reversibility (12% improvement to a bronchodilator or inhaled steroid or oral steroids)
- $\geq$ 20% diurnal variation in PEFR (peak expiratory flow rate) for 3 or more days per week during a 2-week period of monitoring is a diagnostic criteria
- FEV1/FVC <0.7 warrants trial of treatment
- A raised FeNO (fractional exhaled nitric oxide) is a marker of airway inflammation
- In complex cases, assessment by a specialist team might be needed
- In patients presenting with new onset respiratory symptoms during pregnancy, the most common differential diagnosis would be dyspnea of pregnancy (Table 7.4)

Table 7.4 Differential diagnoses of dyspnea in pregnancy

Dyspnea of pregnancy
1. Physiological dyspnea of pregnancy: It is a benign symptom. It is due to physiological respiratory changes in pregnancy. Some gravidas have an increased awareness of the physiological dyspnea caused by progesterone stimulation of the respiratory center and decreased RV and decreased FRC resulting from increased uterine volume.
2. Anxiety
3. Hyperventilation
4. Dysfunctional breathing
5. Respiratory disease: Asthma, pneumonia, thromboembolic disease, interstitial lung disease, pneumothorax, amniotic fluid embolism
6. Cardiac disease: Arrhythmias, ischemic heart disease, cardiomyopathy
7. Endocrine disease: Diabetic acute ketoacidosis, acute thyrotoxicosis
8. Hematological: Chronic anemia, acute hemorrhage
9. Renal disease: Metabolic acidosis secondary to acute renal failure

7.8 Classification of Asthma Severity in Pregnancy (Table 7.5)

Table 7.5 Classification of Severity of Asthma in Pregnancy

Asthma severity (Control†)	Symptom frequency	Night-time awakening	Interference with normal activity	FEV1 or peak flow (predicted percentage of personal best)
Intermittent (well controlled)	2 days per week or less	Twice per month or less	None	More than 80%
Mild persistent (not well controlled)	More than 2 days per week, but not daily	More than twice per month	Minor limitation	More than 80%
Moderate persistent (not well controlled)	Daily symptoms	More than once per week	Some limitation	60–80%
Severe persistent (very poorly controlled)	Throughout the day	Four times per week or more	Extremely limited	Less than 60%

ACOG practice bulletin 2008

7.9 Management of Asthma

- General Principles
  1. Patient's education
  2. Assessment and monitoring of asthma
  3. Avoidance of triggers
  4. Pharmacotherapy
- Treatment of Asthma During Pregnancy
- Management of Asthma During Exacerbation
- Management of Asthma During Labor and Delivery
- Management of Asthma During Postpartum and Lactation

A. *General Principles*
   1. **Patient's Education** [13, 14]
      - Patient education is an integral aspect in the management of asthma.
      - Patient should be educated about the general asthma management and its effect on pregnancy.

- Teach them signs and symptoms of asthma for early recognition, avoidance of triggering factors, and early seeking of medical care.
- Prompt treatment of risk factors like gastroesophageal reflex, allergic rhinitis, sinusitis.
- Women who smoke should be encouraged to quit smoking.
- Educate about the adherence and compliance to treatment
- Should be provided with maintenance therapy and rescue therapy in case of aggravation of symptom.
- Encourage personalized self-management—written action asthma plan is optimal [13, 14].

2. **Assessment and Monitoring of Asthma**
   - Initial assessment of a pregnant patient presenting with acute asthma includes obtaining a brief medical history, performing a physical examination, and examining physiologic measures of airway function and fetal well-being.
   - Pulmonary function, FeNO, ACT (Asthma Control Test) scores, and blood eosinophil counts are important tools for asthma assessment
   - FEV1 is the single best measure of pulmonary function.
   - Monitor with FEV1 or PEFR twice daily. FEV1 ideal is >80% of predicted. PEFR ranges from 380 to 550 L/min. Each woman has her own baseline value, but the personal best value is required.
   - FeNO is an indicator of airway inflammation; studies have found that pregnant women with asthma have the same FeNO as before, which is associated with asthma control. Adjusting treatment of asthma in pregnancy according to FeNO can reduce acute attacks and neonatal admission rate [10, 13].
3. **Avoidance of Triggers**
   - Avoiding exposure to environmental triggers has been widely considered an important component in the management of asthma
   - If food allergy is confirmed, avoidance of food allergens can reduce asthma exacerbation. It is believed that food allergens/additives (such as sulfites) and strenuous exercise, which trigger asthma symptoms, should be avoided.
   - The use of allergen immunotherapy, or "allergy shots," has been shown to be effective in improving asthma in patients with allergies. Anaphylaxis is a risk of allergen injections, especially early in the course of immunotherapy when the dose is being escalated and anaphylaxis during pregnancy has been associated with maternal death, fetal death, or both.

- In a patient who is receiving a maintenance or near-maintenance dose, not experiencing adverse reactions to the injections and apparently deriving clinical benefit, continuation of immunotherapy is recommended. In such patients, a dose reduction may be considered to further decrease the chance of anaphylaxis.
- Risk–benefit considerations do not usually favor beginning allergen immunotherapy during pregnancy [11].

7.9.1 Pharmacotherapy

- The principles of medication for asthma in pregnancy are similar to those of nonpregnant patients
- The main goal of management is to eliminate episodes of maternal hypoxia with optimal asthma control.
- A multidisciplinary management approach is recommended during pregnancy involving obstetricians, respiratory specialists, primary care physicians, asthma educators, nurses, pharmacists, and midwives in antenatal asthma management.
- A written asthma control plan should be developed for each newly diagnosed patient, to assist patient with self-monitoring, regular follow-up, and adjusting treatment according to patient control level to achieve and maintain asthma control.
- "Step-up" therapy is recommended if patient is not improving (Table 7.6).
- The GINA guidelines recommend that asthma control levels should be assessed monthly. Step-down treatment is not a priority in order to avoid acute exacerbation of asthma [14].
- GINA guidelines and Cochrane reviews suggest that poor asthma control and acute exacerbations during pregnancy are riskier than taking asthma medications. Pharmacological medications are widely being considered "safer" for a pregnant woman and her fetus than uncontrolled asthma (Evidence A) [13, 14].

Table 7.6 Step therapy during pregnancy [3, 6, 8, 11]

	Type of asthma	Preferred treatment	Alternative treatment
Quick relief	All patients	Short-acting bronchodilator: 2–4 puffs short-acting inhaled beta2-agonist as needed for symptoms	
Step1	Mild-intermittent	No daily medications, albuterol as needed	
Step 2	Mild persistent asthma	Low-dose ICS	Cromolyn, LTRA, or theophylline
Step 3	Moderate persistent	Low-dose ICS + LABA Or medium-dose ICS or (if needed) medium-dose ICS + LABA	Low-dose /medium-dose ICS + LTRA / theophylline
Step 4	Severe persistent	High-dose ICS + LABA	High-dose ICS + Theophylline
Step 5	Very Severe persistent	High-dose ICS + LABA + oral corticosteroid	Omalizumab for allergic patients

Theophylline (serum level 5–12 mcg/mL), *ICS* Inhaled corticosteroid, *LABA* long-acting β2 agonist, *LTRA* leukotriene receptor antagonist

7.10 Asthma Medications in Pregnancy

Medications for asthma are categorized into:

- *Rescue agents/broncho dilators*: Rescue agents are used "as-needed basis" to treat acute bronchospasm and provide symptomatic relief but do not treat the underlying inflammation that causes bronchospasm. Rescue agents include all the inhaled short-acting β2- agonists and inhaled anticholinergics, such as ipratropium. Short-acting β-agonists(SABA) such as albuterol provide quick relief of symptoms.
- *Controller/maintenance agents*/anti-inflammatory agents: They control airway hyperreactivity and treat the underlying inflammation of the airway. Maintenance agents aim to prevent asthma symptoms and exacerbations. Controller therapy includes inhaled corticosteroids, systemic steroids, long-acting inhaled β2-adrenergic agonists (LABA). Less commonly used maintenance agents include mast cell stabilizers, leukotriene receptor antagonists (LTRA) and theophylline. The inhaled steroids are the keystones of asthma maintenance therapy.

7.10.1 β2-Agonists

Short-acting inhaled β2-adrenergic agonists (SABA)—Salbutamol also known as Albuterol, terbutaline, metaproterenol, pirbuterol

Long-acting inhaled β2-adrenergic agonists(LABA)—Salmeterol, formoterol

- SABAs are effective bronchodilators for quick-acting relief of asthma symptoms
- Inhaled albuterol is the first-choice SABA for pregnant women in view of available safety data, although other agents also may be appropriate.
- SABA do not increase the risk of congenital anomalies or adverse perinatal outcomes.
- LABA are considered for use in moderate-severe asthma, in combination with ICS therapy, only if asthma cannot be controlled by medium-dose steroids in addition to SABAs.

7.10.2 Inhaled Corticosteroids (ICS)

- For those with mild, intermittent asthma, no controller therapy is indicated. Use of inhaled corticosteroids is the first-line controller therapy for persistent asthma during pregnancy.
- ICS are the mainstay of treatment for asthma and appear to be safe in pregnancy
- Inhaled anti-inflammatory treatment has been shown to decrease the risk of an acute attack of asthma in pregnancy and the risk of readmission following an asthma attack (Evidence A).
- Budesonide is the preferred inhaled corticosteroid (FDA category B drug) for use during pregnancy. However, there are no data indicating that the other inhaled corticosteroid (Category C) preparations are unsafe during pregnancy. Therefore, the use of any inhaled corticosteroids may be continued in patients whose asthma was well controlled by these agents before pregnancy (Table 7.7)

Table 7.7 Categorization of inhaled corticosteroids by dose—adults [12]

Inhaled corticosteroid	Low dose	Medium	High dose
Beclometasone pMDI	100 mcg 2 puffs twice a day	200 mcg 2 puffs twice a day	200 mcg 4 puffs twice a day
Beclometasone DPI	200 mcg 1 puff twice a day	200 mcg 2 puffs twice a day	n/a
Budesonide DPI	100 mcg 2 puffs twice a day	200 mcg 2 puffs twice a day	400 mcg 2 puffs twice a day
Ciclesonide pMDI	80 mcg 2 puffs once a day	160 mcg 2 puffs once a day	160 mcg 2 puffs twice a day
Fluticasone pMDI	50 mcg 2 puffs twice a day	125 mcg 2 puffs twice a day	250 mcg 2 puffs twice a day
Fluticasone DPI	100 mcg 1 puff twice a day	250 mcg 1 puff twice a day	500 mcg 1 puff twice a day
Mometasone DPI	200 mcg 1 puff twice a day	400 mcg 1 puff twice a day	n/a

7.10.3 Systemic Corticosteroids

Oral: Prednisone
Intravenous: methylprednisolone, hydrocortisone

- Systemic corticosteroid should be reserved for the maintenance therapy of severe persistent asthma not controlled with high-dose ICS [6, 8, 12]. Prednisolone remains the steroid of choice throughout pregnancy (10% delivered to the placenta—much lower than dexamethasone (33%) and hydrocortisone (15%). Prednisone may be given 40–60 mg per day in one or two divided doses for 3–10 days.
- Risk of isolated cleft lip, with or without cleft palate, can occur on maternal exposure in the first trimester. Preterm birth, low birth weight, and preeclampsia can also complicate asthmatic mothers.
- In the setting of severe asthma or a severe exacerbation, the benefits of controlling a life-threatening disease make systemic steroid use (even in the first trimester) justifiable.

7.10.4 Theophylline

- GINA guidelines indicate that low dose theophylline is considered as an alternative, but not a preferred treatment for mild persistent asthma and moderate-to-severe asthma, during pregnancy [14].
- Blood concentration should be maintained at 5–12 μg/ml in pregnant women. When serum theophylline is higher than 20 μg/ml, the risk of theophylline toxic reactions will increase .
- Theophylline does not appear to have teratogenicity. Theophylline use has no or minimal effects on fetal growth and reduces perinatal complications (FDA Category C drug) when maternal asthma is adequately controlled [10, 12, 14].
- Theophylline may be beneficial in only selected patients as second- or third-line alternative drug.

7.10.5 Leukotriene Receptor Antagonists (LTRAs)

- LTRAs includes zafirlukast and montelukast.
- LTRAs are only recommended for patients who had a favorable response to them before becoming pregnant. They are generally taken in combination with other asthma medications.
- They are an alternative to ICSs and are not preferred as a treatment option in mild persistent asthmatics during pregnancy.
- During pregnancy there is no increased risk for major birth defects.

7.10.6 Omalizumab

- Omalizumab is a recombinant anti-IgE monoclonal antibody that works by binding and neutralizing the effects of IgE in basophils and mast cells, thereby preventing downstream allergic inflammation.
- Due to possible anaphylaxis, this therapy should not be initiated in pregnancy though sometimes may be continued if already in progress following multidisciplinary discussion.
- It is an FDA category B drug [7].

7.10.7 Anti-Interleukin-5/IL-5 Receptor Monoclonal Antibodies [10, 14]

Anti-Interleukin(IL)-5 monoclonal antibodies: Mepolizumab and reslizumab

Anti IL-5 receptor (IL5R) monoclonal antibody: Benralizumab

- They have been approved as add-on maintenance treatment program for patients with uncontrolled, persistent eosinophilic asthma.
- Use of anti-IL-5/IL-5R monoclonal antibody therapy in pregnancy does not have safety data; however monoclonal antibodies can cross the placenta during the third trimester.

7.10.8 Acute Asthma in Pregnancy/Labor [6, 12]

Acute severe asthma in pregnancy is an emergency condition.

Diagnosis of acute severe asthma is made as per British thoracic society guidelines [12] (Table 7.8).

Table 7.8 Levels of severity of acute asthma attacks in adults [12]

Acute severe asthma	Any one of: PEF 33–50% best or predicted Respiratory rate ≥25/min Heart rate ≥110/min Inability to complete sentences in one breath	
Life-threatening asthma	Any one of the following in a patient with severe asthma:	
	Clinical signs Altered conscious level Exhaustion Arrhythmia Hypotension Cyanosis Silent chest Poor respiratory effort	**Measurements** PEF <33% best or predicted SpO2 < 92% PaO2 < 8 kPa "normal" PaCO2 (4.6–6.0 kPa)
Near-fatal asthma	Increased PaCO2 and/or requiring mechanical ventilation with increased inflation pressures	

7.10.9 Treatment of Acute and Severe Asthma

A medical emergency and critical care unit must be involved.

- Treatment should include the following:
  - High flow O2, to maintain SPO2 94–98%
  - Repeated nebulization with beta-2 agonists and ipratropium bromide can be added.
  - IV hydrocortisone 100 mg and/or Tab. Prednisolone 40-50 mg × 5 days.
  - Chest X ray to rule out pneumonia or pneumothorax or if there is no improvement.

7.11 Prepregnancy Care

- Reassure women with asthma that most asthma medications have a good safety profile and can be continued during pregnancy.

7.12 Antenatal Care

- Pregnant asthmatic women should be treated in a manner similar to nonpregnant asthmatic women
- The ultimate goal of asthma management in pregnancy is to maintain adequate oxygenation in the fetus by preventing hypoxic episodes in the mother
- The principles of pharmacological treatment of asthma during pregnancy should be the same as for nonpregnant women. Doses of ICS should be the minimum necessary to control symptoms and maintain normal or best lung function
- Identify and manage common coexisting conditions such as allergic rhinitis, sinusitis, and gastroesophageal reflux that can aggravate asthma and compromise asthma. Encourage women to stop smoking and avoid triggers.
- Routine booking appointment/antenatal care. Serial growth scans to assess fetal well-being.
- Assessing asthma control at each visit. Reassurance regarding asthma medications to ensure compliance.
- Self-management, education, and provision of an asthma action plan
- Assess need for influenza vaccination
- Arrange respiratory physician review as indicated. Women with moderate or severe persistent asthma or who are identified as very poorly controlled should be managed in close consultation with a respiratory physician. Manage exacerbations promptly and aggressively.
- Arrange an antenatal anesthetic team referral for all women with severe and/or uncontrolled asthma for planning labor analgesia and peripartum anesthesia.

7.13 Intrapartum Care

- Acute exacerbations are rare in labor
- β2 agonists and SABA inhalers can be continued, without any risk to the baby.
- If before delivery, oral corticosteroids of 7.5 mg/day was taken >2 weeks, then parenteral hydrocortisone 100 mg 8–12th hourly must be given to avoid the stress of labor
- Oxygen therapy if SPO2 < 94%
  - Continuous fetal monitoring should be considered
  - Prostaglandin E2 and oxytocin are safe to be used
  - 15-methyl PG F2 alpha is contraindicated due to its bronchoconstriction property
  - Epidural analgesia is helpful and Opiates should be avoided
  - Regional must be preferred over general anesthesia, to avoid the postoperative chest complications
  - Cesarean section to be done for obstetric indications

7.14 Postpartum Care

- Prostaglandin E1 (misoprostol) may be used for the management of postpartum hemorrhage
- Ensure that asthmatic women have their asthma medications continued in postpartum
- Breastfeeding should be encouraged as it may reduce the risk of childhood asthma, especially in children with a family history of atopy
- No contraindication to breastfeeding with any asthma medications
- Review asthma management

Key Points

1. Optimal asthma control during pregnancy is the aim of asthma management, to avoid the flare-ups.
2. It is more ideal and safer for these pregnant women to be treated with medications than to suffer asthma symptoms and exacerbations.
3. Management plans involve regular assessment of asthma control, trigger avoidance, patient education, and institution of step-wise therapy approach.
4. Beta2-agonists and ICS constitute the mainstays of therapy.
5. Most asthma medicines can be used during pregnancy and lactation.

References

1. Jamson J, Fauci AS, Kasper DL, Hauser SL, Longo DL, Loscalzo L. Harrison's manual of medicine. 20th ed. Mc Graw Hill Publication; 2019.
2. Kwon HL, Belanger K, Bracken MB. Asthma prevalence among pregnant and childbearing-aged women in the United States: estimates from national health surveys. Ann Epidemiol. 2003;13(5):317–24.
3. Goldie MH, Brightling CE. Asthma in pregnancy. Obstet Gynaecol. 2013;15:241–5.
4. Murphy VE. Managing asthma in pregnancy. Breathe. 2015;11:258–67.
5. Murphy VE, Namazy JA, Powell H, et al. A meta-analysis of adverse perinatal outcomes in women with asthma. BJOG. 2011;118:1314–23.
6. GMEC Asthma Care in Pregnancy guideline Final V1.0 18.10.2019.
7. Blackburn HK, Allington DR, Procacci KA, et al. Asthma in pregnancy. World J Pharmacol. 2014;3(4):56–71.
8. Williams textbook of obstetrics, 25th ed. McGraw Hill Publication. Chapter 4 – Maternal physiology, pp. 64–5, Chapter 51 – Pulmonary disorders, pp. 988–92.
9. Bonica JJ. Principles & practice of obstetric analgesia & anasthesia. Philadelphia: FD Davis; 1967. p. 24.
10. Wang H, Li N, Huang H. Asthma in pregnancy: pathophysiology, diagnosis, whole-course management, and medication safety. Can Respir J. 2020;2020:9046842, 10 pages. https://doi.org/10.1155/2020/9046842.
11. Asthma in pregnancy. ACOG Practice Bulletin No. 90. American College of Obstetricians and Gynecologists. Obstet Gynecol. 2008;111:457–64.
12. SIGN 158 British guideline on the management of asthma. 2019.
13. Cochrane database of systemic reviews. Interventions for managing asthma in pregnancy Version published: 21 October 2014. https://doi.org/10.1002/14651858.CD010660.pub2
14. Global Initiative for Asthma. Global strategy for asthma management and prevention; 2020. Available from: http://www.ginasthma.org

Epilepsy in Pregnancy

8

Deepti Vibha and Richa Sharma

Any medical disease during pregnancy is fraught with additional apprehension about the additional effect of the medical condition on the mother and baby. The clinical approach and decisions might change depending upon whether it is the first clinical presentation during pregnancy or had been a medical problem, now having associated pregnancy. Important considerations in the care of women with epilepsy (WWE) that must be taken before and during pregnancy include teratogenic risk, change of antiepileptic drug (AED) concentrations during pregnancy, postpartum, and lactation. This chapter attempts to describe the disease burden of epilepsy in WWE, preconception counseling, clinical features, obstetrical management, and follow-up.

8.1 Epidemiology

Approximately 24,000 women with epilepsy become pregnant each year. In the majority of women with epilepsy, pregnancy has *no effect* on their seizure frequency. Therefore, if seizures are well controlled, they are likely to remain so during pregnancy. However, in approximately 20–35% of pregnancies in women with epilepsy, an increased seizure frequency occurs during pregnancy. Women with epilepsy (WWE) should be counseled that seizure freedom for at least 9 months prior to pregnancy is probably associated with a high rate (84–92%) of remaining seizure-free during pregnancy (Level B).

D. Vibha (✉)
Department of Neurology, All India Institute of Medical Sciences, New Delhi, Delhi, India

R. Sharma
Department of Obstetrics and Gynecology, UCMS–GTB Hospital, New Delhi, Delhi, India

R. Sharma, A. Kumar (eds.), *Systemic Disorders in Pregnancy*,
https://doi.org/10.1007/978-981-96-4876-4_8

Table 8.1 Etiology of epilepsy in adults

Head Trauma
Alcohol
Drug-induced withdrawals
Cerebral infection
Brain tumors
Biochemical abnormality
Arteriovenous malformations
Idiopathic (*diagnosis of exclusion*)

These causes should be ruled out in a new onset seizure disorder in pregnant women

While there is no systematic country or statewide registries of WWE in India, a few hospitals and community-based registries from India have published data on safety of AEDs and teratogenic effects of AEDs in Indian population. In a hospital-based study from North India, it was found that a significantly higher (p value = 0.02) number of women were using more than two antiepileptic drugs simultaneously, in recent study period (5-year period from 2011 to 2015 (n = 177)) as compared to the earlier study period (years 1987–1994 (n = 219)). There was a significantly higher incidence (p value = 0.001) of small for gestational age babies in a recent study period group.

The risk of major congenital malformations (MCM) was studied in the registry in South India and this center was also a part of a longitudinal, prospective cohort-based EURAP international registry. This registry had 7355 pregnancies, which were exposed to one of the eight antiepileptic drugs for which the prevalence of MCM was studied. The occurrence of MCM was 10·3% for valproate, 6·5% for phenobarbital, 6·4% for phenytoin, 5·5% for carbamazepine, 3·9% topiramate, 3·0% for oxcarbazepine, 2·9% for lamotrigine, and 2·8% for levetiracetam (Table 8.1). The prevalence of major congenital malformations increased with the dose at time of conception for carbamazepine ($p = 0{\cdot}0140$), lamotrigine ($p = 0{\cdot}0145$), phenobarbital (p = 0·0390), and valproate ($p < 0{\cdot}0001$). Studies targeting home-based care versus routine clinic-based care are also underway.

8.2 Classification of Seizures During Pregnancy (Fig. 8.1)

Seizures in pregnancy can occur in three scenarios: (1) uncontrolled preexisting seizures; new onset seizures; pregnancy-related conditions, especially the eclampsia. Women with risk of eclampsia may have some evidence of preeclampsia, which should be monitored and prevented in advance.

8.2.1 Uncontrolled Preexisting Seizures

The frequency of seizures during pregnancy in women with epilepsy was similar to the seizure frequency of nonpregnant women with epilepsy in a recent cohort from the USA. However, earlier studies have found increase in seizure frequency during pregnancy and the postpartum period, the recent studies showing nearly similar

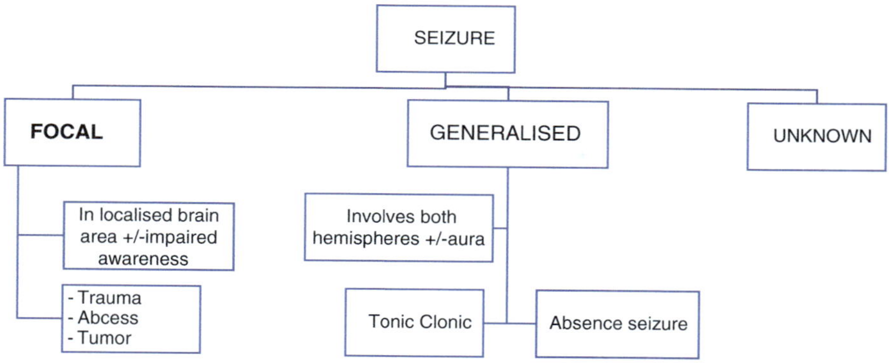

Fig. 8.1 Classification (as per International league against epilepsy)

frequencies has been attributed to increased awareness, newer antiepileptic drugs, and better drug monitoring. The prediction models during pregnancy have taken into account the age at first seizure, classification of seizure type, dose of AEDs, seizure frequency, seizures in prior pregnancy as variables for predicting probability of seizures during pregnancy.

8.2.2 New Onset Epilepsy During Pregnancy

In a hospital-based study from China, about only 2.1% patients had their first seizure during pregnancy. Most of the new onset seizures occurred in the second and third trimester. However, the teratogenic effects were most frequent in those having seizures in the first trimester. The prevalence has ranged from 3.4% to 10.5% in other studies. Most of these seizures were provoked seizures, and few with structural lesions in the imaging.

8.2.3 Pregnancy-Related Conditions Causing Seizures

This condition is given the special diagnosis of eclampsia. Eclampsia is defined as the occurrence of seizures during gestational hypertension (> 20 week) with proteinuria (>300 mg/24 h). It is seen in 5–10% of pregnant women. The seizures may occur prepartum (45%), and during partum (5%) and postpartum (50%) period (Fig. 8.2). The clinical features in addition to seizures include visual disturbances

Seizure frequency during Pregnancy	increase in 20-30% of women
	no change in 50%
	decreased frequency in 15%

Fig. 8.2 Seizure frequency during pregnancy

(50%), headache (19%), or pain in abdomen (19%) and signs of preeclampsia (arterial hypertension or proteinuria) (38%).

The mechanism of seizure may be brain edema due to rapid increase in arterial hypertension, or release of excitatory cytokines. MRI brain typically shows vasogenic edema in parietooccipital area. The management is unique in this situation. It consists of magnesium sulfate and it has been shown to be more effective in decreasing seizure recurrence than diazepam or phenytoin [1]. It acts via decreasing peripheral vascular resistance, reducing vasogenic edema, and centrally inhibits NMDA receptors, providing anticonvulsant activity by increasing the seizure threshold.

8.3 Clinical Features

The clinical features that aid in the diagnosis of seizures typically consists of episodes of generalized or focal abnormal movements with or without loss of consciousness. The scheme of classification should follow the International League Against Epilepsy (ILAE). The correct classification will help in proper selection of investigations as well as treatment. It will also help in better counseling patients about chance of recurrence, precautions to be taken, and prognosis. A complete knowledge of impact of epilepsy and drugs on mother and child is very important to manage the course of pregnancy and childbirth (Table 8.2).

Table 8.2 Effects of epilepsy on pregnancy

Fetal malformation
Convulsions
Miscarriage
Hemorrhage
PIH
Abruption
Intrauterine death
Preterm birth
Increased cesarean rate
Maternal death
Seizure disorder in offspring
SUDEP Epilepsy is the second most common cause of SUDEP (Sudden unexplained death in pregnancy) after amniotic fluid embolism

8.4 Diagnosis

The diagnosis is mostly clinical. To confirm the etiology of seizures, further investigations may be ordered. A CT head is contraindicated in pregnancy and an MRI brain without contrast should be sufficient most of the times to exclude a structural lesion. In India, the commonest causes of focal seizures are neurocysticercosis, perinatal hypoxia, and post head trauma. The situations exclusive to pregnancy state in which MRI brain is helpful are posterior reversible encephalopathy syndrome (PRES) and cerebral venous thrombosis (CVT). An electroencephalogram (EEG) is a simple, safe, and noninvasive test, which may also be helpful in pregnancy to classify seizure type, especially a patient with generalized epilepsy who had not been classified earlier or has had first episode during pregnancy. The acute symptomatic seizures during pregnancy due to metabolic derangements, eclampsia, or associated neurological infections may warrant specific investigations.

8.5 Treatment

The occurrence of seizure during pregnancy can occur in the following scenarios:

8.6 History of Epilepsy with Recurrence of Seizure in Pregnancy

The most common cause here is drug default followed by change in drug levels during pregnancy leading to subtherapeutic drug levels. Although the American Academy of Neurology (AAN), 2009 guidelines recommend routine monitoring of drug levels and adjustment of doses, this facility is not available routinely and for all AEDs in India. More often, a preemptive adjustment of drug levels is based on seizure control, especially for AEDs for which level monitoring is not available. However, a recent study also found that there was no evidence to suggest that regular monitoring of serum AED levels in pregnancy improved seizure control or affects maternal or fetal outcomes. In face of these conflicting evidence and lack of monitoring facilities, it is best to individualize treatment. The titration of the dose should be ideally done in the prepregnancy period.

8.7 Seizure for the First Time in Life During Pregnancy

Seizure occurring for the first time in pregnancy is fraught with challenges of the underlying diagnosis depending upon the period of gestation. While MRI may be done in any trimester of pregnancy to ascertain any underlying lesion causing seizure, those occurring in a setting of preeclampsia does not warrant imaging. The choice of drug depends upon the type of seizure and the underlying etiology.

Single seizure occurring in the setting of metabolic abnormality (uremic or hepatic encephalopathy, hyponatremia, septic encephalopathy) does not warrant long-term AED administration.

8.8 First Time or Recurrence of Seizure in Pregnancy with Repeated Seizures and Encephalopathy

Any convulsive activity persisting for more than 5 min should be managed as status epilepticus. The causes of seizures with encephalopathy in pregnancy may be eclampsia, most commonly, to Posterior Reversible Encephalopathy Syndrome (PRES), reversible vasoconstriction syndrome (RCVS), metabolic abnormalities like uremia, hyperammonemia, sepsis, hyponatremia, hypomagnesemia, hypocalcemia. Underlying secondary causes predisposed in pregnancy may be cerebral venous sinus thrombosis and hypertensive encephalopathy. It may also be unrelated to pregnancy like cerebral infection, encephalitis, acute autoimmune or demyelinating syndromes, space occupying lesions, etc.

8.9 Preconception Precautions and Counseling

The medical management of epilepsy in women of childbearing age includes counseling regarding premarital and preconceptual, in addition to during pregnancy. It is known in Indian society that marriage is more difficult when it comes to WWE. WWE are usually brought to medical attention the first time when marriage is contemplated, in an effort to "cure" epilepsy before marriage. This further reflects in lack of AED adherence after marriage and during planning conception.

Following women are excluded from epilepsy [Evidence level 2]

- *If she is convulsions free since last 10 years*
- *If she is off antiepileptic drugs since last 5 years*

It is important to counsel the patient and their families about the increased risk of recurrence of seizure during pregnancy than the teratogenic effects of the AEDs per se. It is also important to optimize the AEDs and add folic acid 4–5 mg/day prophylaxis before the patient plans conception. Antiepileptics interfere with folate metabolism leading to folic acid deficiency further resulting in congenital malformation (Table 8.3 and Fig. 8.3).

Table 8.3 Antiepileptics drugs: Doses and adverse effects

Drugs	Dose	Maternal effects	Fetal effects	Malformation
Valproate	500–2000 mg in three divided doses	Drowsiness, ataxia, alopecia, thrombocytopenia	Neural-tube defects, clefts, cardiac anomalies-associated developmental delay, ADHD	7–10% with monotherapy Higher with polytherapy
Phenytoin	150–300 mg on two divided doses	Gingival hyperplasia, megaloblastic anemia, nystagmus, hirsutism	Fetal hydantoin syndrome: craniofacial anomalies, fingernail hypoplasia, growth deficiency, developmental delay, cardiac anomalies, clefts	5–11%
Carbamazepine; oxcarbazepine	600–1200 mg per day in three divided doses	Drowsiness, leukopenia, slight hepatotoxicity, ataxia	Fetal hydantoin syndrome, as above, spina bifida	2–5%
Phenobarbital	60–180 mg daily at night	Drowsiness	Clefts, cardiac anomalies, urinary tract malformations	6–20%
Lamotrigine	300–500 mg in two divided doses	–	Increased risk for clefts	Up to 2% (four- to tenfold higher than expected)
Topiramate	100 mg per day	–	Clefts	2–3% (15- to 20-fold higher than expected)
Levetiracetam	1000–3000 mg in two divided doses	–	Theoretical: skeletal abnormalities; impaired growth in animals	1–3%

Lower seizure threshold Increased nausea vomiting (due to low compliance)
Lower gut motility (lower absorption)
Increased drug clearance
Labour
Sleep deprivation
Hyperventilation during pain
Hypoglycaemia

Fig. 8.3 Reasons for increased frequency of seizure in pregnancy

Table 8.4 AEDs protein binding and teratogenicity

Antiepileptic drug	Protein binding	Teratogenicity[a]
Phenobarbital	Low	High
Phenytoin	High	Intermediate
Carbamazepine	High	Intermediate
Oxcarbazepine	Low	Low
Eslicarbazepine	Low	Unknown
Valproate	High	Very high
Clobazam	High	Unknown
Gabapentin	Low	Low
Lamotrigine	Low	Low
Topiramate	Low	Intermediate
Levetiracetam	Low	Low
Brivaracetam	Low	Unknown
Zonisamide	Low	Low
Lacosamide	Low	Unknown
Perampanel	High	Unknown

[a]Low: <3%; intermediate: 3.1% to 6%; high: 6.1% to 9%; very high: >9%.

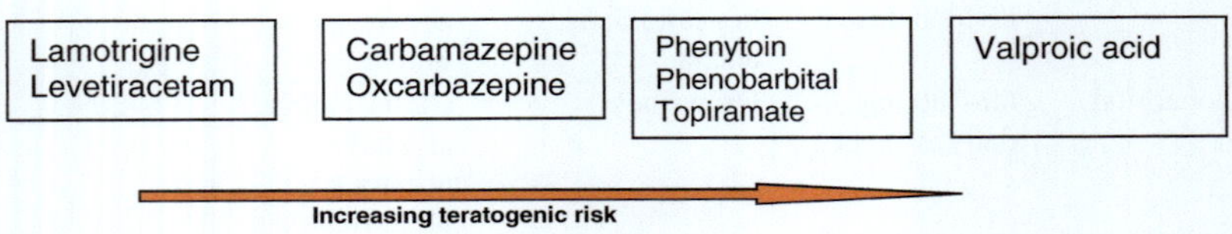

Fig. 8.4 Teratogenic risk profiles of antiseizure medications

Any antenatal women coming with history of convulsions should be regarded and treated as eclampsia.

Differential diagnosis includes any cardiac, metabolic, neuropsychiatric, and intracranial pathologies. Diagnosis of epilepsy requires complete neurological assessment.

Phenytoin and phenobarbital increase the major malformation rate two- to three-fold above baseline while valproate is teratogenic in a dose-dependent manner (Table 8.4 and Fig. 8.4).

Nearly 2/3rd women do not have worsening of epilepsy during pregnancy, but if convulsions had occurred in last year then close supervision is mandatory.

The AEDs taken in the prepregnancy period should be continued as such throughout pregnancy and puerperium. In the event of a breakthrough seizure, compliance, drug levels, and sleep deprivation (can trigger seizures) need to be checked. Even with changes in serum levels of AED during pregnancy, there is no guideline recommending regular monitoring of drug levels or escalating the dose in well-controlled epilepsy (Fig. 8.5).

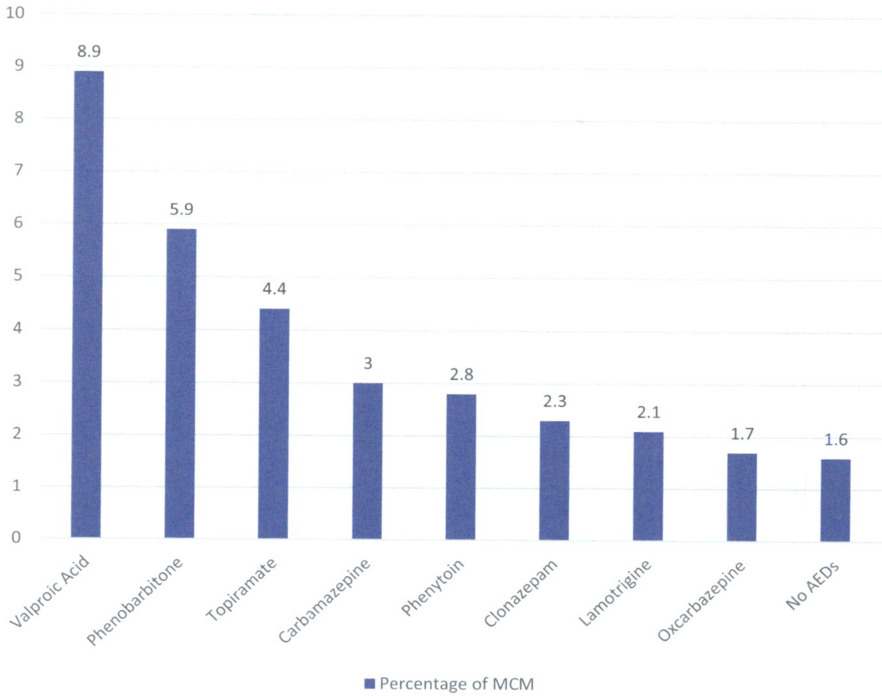

Fig. 8.5 Major congenital malformations (MCM) with various antiepileptic drugs (AEDs)

Antepartum

- Routine serum antiepileptic drug monitoring during pregnancy is not recommended.
- Routine oral vitamin K is not recommended to prevent hemorrhagic disease of the newborn or postpartum hemorrhage.
- Level II USG at 18–20 weeks gestation to rule out anomalies, mainly NTDs and cardiac defects.
- Serial growth scans to pick up and manage fetal growth restriction.
- Regular monitoring of risk factors for convulsions—compliance, stress, insomnia, etc.
- If convulsions are well controlled, then early termination of pregnancy is indicated for obstetric indications only.
- Timing and mode of delivery has to be individualized.
- Elective cesarean delivery is considered if there are recurrent and prolonged convulsions, significant deterioration, and in cases of status epilepticus.

Peri-delivery seizures that are longer than 30 s should be terminated with a benzodiazepine. In delivery planning, this should be documented, and drugs should be easily accessible. Women with a very high risk of seizures at this time can be managed with additional clonazepam or clobazam around the time of delivery.

8.9.1 Intrapartum

There is low risk of convulsions in labor

- Regular monitoring of risk factors for convulsions like stress, dehydration, sleep deprivation, etc.
- Adequate analgesia.
- For high-risk cases of seizures, consider long-acting benzodiazepine, e.g.,. clobazam.
- Continue antiepileptic drug in labor.
- Can consider alternative parenteral drugs, if previous AAD is intolerant (Fig. 8.6).

8.9.2 Maternal and Neonatal Outcome

The effects of epilepsy and AEDs on the newborn depend on the epilepsy syndrome, the seizure controls, and the AED(s) that the mother is taking. Therefore, in patients with well controlled epilepsy who are on a single drug and had uneventful antenatal period, the outcomes of pregnancy are usually uneventful. Despite the secretion of AEDs in variable amount in the breast milk depending upon the protein binding of the AED, breastfeeding is superior to the mild exposure of AED transmitted via breast milk. This has been supported by large community-based registries.

All babies should be given inj.1 mg vitamin K (IM) to protect them from hemorrhagic disease of the newborn.

Postpartum

Antiepileptics to continue and should be tapered if dose is increased in antenatal period on advice of the concerned speciality.

Breastfeeding is not contraindicated but the drugs cross into the breastmilk, so signs for neonatal sedation, jitteriness, convulsions should be looked for, these symptoms and signs are more with carbamazepine and valproate.

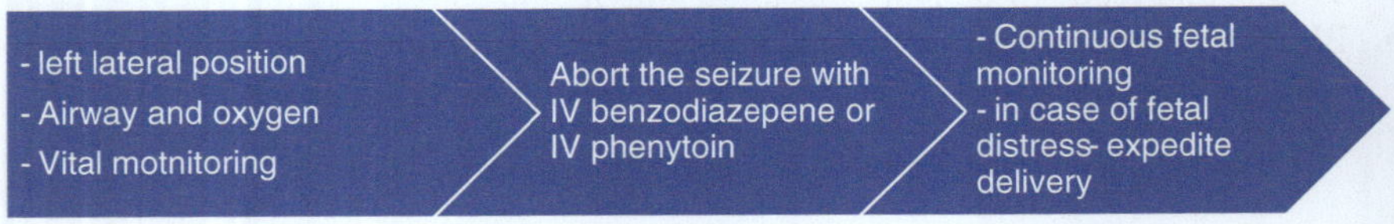

Fig. 8.6 Management of epileptic seizures in labor

Contraception: IUDs or DMPA to be preferred whereas, OCPs, POPs, vaginal rings should be avoided as they are less effective with enzyme inducing antiepileptics drugs.

Prolonged follow-up as there is an increased risk of postpartum depression.

Status Epilepticus (SE)

Seizure activity that is ongoing and lasts for more than 30 min or recurrent seizure without full recovery of consciousness between episodes is defined as status epilepticus (Fig. 8.7 and Table 8.5).

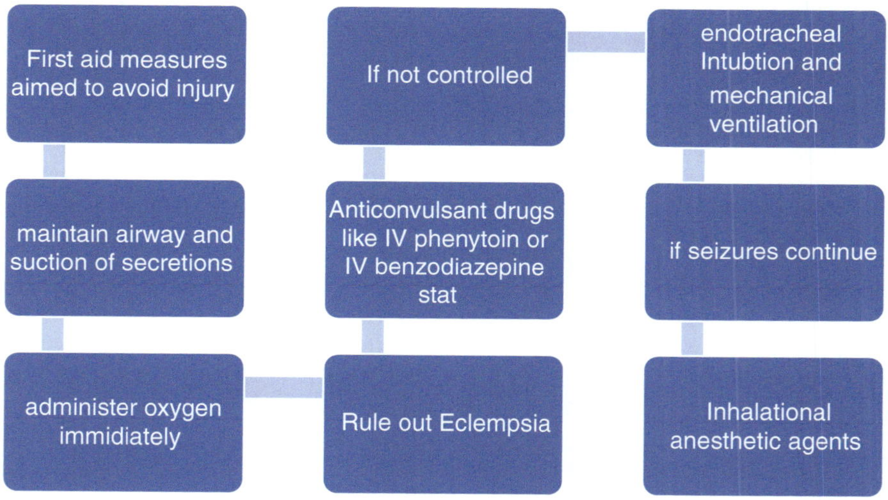

Fig. 8.7 Management of status epilepticus according to the American Epilepsy Society Guidelines, 2016

Table 8.5 Timeline and suggested action

Timeline	Action
0–5 min	Stabilize the patient (Airway, breathing, circulation, disability) Finger stick glucose IV access and blood work
5–20 min	Benzodiazepine administration Intramuscular Midazolam (10 mg if >40 kg) Intravenous Lorazepam (0.1 mg/kg, maximum 4 mg/dose) IV Diazepam (0.15–0.2 mg/kg/dose, maximum 10 mg) If not, intranasal or buccal midazolam
20–40 min	Second AED IV Fosphenytoin (20 mg/kg, maximum 1500 mg) IV Valproate (40 mg/kg, maximum 3000 mg/dose) IV Levetiracetam (60 mg/kg, maximum 4500 mg/dose) If nonavailable, IV Phenobarbitone (15 mg/kg)
40–60 min	Third therapy phase Repeat second line or anesthesia induction with EEG monitoring

8.10 Conclusion

Epilepsy in pregnancy requires coordination of the treating obstetrician and neurologist. The hormonal effect of pregnancy and the implications of treatment on the fetus make it a special situation. The paucity of data is due to exclusion of this group from most clinical trials. However, with pregnancy registries across the world as well as in India, and with the advent of better diagnostic and treatment modalities, the management and outcomes have become more efficient. It is crucial for the obstetrician to identify warning signs of differentials like CVT and PRES, which require timely and specific management may change outcomes.

Bibliography

1. The Eclampsia Trial Collaborative Group. Which anticonvulsant for women with eclampsia? Evidence from the Collaborative Eclampsia Trial. Lancet. 1995;345:1455–63.

9 Cholestasis of Pregnancy

Uma Pandey and Ruchi Birendra

Intrahepatic cholestasis of pregnancy (IHCP) is the most common multifactorial hepatic disorder of pregnancy, which mainly manifests in the second or third trimester (after 30 weeks). About 1.5%–4% of otherwise healthy pregnancies are affected by intrahepatic cholestasis during pregnancy [1]. It is characterized by intense pruritus without any primary skin rash with elevated levels of bile acid and transaminases with or without increased serum bilirubin in the absence of any alternative cause, and the condition resolves 2–3 weeks after delivery [2]. The maternal outcome is good, but it is associated with very adverse fetal complications like preterm delivery, meconium staining of amniotic fluid, fetal bradycardia, fetal distress, and, most unfortunately, fetal demise, so timely diagnosis and treatment are needed. The deleterious effect on the fetus is directly proportional to the total bile acid (TBA) level with the risk of stillbirth above TBA serum concentration of 100 μmol/L or more. Meta-analysis suggests that most women with IHCP can probably be reassured that the risk of stillbirth is equivalent to that of pregnant women in the general population, as most women have bile acids below this threshold [3]. The therapy's primary goal is to relieve pruritus, normalize maternal biochemistry, and prevent fetal complications. Ursodeoxycholic acid (UDCA) is used for medical management, but it is advisable to deliver around 37–38 weeks or even earlier if fetal compromise is detected. Pruritus Gravidarum is the term used for pruritus without skin rash occurring in the first trimester of pregnancy [4]·

U. Pandey (✉) · R. Birendra
Department of OBG, BHU, Varanasi, Uttar Pradesh, India

R. Sharma, A. Kumar (eds.), *Systemic Disorders in Pregnancy*,
https://doi.org/10.1007/978-981-96-4876-4_9

9.1 Incidence

In 1987, Wilson reported the first case of ICP in African American patients. The incidence of cholestasis varies according to ethnic background and geographical location. Reproductive hormones, particularly estrogen, and genetic predisposition are considered to be the leading causes of ICP development [5]. ICP is very common among northern Europe and south America and Asian women are twice more prone than white European women [6]. It is uncommon in North America (1 in 1000 pregnancies). It complicates 1.2–1.5% of the Indian–Asian population and 5% of the Araucanian-Indian origin [7]. ICP is encountered in 1–4% of Polish population. In Andean natives, its incidence is as high as 25%. Worldwide, the Mapuche Indians (Indigenous inhabitants of present-day south-central Chile and southwestern Argentina) have the highest incidence, where cholestasis has been reported to complicate >27% of pregnancies [8]. It is the second most common cause of jaundice in pregnancy.

9.2 Risk Factor

Risk factors are as follows:

- Genetic predisposition manifested by mutations in bile transporter proteins.
- Multidrug resistance protein 3 (MDR3), involved in the biliary secretion of phospholipids, and multidrug resistance-related protein 2 (MRP2) are assigned a major role in the pathogenesis of ICP [9]. MDR3 mutation is also related to the severity of the disease. Mutations may also affect the bile salt export pump (BSEP) protein-encoding gene. Other rare mutations within the FIC1 gene (ATP8B1) present within the bile duct membrane and the FXR gene (NR1H4) were also detected in Caucasian patients diagnosed with ICP. Steroid hormones or their metabolites may cause mutations in these genes [10].
  The increased incidence in multiple gestations or patients treated with oral contraceptives points toward the involvement of sex steroids in the pathogenesis of ICP. Further concentrations of sex hormones increase as the pregnancy advances and subsequently fall after birth, which coincides with the natural history of the disease. However, the exact mechanism of sex hormones to the development of ICP has not been fully explained as of yet. The cholestasis effects were demonstrated for 17-β-D-estradiol and sulfated metabolites of progesterone [10].

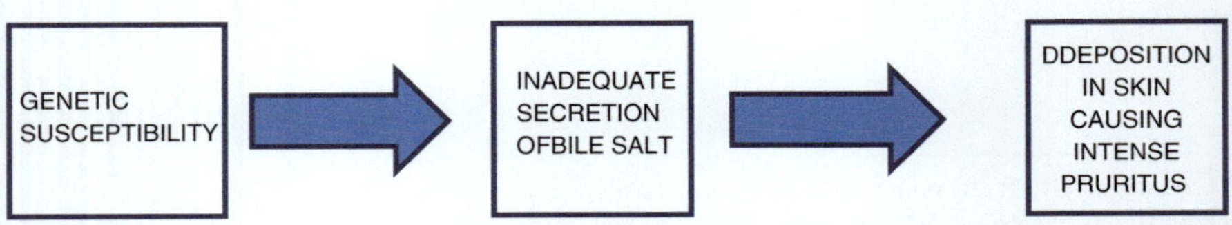
GENETIC SUSCEPTIBILITY
INADEQUATE SECRETION OFBILE SALT
DDEPOSITION IN SKIN CAUSING INTENSE PRURITUS

- Several studies confirmed the damaging effects of gestational hormones on the function of hepatobiliary transport proteins involved in the excretion of bile acids into the hepatic bile ducts. This may lead to changes in the ratio of hydrophilic and hydrophobic bile acids being disturbed to favor hydrophobic acid, which results in the impairment of water-soluble bile acids being transported across the placenta and excreted by maternal kidneys. Normally, bile acids are transported from the fetus to the mother, whereas in cholestatic pregnancy, trans-placental transport occurs in the opposite direction. As a result, levels of bile acids are increased in both the mother and the fetus, which is associated with the induction of oxidative stress, thus leading to damage to liver cells and other tissues [10]
  - Multifetal gestation [6]
  - Advanced maternal age [6]
  - HCV infection [6]
  - H/O gallstones [6]
  - History of cholestasis in previous pregnancy (40–60%) [4]
  - Family history (14%) [6]
  - Oral progesterone treatment to prevent preterm labor [6]
  - Diet deficient in selenium and vitamin D levels [6]
  - Winter season [6]

9.3 Classification

A pregnant female presenting with abnormal liver function should be investigated as with any nonpregnant female [2]. A detailed history, including drug history or history of liver or gall bladder disease, physical examination, and standard serological workup should be performed. After initial evaluation, these patients are divided into three groups [11].

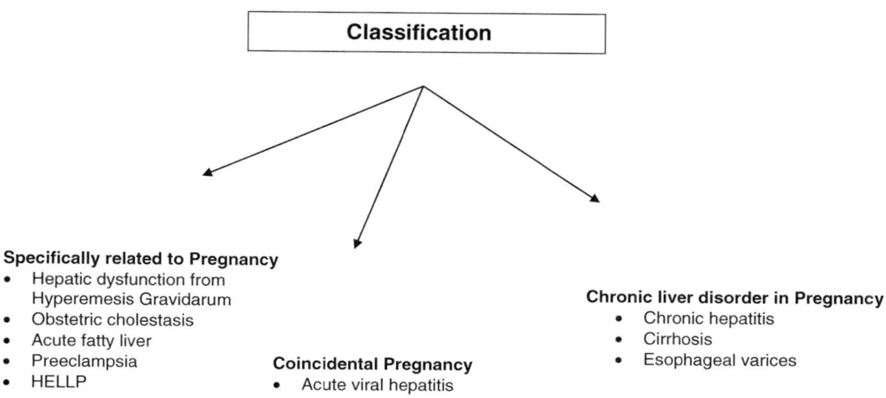

9.4 Clinical Features

ICP usually presents with pruritus in the third trimester (after 30 weeks). However, there have also been a few case reports in the first trimester [4]. Pruritus usually begins on the palmar aspect of the palms and soles, worsening during the night, leading to disturbed sleep or sometimes intractable enough to cause psychological suffering and even suicidal thoughts in the mother [4]. However, all body parts may be affected. Usually, 3 weeks separate the beginning of pruritus from the increase of liver enzymes and blood bilirubin [12]. Primary skin lesions are absent, but secondary excoriation marks, pigmented lesions that resemble prurigo, and abrasions secondary to women's response to pruritus may be observed [6]. Jaundice is not the presenting feature, but mild jaundice may develop within 4 weeks of the appearance of itching in 10–15% of cases [10]. If jaundice is the presenting complaint, further evaluation for alternative causes is mandatory [2]. Postnatal resolution of pruritus and abnormal liver function tests (LFTs) is the characteristic of cholestasis [7]. The incidence of gallstone formation and cholecystitis is higher in women with a history of ICP [4].

Rarely, patients may present with abdominal pain, nausea, poor appetite, weight loss, pale stools, dark urine, or sleep deprivation. Steatorrhea due to fat malabsorption may develop [8]. Steatorrhea may be severe enough to cause vitamin K deficiency, leading to prolonged prothrombin time, which may manifest as bleeding into the fetal central nervous system [10]. Several studies have reported higher rates of GDM and Preeclampsia in cases complicated by ICP [8]. Therefore, patients should be screened for these conditions.

9.5 Diagnosis and Treatment

In patients presenting with pruritus, LFT and TBA estimation should be done. However, elevation of serum bile acids alone cannot be used to diagnose; the patient must also have clinical symptoms. ICP is the diagnosis of exclusion. It is diagnosed in a patient with a history of pruritus without rash, with abnormal liver function tests with elevated fasting bile acids after excluding other causes of itching and abnormal liver function tests [7].

Women in whom pruritus persists with normal liver biochemistry should have LFTs repeated every 1–2 weeks, as the onset of pruritus may precede abnormal liver biochemistry [7]. Serum bile acids should be tested at least weekly from 32 weeks gestation in women with proven intrahepatic cholestasis of pregnancy to identify those with concentrations > – 40 μmol/L at increased risk of unfavorable pregnancy outcomes [13].

The upper limit of normal throughout pregnancy is 25% lower than the nonpregnant level except ALP[9]. Differential diagnosis includes drug-induced liver injury, viral hepatitis, and autoimmune liver disease. Additional tests may include a viral screen for hepatitis A, B, C, Epstein–Barr virus, cytomegalovirus, a liver autoimmune screen (anti-smooth muscle and anti-mitochondrial antibodies), and a liver ultrasound [14].

Although fasting bile acids are the most sensitive and specific for the diagnosis and monitoring of cholestasis [6], RCOG guideline recommends that cholestasis may be diagnosed in a woman with typical pruritus and abnormal LFT in the absence of fasting bile acid testing provided there is resolution of both following delivery.

With regard to other liver function tests, alkaline phosphatase is not useful in diagnosis as it is elevated in normal pregnancy. The elevation in transaminases associated with ICP is less than two times the upper limit of normal, which differentiates it from other liver diseases [8]. Bilirubin is raised in only 10% of women, and gamma-glutamyl transferase is usually normal [6]. Consult a hepatologist if you experience severe, early, or atypical ICP symptoms [15].

Once obstetrics cholestasis is diagnosed, LFTs should be repeated weekly until delivery. However, none of the methods of antenatal fetal monitoring can predict poor fetal outcomes [7]. Even a reactive CTG does not guarantee fetal well-being, and fetal death is usually sudden [7]. The mother should be asked to monitor fetal movements and to attend the hospital for Cardiotocogram (CTG) monitoring if there are any concerns. The Society for Maternal–Fetal Medicine and EASL (European Association for the Study of the Liver) Clinical Practice Guidelines [13] recommend delivery at 36 0/7 and 35 weeks of gestation, respectively, for patients with TBA $\geq$ 100 μmol/L, given that the risk of stillbirth increases substantially around this gestational age (GRADE 1B) and delivery between 36 0/7 and 39 0/7 weeks of gestation for patients with TBA of <100 μmol/L (GRADE 1C). This recommendation is based on recent studies that have shown that the risk of stillbirth is not as high as was previously thought in women with cholestasis of pregnancy with low bile acids [16].

9.6 Management

Due to the lack of high quality RCTs, the optimal management of IHCP is controversial. But however, risk of adverse perinatal outcomes can be minimized by drugs, fetal monitoring, and elective late preterm and early-term delivery [7].

9.7 Drugs

1. Topical Emollients

Calamine lotion and aqueous cream with menthol. But there is no trial to support or refute the use of these products

2. UDCA

UDCA is used as first-line therapy in doses of 10–15 mg/kg of body weight. The starting dose is 300 mg BD but can be increased to 600 mg BD (max dose 1.5–2 g/day). Although UDCA is not licensed for ICP, but US FDA states that while the effects during the first trimester are unclear, there is no evidence of adverse fetal outcomes. Women should be informed of the lack of robust data regarding protection against stillbirth and the safety of the fetus or neonate [7]. Several studies, including multiple meta-analyses, report that UDCA significantly improves itching and serum bile acid levels and may potentially reduce adverse perinatal outcomes. Symptoms improve within 1–2 weeks, and a decrease in bile acids occurs after 2 weeks. UDCA is a naturally occurring hydrophilic bile acid that disrupts micelles in the intestine and decreases the rate at which cholesterol is absorbed. It concentrates in hepatocytes and decreases hepatic cholesterol synthesis, secretion, and reabsorption. Due to enterohepatic circulation, UDCA becomes the primary circulating bile acid. Thus, UDCA, a hydrophilic nontoxic bile acid, replaces cholic acid, the hydrophobic toxic bile acid thought to be implicated in adverse outcomes [8]. Mild to moderate gastrointestinal disturbance is rarely associated with it. However, PITCHES TRIAL, a double-blind, multicenter, randomized, placebo-controlled trial, showed that treatment with ursodeoxycholic acid does not improve pregnancy outcomes for women with intrahepatic cholestasis [17]. In randomized controlled trials, ursodeoxycholic acid was found to reduce stillbirths and preterm births, indicating its clinical benefits [18].

3. Dexamethasone

Dexamethasone was shown to improve symptoms and total bile levels in a study of a small cohort of Finnish women by inhibition of placental estrogen, which was, however, not supported by subsequent studies [8]. It may be used to promote lung maturity if needed.

4. Rifampicin

A case report of the utility of Rifampicin is present [8]. Rifampicin, an effective second-line treatment for primary biliary cirrhosis, is a choleretic antibiotic shown to reduce pruritus and enhance bile acid excretion in primary biliary cirrhosis when used in conjunction with UDCA. Dual therapy of UDCA and rifampicin, can decrease serum bile acids by 50% in IHCP. However, more studies are required to establish its use in pregnancy [6].

5. Others
   - Vitamin K: ICP may reduce the absorption of vitamin K, leading to an increase in prothrombin time, which may result in Postpartum Haemorrahge (PPH), so vitamin K should be considered at the dose of 10 mg [10].
   - Cholestyramine and S-adenosyl-L- methionine are no longer considered as first-line treatments in ICP.

9.8 Maternal and Fetal Complications and Their Management

The maternal outcome is usually good as the symptoms subside spontaneously following delivery, along with normalization of serum liver tests. If abnormalities persist, then other underlying chronic liver diseases like primary biliary cirrhosis, primary sclerosing cholangitis, or chronic hepatitis C should be suspected.

ICP is strongly linked with adverse perinatal outcomes [6] and a positive correlation has been seen between TBA concentration and fetal complication, with fetal complication rising by 1–2% for every 1 μmol/L increase in bile acids above 40 μmol/L [6].

Bile acid also causes increased myometrial contractility and increased sensitivity to oxytocin [6], thus increasing the risk of premature delivery by 20–60% [10].

Babies born at any period of gestation from IHCP women are at risk of respiratory distress syndrome [6]. The increased risk can be because of both spontaneous and iatrogenic preterm delivery. Various animal models have demonstrated causative relationships. One model hypothesized that elevated bile acid levels damage alveolar enzyme function, resulting in decreased surfactant levels and subsequent RDS [8]. In another model, bile acids were shown to cause severe chemical pneumonitis and pulmonary edema [8].

High levels of circulating bile acids have been implicated in causing meconium staining of amniotic fluid by causing increased gut motility [6] and anal sphincter relaxation. Serum bile acid concentrations of 100 μmol/L and more are associated with an increased risk of stillbirth [10] [19]. Stillbirth seen in cholestasis is because of the direct effect of bile acid on the fetal heart and not due to chronic uteroplacental insufficiency [8]. Bile acids have been implicated to cause cardiac arrhythmia in an in vitro model of the fetal heart. Bile acids are also known to cause marked vasoconstriction of placental veins, thus explaining the acute anoxia causing fetal death [6].

9.9 Prevention or Pre-conceptional Precaution/Counseling

ICP is familial in nearly one-fifth of cases and chances of recurrence is 90% in subsequent pregnancies. However, many studies have shown that in the majority of cases, ICP does not affect the outcome of future pregnancy. Therefore, appropriate counseling of all women with a history of ICP should be done [20].

9.10 Differential Diagnosis

Differential diagnosis includes other causes of pruritus and abnormal LFTs [20–22]

	Hyperemesis gravidarum	Preeclampsia, eclampsia, and HELLP	Viral hepatitis, EBV, CMV, HSV	Acute fatty liver of pregnancy	Chronic liver disease	Cholestasis of pregnancy
Onset	Early	Mid to late	Variable	Late	Early	Late
Clinical findings	Severe nausea and vomiting	Hypertension, headache, convulsions, features of hemolysis	Prodromal symptom jaundice, fever	Nausea, vomiting, abdominal pain, hypertension, jaundice, encephalopathy	Decompensated disease due to portal hypertension, variceal bleed and premature delivery	Pruritus, jaundice
Laboratory tests	Hypokalemia, hyponatremia, low urea, ketosis, metabolic hypochloremic alkalosis	Elevated liver enzyme, low platelet, decreased hemoglobin, abnormal peripheral blood smear, low haptoglobin	Elevated liver enzymes	Elevated liver enzymes, elevated bilirubin, abnormal coagulation, decreased serum glucose level, increased uric and creatinine level	Deranged serum creatinine, bilirubin, and INR	Elevated bile acid and transaminases
Recurrence	Yes (15–20%)	Yes (4–19%)	No	Yes (in case of certain mutant allele recurrence is >25%)	Yes	Yes (90%)

9.11 Prognosis or Long-Term Effect and Follow-Up

- ICP is considered a transient disease without long-term morbidity. Hepatocellular damage resolves after pregnancy in nearly all cases.
- LFT and TBA levels must be repeated at 6 weeks postpartum to ensure complete resolution [6]. If it remains elevated, an alternative cause for hepatic dysfunction should be sought.
- The recurrence rates are high (up to 90% in some cases). Moreover, when ICP recurs, it tends to be more severe and occurs at an earlier gestational age in subsequent pregnancies.
- ICP may be misdiagnosed or coexist with other pregnancy issues, such as pre-eclampsia or the rare but catastrophic HELLP syndrome. Clinicians should consider this possibility when diagnosing atypical or early-onset ICP with rapidly declining liver function [5].
- An increased risk of liver and biliary tree cancer, immune-mediated disease, cardiovascular disease, and maternal diabetes is seen in women with ICP [6].
- The incidence of hepatobiliary diseases, including hepatitis C, chronic hepatitis, hepatic fibrosis, and gallstones, is also increased in women with a history of ICP.
- Children are at increased risk of metabolic disease later in life (Fig. 9.1).

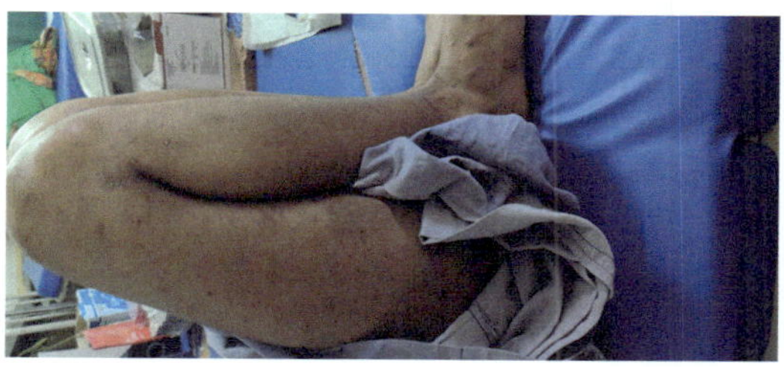

Fig. 9.1 A picture taken at Sir Sundar Lal Hospital (SSH), Banaras Hindu University (BHU) shows excoriation due to intense pruritus

References

1. Hobson S, Gandhi S, Sobel M. Intrahepatic cholestasis of pregnancy. C Can Med Assoc J. 2022;194(48):E1650.
2. Tran TT, Ahn J, Reau NS. ACG clinical guideline: liver disease and pregnancy. Am J Gastroenterol. 2016;111:1–19. https://doi.org/10.1038/ajg.2015.430.
3. Ovadia C, Seed PT, Sklavounos A, Geenes V, Di Illio C, Chambers J, et al. Association of adverse perinatal outcomes of intrahepatic cholestasis of pregnancy with biochemical markers: results of aggregate and individual patient data meta-analyses. Lancet. 2019;393(10174):899–909.
4. Ghosh S, Chaudhuri S. Intra-hepatic cholestasis of pregnancy: a comprehensive review. Indian J Dermatol. 2013 Jul;58(4):327.
5. Myszkowski S, Ayuk PTY. Intra-hepatic cholestasis of pregnancy: management challenges. Case Rep Women's Health. 2024;41(December 2023):e00576. Available from: https://doi.org/10.1016/j.crwh.2023.e00576
6. Geenes V, Williamson C, Chappell LC. Intrahepatic cholestasis of pregnancy. Obstet Gynecol. 2016;18:273–81.
7. Green–top Guideline No. 43. Obstetric Cholestasis. R Coll Obstet Gynaecol. 2011:43.
8. Smith DD, Rood KM. Intrahepatic cholestasis of pregnancy. Clin Obstet Gynecol. 2019;63(1):134.
9. Xiao J, Li Z, Song Y, Sun Y, Shi H, Chen D, et al. Molecular pathogenesis of intrahepatic cholestasis of pregnancy. Can J Gastroenterol Hepatol. 2021;2021:1.
10. Piechota J, Jelski W. Intrahepatic cholestasis in pregnancy: review of the literature. J Clin Med. 2020;9:1361.
11. Theodoridis T, Kraemer J, Cunningham FG, Leveno KJ, Bloom SL, Haulh JC, Gilstrap LC, Wenstrom KD, editors. Abortion. Williams Textbook of Obstet_rics. 25th ed. New York: McGraw-Hill; 2005. p. 7823–30.
12. Bakhsh HA, Elawad MM, Alqahtani RS, Alanazi GA, Alharbi MH, Alahmari RA. Intrahepatic cholestasis of pregnancy: a case report of third-trimester onset of the disease. Cureus. 2022;14(11):14–6.
13. Williamson C, Nana M, Poon L, Kupcinskas L, Painter R, Taliani G, et al. EASL Clinical Practice Guidelines on the management of liver diseases in pregnancy. J Hepatol. 2023;79(3):768–828. Available from: https://doi.org/10.1016/j.jhep.2023.03.006
14. Mackillop L, Williamson C. Liver disease in pregnancy. Postgrad Med J. 2010;86:160–4.
15. Girling J, Knight CL, Chappell L. Intrahepatic cholestasis of pregnancy: green-top guideline No. 43 June 2022. BJOG Int J Obstet Gynaecol. 2022;129(13):e95–114.
16. Lee RH, Greenberg M, Metz TD, Pettker CM. Society for maternal-fetal medicine consult series #53: intrahepatic cholestasis of pregnancy: replaces Consult #13, April 2011. Am J Obstet Gynecol. 2021;224(2):B2–9. Available from:. https://doi.org/10.1016/j.ajog.2020.11.002.
17. Chappell LC, Bell JL, Smith A, Linsell L, Juszczak E, Dixon PH, et al. Ursodeoxycholic acid versus placebo in women with intrahepatic cholestasis of pregnancy (PITCHES): a randomized controlled trial. Lancet. 2019;394(10201):849–60.
18. Ovadia C, Sajous J, Seed PT, Patel K, Williamson NJ, Attilakos G, et al. Ursodeoxycholic acid in intrahepatic cholestasis of pregnancy: a systematic review and individual participant data meta-analysis. Lancet Gastroenterol Hepatol. 2021;6(7):547–58.
19. Palmer KR, Xiaohua L, Mol BW. Management of intrahepatic cholestasis in pregnancy. Lancet. 2019;393(10174):853–4. https://doi.org/10.1016/S0140-6736(18)32323-7.
20. James D, Steer P, Weiner C, et al. High-risk pregnancy: management options. 5th ed. Cambridge University Press; 2017. Online ISBN: 9781108664677.
21. Faulkes RE, Chauhan A, Knox E, Johnston T, Thompson F, Ferguson J. Review article: chronic liver disease and pregnancy. Aliment Pharmacol Ther. 2020;52(3):420–9.
22. Verma D, Saab AM, Saab S, El-Kabany M. A systematic approach to pregnancy-specific liver disorders. Gastroenterol Hepatol. 2021;17(7):322–9.

Thyroid Disorder in Pregnancy

10

Komal Chavan and Dinesh Wade

Thyroid disorders are among the most common endocrine diseases in pregnancy. Providers will frequently be called upon to diagnose, treat, and monitor women with these conditions. Undiagnosed or uncontrolled thyroid conditions may lead to perinatal morbidity and even mortality. Both thyrotoxicosis and hypothyroidism are associated with adverse pregnancy outcomes. There also is concern about the effect of overt maternal thyroid disease on fetal development. In addition, medications that affect the maternal thyroid gland can cross the placenta and affect the fetal thyroid gland. The association between subclinical hypothyroidism and pregnancy complications is less clear. Treatment for overt hypothyroidism with thyroid replacement is universally recommended, which decreases risks of complications. Despite the morbidity of thyroid disorders, there is no clear evidence for the benefit of universal screening in pregnancy. To evaluate thyroid hormone levels during gestation, gestational age-specific values should be used. When hyperthyroidism is treated, the goals of therapy are to achieve a subclinical hyperthyroid state and monitor fetal development. Care must be taken so as not to induce a state of maternal hypothyroidism during pregnancy, since such a diagnosis is also associated with adverse outcomes for both mother and infant [1].

The suggested total daily iodine ingestion for pregnant women is 229 μg/day, and for lactating women it is 289 μg/day; prenatal vitamins should contain 150 μg of iodine in the form of potassium iodine.

The normal thyroid gland is able to compensate for the increase in thyroid hormone demands by increasing its secretion of thyroid hormones stored as colloid and maintaining them within normal limits throughout gestation.

K. Chavan (✉)
VN Desai Hospital, Mumbai, India

Chavan Maternity & Nursing Home, Mumbai, India

D. Wade
Progenesis Fertility Center, Pune, India

R. Sharma, A. Kumar (eds.), *Systemic Disorders in Pregnancy*,
https://doi.org/10.1007/978-981-96-4876-4_10

Thyroid Function Tests

TSH below 2.5 mIU/L in the first trimester, and less than 3.0 mIU/L in the second and third trimesters, is the upper limit of normal.

According to population, trimester-specific reference ranges of serum TSH and FT4 should be used, but if it is not available then the cutoff for serum TSH in the first trimester is 2.5 mIU/L and 3.0 mIU/L in the second and third trimesters [2] (American Thyroid Association and the Endocrine Society) [3].

.

10.1 Hyperthyroidism

Hyperthyroidism is relatively uncommon during pregnancy, affecting 0.1–0.4% of all pregnancies [4]. The two most common etiologies of hyperthyroidism encountered during pregnancy are Graves' disease and gestational transient thyrotoxicosis (GTT). The majority of pregnant patients with Graves' disease will enter pregnancy with a known history of thyroid disease [5].

The remaining etiologies of hyperthyroidism in pregnancy are all relatively uncommon.

10.1.1 Gestational Hyperthyroidism

Also known as gestational thyrotoxicosis, transient hyperthyroidism of HG, and transient nonautoimmune hyperthyroidism of early pregnancy, this condition is defined as transient hyperthyroidism in the first trimester of pregnancy. Common causes are HG, multiple gestation, molar pregnancy, hyperplacentosis.

10.1.2 Transient Hyperthyroidism of Hyperemesis Gravidarum

Hyperemesis Gravidarum leads to frequent hospital visits due to severe nausea and vomiting, beginning at 4–8 weeks gestation. There is weight loss, ketonuria, altered liver function tests, and hypokalemia due to vomiting and dehydration.

FT4 and TT4 levels can rise 4–6 times the base line, in 40% women TT3 and free triiodothyronine (FT3) values can be elevated [5]. The TT3/TT4 ratio <20, while in Graves' hyperthyroidism ratio >20.

Routine monitoring of thyroid function tests is not required because the symptoms tend to be transient.

The cause of the elevations of thyroid hormones in patients with HG is the endocrine effect of hCG [6]. Most likely, high levels of hCG—a known stimulator of the TSH receptor—play an important role, as does the prolongation in its biologic activity seen in twin pregnancies.

Obstetric outcome is not affected by gestational hyperthyroidism. Birth weight may be slightly lower, but not significantly different, compared with fetuses of control mothers and is related to maternal weight loss. Gestational trophoblastic diseases, partial and complete hydatidiform moles, and choriocarcinoma are other causes of hyperthyroidism early in pregnancy.

10.2 Hypothyroidism

Hypothyroidism is diagnosed if the serum TSH >5 mIU/L [7].

Patients who also have a low serum FT4 would be considered to have overt disease.

Patients with a normal range FT4 are classified as having subclinical hypothyroidism.

10.2.1 Classification of Hypothyroidism

10.2.1.1 Primary Hypothyroidism

- Autoimmune (Hashimoto) thyroiditis
- Surgical or 131I induced
- Post–thyroid ablation therapy
- Congenital disease
- Drug-induced, e.g., lithium, amiodarone, iodine excess, antithyroid
- Head and neck radiation for nonthyroid malignancy

10.2.1.2 Secondary Hypothyroidism

- Pituitary gland or hypothalamus disorders
- Autoimmune hypophysitis—Sheehan syndrome

Primary hypothyroidism is classified as

1. *Subclinical hypothyroidism* (FT4 is normal but raised TSH)
2. *Clinical hypothyroidism* (reduced level of T4, normal FT4 and serum TSH >10 mIU/L)
3. *Isolated Hypothyroxinemia*

Subclinical Hypothyroidism

Subclinical hypothyroidism (SCH) diagnosed in the first trimester of pregnancy has been associated with maternal, fetal, and neonatal complications. The most commonly reported complications are pregnancy loss, preterm delivery, and preeclampsia [8].

Laboratory tests diagnostic of subclinical hypothyroidism are an elevated serum TSH in the presence of normal trimester-specific FT4 levels. The recommended serum TSH upper limit of normal, if gestation-specific reference ranges are not available, is 3.5 mIU/L in the first trimester and up to 4 mIU/L in the second and third trimesters [9].

Clinical or Overt Hypothyroidism
If there is raised serum TSH and low FT4 or if serum TSH > 10 mIU/L.

symptoms are tiredness, cold intolerance, fatigue, muscle cramps, constipation, irregular menses, infertility, and deepening of the voice.

Skin is dry and cold, delayed deep tendon reflexes, bradycardia, periorbital edema.

Atrophic thyroiditis or *primary myxedema* or *chronic thyroiditis without goiter*—occurs in 20% of chronic thyroiditis without goiter.

Serum thyroid antibodies—TPOAbs, also known as *antimicrosomal antibodies*—are elevated in almost 95% of patients with autoimmune hypothyroidism.

Isolated Hypothyroxinemia
If a women has normal TSH & low FT4 and residing in a geographical area having sufficient dietary intake of iodine.

10.2.2 Treatment of Hypothyroidism in Pregnancy

- Drug of choice is L-Thyroxine
- Normalization of Thyroid Function Test (TFTs) must be achieved in prepregnancy or in early trimester of pregnancy [10].
- Dose of L-thyroxine is 2–2.4 μg/kg per day during pregnancy, which is higher than in nonpregnant women (1.7–2 μg/kg per day)
- Women planning conception should have TSH <2.5 mIU/L
- In pregnancy <20 weeks, TSH must be repeated every 2–6 weeks
- Repeat TSH at 24–28 weeks and 32–34 weeks gestation
- Soon after delivery, prepregnancy dose should be started

10.2.3 Patients with Known Thyroid Cancer Before Pregnancy

Pregnancy does not appear to be a risk factor for recurrences in women with a previous history of treated thyroid cancer and no evidence of residual disease.

Women on suppressive T4 therapy, should continue the same, adjusting the L-thyroxine to maintain normal TSH and TFT4 [11].

Postpartum Thyroid Dysfunction A variant of Hashimoto or chronic thyroiditis and most common cause of thyroid dysfunction in postpartum period. *Postpartum thyroiditis* (PPT) is defined as transient thyroid dysfunction in the first year after delivery in women who were euthyroid before pregnancy on no thyroid therapy [12]. PPT should be considered if thyroid disorder occurs within 1 year of delivery or abortion.

Women having high titers of TPOAb in the first trimester, family or personal history of thyroid disease, presence of goiter, smoking, diabetes, other autoimmune diseases are prone for PPT.

Evaluation should be done at 3, 6, and 12 months postdelivery. Firm and non-tender goiter, tachycardia, increased TFTs and thyroid antibodies (TPOAbs), and negative titers of TRAb.

Presentation of PPT is characterized by:

1. An episode of hyperthyroidism (1–3 months), followed by hypothyroidism (3–7 months) and reverting to euthyroidism (after the seventh month).
2. Hyperthyroidism (1–4 months) to euthyroidism.
3. Hypothyroidism (3–7 months) to a euthyroid state.
4. Permanent hypothyroidism after the hypothyroid phase [12].

It is recommended that a diagnosis of the late postpartum period (8–12 months) is associated with the risk of developing Graves' disease de novo.

- Treatment of hyperthyroid symptoms

β-adrenergic blockers—propranolol 10–40 mg every 6 hourly or atenolol 25–50 mg every 24 hourly. Since hyperthyroxinemia is secondary to acute thyroid gland injury and release of hormones, antithyroid drugs are not useful.

- For hypothyroid symptoms

Small amounts of L-thyroxine (50 μg/day) will control symptoms and women desiring conception should continue L-thyroxine therapy.

References

1. Krassas GE, Poppe K, Glineor D. Thyroid function and human reproductive health. Endocr Rev. 2010;31:702.
2. Alexander EK, Pearce EN, Brent GA, et al. 2017 guidelines of the American Thyroid Association for the diagnosis and management of thyroid disease during pregnancy and the postpartum. Thyroid. 2013;23(11):1479–83.
3. Lee RH, Spencer CA, Mestman JH, et al. Free T4 immunoassays are flawed during pregnancy. Am J Obstet Gynecol. 2019;200:260.e1.
4. Cooper D, Laurberg PP. Hyperthyroidism in pregnancy. Lancet Diabetes Endocrinol. 2013;1:238–49.
5. Marx H, Amin P, Lazarus JH. Hyperthyroidism and pregnancy. BMJ. 2008;336:663–7.
6. Niebyl JR. Nausea and vomiting in pregnancy. N Engl J Med. 2010;363:1544.
7. McClain M, Lambert-Messerlian G, Haddow JE. Sequential first- and second-trimester TSH, free thyroxine, and thyroid antibodymeasurements in women with known hypothyroidism: FaSTER trial study. Am J Obstet Gynecol. 2008;199:129.e1.
8. Cleary-Goldman J, Malone FD, Lambert-Messerlian G, et al. Maternal thyroid hypofunction and pregnancy outcome. Obstet Gynecol. 2008;112:85.

9. De Groot L, Abalovich M, Alexander EK, et al. Management of thyroid dysfunction during pregnancy and postpartum: an Endocrine Society clinical practice guideline. J Clin Endocrinol Metab. 2012;97:2543–65.
10. Negro R, Formoso G, Mangieri T, et al. Levothyroxine treatment in euthyroid pregnant women with autoimmune thyroid disease: effects on obstetrical complications. J Clin Endocrinol Metab. 2006;91:2587.
11. Mazzaferri E. Approach to the pregnant patient with thyroid cancer. J Clin Endoc Metab. 2011;96:265–72.
12. Stagnaro-Green A, Schwartz A, Gismondi R, et al. High rate of persistent hypothyroidism in a large scale prospective study in postpartum thyroiditis in southern Italy. J Clin Endocrinol Metab. 2011;96:652–7.

Pregnancy in Women with Congenital Heart Disease

11

Mukta Agarwal, Shaheen Ahmad, and Simran Simran

Congenital heart disease (CHD) is a condition that affects around 0.8% of newborn infants worldwide. Due to recent medical and surgical improvements, more than 85% of these infants now survive into adulthood [1, 2]. Most treatments have not successfully cured the problem, and around 50% of adults with congenital heart disease will need additional surgery and are at risk of arrhythmia, heart failure, and premature death if not appropriately controlled. Women with innate heart conditions encounter extra obstacles when pregnant.

Cardiovascular Change During Pregnancy

Pregnancy induces diverse physiological alterations in the cardiovascular system. During the first trimester, the heart must pump up to 50% more blood to sustain the developing fetus. Furthermore, there is a 30–40% reduction in vascular resistance [3–5]. During the first and second trimesters, there is an increase in blood flow, leading to an expansion in plasma volume and a rise in heart rate of approximately 10–20%. These modifications are heightened even further during delivery. Following childbirth, there is a transient rise in fluid volume, potentially causing a short period of volume overload during the initial days after delivery.

During pregnancy, alterations in blood circulation impact the heart's functionality. The alterations result in an enlargement of the left ventricle at the end of diastole, whereas its size remains constant during systole [6]. This results in an elevated stroke volume, leading to an increase in ventricular outflow tract velocity, which may present as a hyperkinetic state. A similar outcome is probable in the right

M. Agarwal (✉) · Simran Simran
Department of Obstetrics and Gynaecelogy, AIIMS, Patna, India
e-mail: drmuktaa@aiimspatna.org

S. Ahmad
Interventional Cardiologist, Zulekha Hospital, Dubai, UAE

R. Sharma, A. Kumar (eds.), *Systemic Disorders in Pregnancy*,
https://doi.org/10.1007/978-981-96-4876-4_11

ventricle; however, there is limited evidence to confirm this. Stroke volume increases and afterload decreases explain why regurgitant lesions rarely worsen during pregnancy (Fig. 11.1).

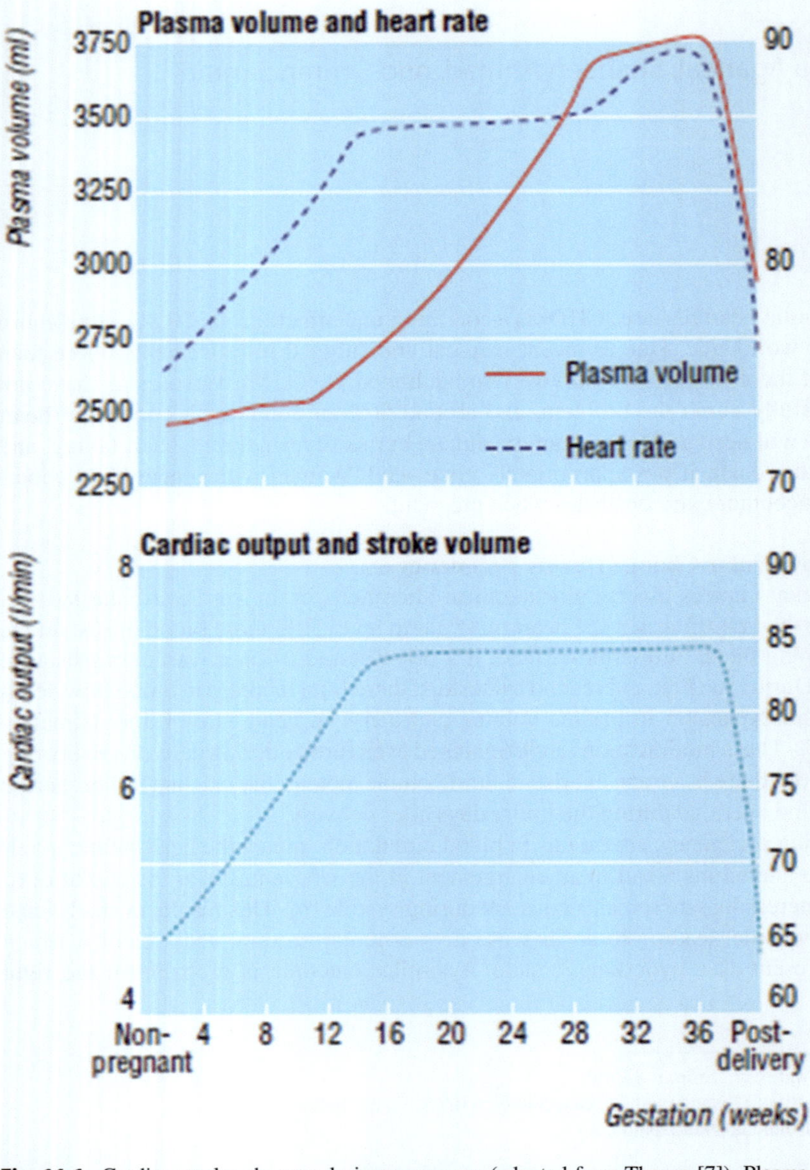

Fig. 11.1 Cardiovascular changes during pregnancy (adapted from Thorne [7]). Plasma volume and cardiac output increase steadily until the end of the second trimester, when cardiac output reaches a plateau at 30–50% above prepregnancy levels. Obstructive heart lesions (such as aortic or mitral valve stenosis), which limit cardiac output, are particularly compromised during pregnancy. The increase in blood volume may precipitate heart failure. Cyanosis often worsens during pregnancy as pregnancy-related systemic vasodilation may lead to increased right to left shunting

11.1 Introduction About Congenital Heart Disease

11.1.1 Pulmonary Hypertension

Pulmonary hypertension (PH) is a disease with multiple etiologies. Diagnosis involves monitoring the average pressure in the pulmonary artery, which must exceed 25 mmHg in a right cardiac catheterization. Pulmonary arterial hypertension (PAH) is distinguished by a left ventricular filling pressure below 15 mmHg and a pulmonary vascular resistance exceeding 3 Wood units [8]. Untreated idiopathic pulmonary hypertension can result in death within an average of 2.8 years. PAH is frequently seen in women and may manifest for the first time during pregnancy [9].

11.1.2 Maternal and Fetal Risk

Advancements in treatments and a collaborative team approach have enhanced results for patients with pulmonary arterial hypertension (PAH). Nevertheless, pregnancy remains a substantial threat to women with PAH, with fatality rates varying from 16% to 30% [10, 11]. Avoiding pregnancy is advised, and abortion should be considered if it happens. Patients with moderate pulmonary vascular disease may also experience exacerbated symptoms during pregnancy. Higher rates of fetal and neonatal death also occur (Table 11.1).

11.1.3 Management

When a pregnant patient presents with new PH, it is crucial to follow the usual diagnostic algorithm. Echocardiography plays a vital role in the diagnosis, and other diagnostic measures should be planned based on the PH guideline. In cases of diagnostic uncertainty, invasive right heart catheterization is recommended to assist in making significant therapeutic decisions. However, this procedure should only be performed in a specialized center. If the condition is familial, it is appropriate to consider genetic counseling.

When caring for a pregnant patient with pulmonary hypertension, a team of experts from different fields is required. The care plan should be tailored to the patient's needs, but regular follow-up visits are essential, especially during the third trimester (often on a weekly basis). During each visit, a thorough evaluation, including oxygen saturation and RV function assessment, should be conducted.

Table 11.1 Causes of mortality

Maternal death	Fetal and neonatal death
1, Pulmonary hypertensive crisis	1. Premature birth
2. Pulmonary thrombosis	2. Decreased maternal cardiac output
3. Right heart failure	3. Low oxygen levels

Symptomatic patients may require bed rest, and additional risk factors such as air travel should be avoided. Anticoagulation therapy should be considered since thromboembolism is a significant risk. Patients with heart failure may need diuretics, and iron deficiency should be treated.

Pregnancy can be high risk for patients with pulmonary arterial hypertension (PAH), and it is important to adopt a proactive approach to commencing advanced therapies. Risk stratification should be performed as in nonpregnant patients. Although there is no evidence of benefit comparing a stepwise approach versus early combination therapy in pregnant patients, the latter is often preferred according to guidelines. Bosentan and other endothelin receptor antagonists are associated with embryopathy and should be discontinued unless doing so would greatly increase maternal risk. An individualized approach is required, and many units start therapy with oral sildenafil. Patients with true vasodilator responsiveness who are well-controlled on calcium channel blocker (CCB) therapy may be at lower risk, and this therapy should be continued, along with all IV therapies.

11.1.4 Delivery

The pregnant cardiac team must establish a comprehensive birth plan, which involves selecting the optimal method and timing of delivery as well as arranging for any required intensive care and mechanical assistance postdelivery. Regional anesthesia is generally favored over general anesthesia [12]. Precise control of fluid levels and maximizing right ventricular performance are essential for a positive result. Patients are at a heightened risk for an extended period after giving birth, and tailored counseling should be given to address the necessity of continued treatments and the prevention of future pregnancies. Continuing therapy during the early postpartum period is crucial.

11.2 Eisenmenger Syndrome

11.2.1 Maternal and Fetal Risk

Patients with Eisenmenger syndrome need special attention because of the added complexities of cyanosis, right-to-left shunting, and paradoxical embolism. Pregnancy causes systemic vasodilation, which results in an increase in the right-to-left shunt and a decrease in pulmonary flow. This leads to heightened cyanosis and reduced cardiac output. Maternal mortality rates are elevated, varying between 20% and 50%, so termination of pregnancy should be considered [13]. Nevertheless, it is important to consider that abortion also has associated hazards. Maternal carbon monoxide exposure and cyanosis elevate the risks of fetal and neonatal complications, resulting in increased miscarriage rates. Maternal hypoxemia is the most crucial predictor of outcome.

11.2.2 Management

Patients with Eisenmenger syndrome are at increased risk of thrombocytopenia, deficits in vitamin K-dependent clotting factors, and bleeding. Caution should be taken while providing antiplatelet treatment, or low-molecular-weight heparin (LMWH). Although the data supporting the use of advanced treatments is not as extensive, sildenafil and other PDE inhibitors like tadalafil and vardenafil are frequently recommended. If individuals continue to experience symptoms, prostanoids may be included in the treatment plan [14]. Extreme caution is necessary when prescribing medications that could cause abrupt systemic vasodilation or provide a risk of paradoxical air embolism (intravenous treatments). Competent pregnancy heart teams, which should include a pulmonary hypertension specialist, should prescribe advanced therapy for patients with Eisenmenger's syndrome. The rules governing delivery are consistent with those for other forms of public health, as previously stated.

11.3 Cyanotic Heart Disease Without Pulmonary Hypertension

11.3.1 Maternal and Fetal Risk

Cyanotic congenital heart disease is usually managed before pregnancy, although certain instances that are stable cannot be operated on or have been palliated may advance to childbearing age [15]. Over 15% of cyanotic pregnant women experience maternal problems, including heart failure, thrombosis, arrhythmias, and endocarditis. The underlying illness and ventricular function, rather than the saturation level, will determine the mother's outcome. When oxygen saturation during pregnancy exceeds 90%, there is a high likelihood of a favorable fetal outcome, with just a 10% probability of fetal loss. If the oxygen saturation level falls below 85%, there is a significant danger of fetal development limitation, early birth, and fetal mortality. Thus, in such instances, pregnancy should be discouraged due to the low live birth percentage of 12%.

11.4 Specific Congenital Heart Defects [16]

11.4.1 Atrial Septal Defect

11.4.1.1 Maternal and Fetal Risk

Women with a mended atrial septal defect (ASD) in the WHO risk class can often manage pregnancy without complications. Thromboembolic consequences have been documented in 5% of cases with unrepaired ASDs. Unrepaired or closed atrial septal defects in older individuals increase the likelihood of developing atrial arrhythmias [17]. Women with unrepaired ASD may have a higher incidence of preeclampsia and growth limitations during pregnancy.

11.4.1.2 Management

Catheter device closure for a second defect during pregnancy is unusual. Antiplatelet therapy will be necessary if this operation is required. Avoid doing closure to prevent paradoxical embolism. Preventing venous stasis is crucial in circumstances where women have residual shunts. To do this, utilize compression stockings, reduce bed rest, and take precautions to prevent air in intravenous lines.

11.4.2 Ventricular Septal Defect

11.4.2.1 Maternal and Fetal Risk

Ventricular septal defects (VSDs) that are small or have been corrected and do not cause left heart enlargement or ventricular dysfunction pose a minimal risk of problems during pregnancy (mWHO I and II).No evidence suggests heightened obstetric risks.

11.4.2.2 Management

Patients should be monitored once or twice during pregnancy with surveillance for PH.

11.4.3 Atrioventricular Septal Defect

11.4.3.1 Maternal and Fetal Risk

Pregnancy after repairing an atrial septal defect (ASD) is typically well-tolerated, particularly in women categorized as WHO risk class II–III. Reported cases have shown instances of arrhythmias and deterioration of atrioventricular (AV) valve regurgitation. Heart failure (HF) risk is minimal, occurring exclusively in women with severe regurgitation or reduced ventricular function.

Six percent of instances lead to progeny mortality, primarily due to the recurrence of congenital cardiac disease.

11.4.3.2 Management

For best management, it is advised to schedule follow-up appointments at least once every trimester. It is recommended to schedule appointments more frequently, perhaps monthly or biweekly, for individuals with substantial valve regurgitation or decreased ventricular function.

11.4.4 Coarctation of the Aorta

11.4.4.1 Maternal and Fetal Risk

Women who have had their coarctation of the aorta (CoA) corrected and are categorized as WHO risk class II can normally safely become pregnant. Women with unrepaired coarctation of the aorta (CoA), or those with corrected CoA but still experiencing systemic hypertension, residual CoA, or aortic aneurysms, face a higher risk of complications such as dissection. Additional risk factors are aortic dilatation and bicuspid aortic valve. There have been reports of an abundance of hypertensive illnesses, such as preeclampsia and miscarriages.

11.4.4.2 Management

It is crucial to constantly monitor persons with high blood pressure, and follow-up appointments should be scheduled at least every 3 months. Treat individuals with residual coarctation for hypertension and take precautions to avoid placental hypoperfusion. Percutaneous intervention with a covered stent for re-CoA can be considered during pregnancy; however, it should only be done in situations of severe hypertension or when there are risks to the mother or fetus.

11.4.5 Pulmonary Valve and Right Ventricular Outflow Tract Disease

11.4.5.1 Maternal and Fetal Risk

Severe pulmonary valve stenosis (PS) can result in problems such right ventricular (RV) failure and arrhythmias, although it is typically well tolerated. Severe pulmonary regurgitation is an independent predictor of maternal problems, especially in patients with compromised right ventricular function. There is no indication of heightened obstetric risks.

11.4.5.2 Management

Mild and moderate pulmonary stenosis (PS) is categorized as low-risk lesions, falling under WHO risk groups I and II. Typically, two or three follow-up sessions suffice for these circumstances. Patients with severe PS should undergo monthly or bimonthly cardiac examinations that specifically assess the right ventricular function. If symptomatic PS is severe and does not improve with medication treatment and bed rest, percutaneous valvuloplasty may be suitable.

11.4.6 Tetralogy of Fallot

11.4.6.1 Maternal and Fetal Risk

Women who have had surgery to correct tetralogy of Fallot typically tolerate pregnancy successfully, classified as WHO risk class II. Cardiac problems have been seen in approximately 8% of patients who had undergone repair, especially in those who were using cardiac medication before becoming pregnant [18]. Arrhythmias and cardiac failure are the most common complications. Thromboembolism and endocarditis are less frequent but can still happen. Pulmonary regurgitation and right ventricular dysfunction of moderate to severe degree pose risks. Prior pregnancy can lead to a lasting enlargement of the right ventricle and possible long-lasting heart issues. Maternal screening for 22q11 deletion is advised prior to pregnancy due to the heightened risk of progeny issues, including fetal growth limitation.

11.4.6.2 Management

Typically, quarterly follow-up is adequate. Women with severe pulmonary regurgitation should undergo monthly or biweekly cardiac assessment. If right ventricular failure happens during pregnancy, treatment should begin with diuretics and bed rest should be recommended. In exceptional situations, early delivery or transcatheter valve implantation may be options for individuals who do not improve with conservative treatment.

11.4.7 Ebstein's Anomaly

11.4.7.1 Maternal and Fetal Risk

Uncomplicated Ebstein's abnormality in women typically results in good pregnancy tolerance, classified as WHO risk class II. Symptomatic patients with cyanosis and/or heart failure should avoid pregnancy. Tricuspid regurgitation (TR) severity and right ventricle function are the main factors that define the hemodynamic problems. Cyanosis resulting from atrial septal defect (ASD) or patent foramen ovale and arrhythmias triggered by accessory routes are frequently observed. Additionally, there is an increased likelihood of heart failure and premature delivery [19]. Fetal and neonatal outcomes are associated with maternal oxygen saturation and carbon monoxide levels.

11.4.7.2 Management

The health of the fetus and newborn relies on the mother's oxygen saturation and carbon monoxide levels. Pregnant women with severe tricuspid regurgitation and heart failure can typically be treated with medication. Women with interatrial shunting may develop exacerbated cyanosis during pregnancy, heightening their susceptibility to paradoxical embolism. Thus, their condition should be evaluated during every visit.

11.4.8 Transposition of the Great Arteries

11.4.8.1 Maternal and Fetal Risk

Pregnancy hazards for patients with transposition of the great arteries (TGA) are mostly relevant to women who have undergone an atrial (Senning and Mustard) switch rather than an arterial switch. Women who have had an atrial switch operation may experience a higher risk of having arrhythmias and heart failure (WHO risk class III) during pregnancy, although generally tolerating pregnancy well. Irreversible deterioration of right ventricular (RV) function and tricuspid regurgitation (TR) may occur [20, 21]. Women should be discouraged from getting pregnant if their RV function is significantly reduced or if they have severe TR. The incidence of low birth weight and preterm delivery is 38%.

11.4.8.2 Management

Monthly or bimonthly review focusing on systemic RV function and arrhythmia is required. Diuretics and other HF therapies may be required.

11.4.8.3 Arterial Switch Operation

Women who are in good clinical condition and have maintained ventricular function may experience a low-risk pregnancy. Women with an enlarged neo-aorta will require closer monitoring. Although the procedure for TGA is increasingly common, there is a lack of evidence on pregnancy outcomes.

11.4.9 Congenitally Corrected Transposition of the Great Arteries

11.4.9.1 Maternal and Fetal Risk

Individuals with congenitally repaired transposition of the great arteries (TGA), sometimes referred to as atrioventricular and ventriculoarterial discordance, face potential difficulties that are influenced by their functional capacity, ventricular performance, occurrence of arrhythmias, and concurrent conditions such as ventricular septal defect (VSD) and pulmonary valve stenosis. These consequences may involve arrhythmias and cardiac failure categorized as WHO risk class III. Moreover, these individuals have a tendency to develop AV block, and approximately 10% of them may suffer from a permanent decrease in RV function [14, 22]. Counsel patients in New York Heart Association (NYHA) classes III or IV, with ventricular failure (ejection fraction (EF) <40%), or severe TR against pregnancy. Fetal loss is more likely to occur when cyanosis is present, leading to an increased rate of loss.

11.4.9.2 Management

Patients should undergo regular echo surveillance of systemic RV function every 4–8 weeks for follow-up, including with assessment of symptoms and rhythm.

11.4.10 Fontan Circulation

11.4.10.1 Maternal and Fetal Risk

Individuals who have undergone Fontan circulation are more likely to experience reproductive problems. Nevertheless, they can still have a successful pregnancy. These pregnancies are classified as high to extremely high risk (WHO risk class III

Table 11.2 Risk of recurrent disease in offspring of parents with congenital heart disease [25]

	Mother affected		Father affected	
Lesion	Risk of transmission (%)	No. of cases	Risk of transmission (%)	No. of cases
Atrioventricular septal defect	11.6	5/43	4.3	1/23
Aortic stenosis	8.0	36/248	3.8	18/469
Coarctation	6.3	14/222	3.0	9/299
Atrial septal defect	6.1	59/969	3.5	16/451
Ventricular septal defect	6.0	44/731	3.6	26/717
Pulmonary stenosis	5.3	24/453	3.5	14/396
Persistent ductus arteriosus	4.1	39/828	2.0	5/245
Tetralogy of fallot	2.0	6/301	1.4	5/362
Total	5.8	222/3795	3.1	93/2961

or IV). Patients may also suffer from atrial arrhythmias and decline in NYHA class. Patients with saturations below 85%, decreased ventricular function, moderate to severe AV regurgitation, refractory arrhythmia, or protein-losing enteropathy are strongly advised against getting pregnant (mWHO IV). Patients who have undergone Fontan surgery have a 30% chance of experiencing a miscarriage [23]. Antenatal and peripartum hemorrhage frequently occurs and is associated with a higher likelihood of premature birth, small for gestational age infants, and neonatal mortality [24].

Fontan patients should undergo regular monitoring during pregnancy, including monthly check-ups, and in the initial weeks following childbirth. They are also susceptible to thromboembolic problems and may need therapeutic anticoagulation, which must be carefully weighed against the risk of bleeding. Immediate treatment is required if atrial arrhythmias arise, which may include electrical cardioversion. Risk of recurrence of CHD depends upon the type of disease (Table 11.2).

11.4.10.2 Maternal and Fetal Risk

Pregnant women with congenital heart disease who are susceptible to serious cardiovascular events include symptomatic arrhythmia, stroke, pulmonary edema, overt heart failure, or death. The risk level is defined by the cardiovascular system's ability to respond to the physiological changes of pregnancy. The hazards associated with a patient's congenital condition, morphological traits, previous surgeries, and current hemodynamic status are unique to each individual. It is essential to comprehensively evaluate patients with congenital cardiac disease prior to pregnancy to categorize risks, offer guidance, and reach well-informed conclusions.

Women with congenital cardiac disease exhibit a greater frequency of prenatal and neonatal adverse outcomes. Possible events may involve intrauterine growth restriction, early birth, cerebral bleeding, and fetal loss [26]. Other obstetric risk factors increase the likelihood of adverse events, especially in women with poor functional class, cyanosis, and left heart blockage, which limits cardiac output and flow to the placenta [27, 28].

Assessing the mother's status is essential for determining the risk of cardiac problems during pregnancy. This involves analyzing her medical history, functional status, oxygen levels, natriuretic peptide levels, echocardiogram evaluation of heart chambers and valves, intrapulmonary pressures and aortic sizes, physical fitness, and heart rhythm irregularities. For evaluating the risk associated with a particular disease, utilize the modified World Health Organization (mWHO) categorization and adhere to the guidelines for that specific disease. The risk assessment should also take into account additional predictive factors found in research involving large populations like CARPREG [28, 29] and ZAHARA [30, 31] (Table 11.3).

However, the mWHO classification is currently the most accurate system of risk assessment, although it is probably more appropriate for developed, rather than developing, countries.

Predictors of adverse neonatal events are [16]:

- NYHA class III/IV or cyanosis during baseline prenatal visit
- Maternal left heart obstruction
- Smoking during pregnancy
- Maternal oxygen saturation (<90%)
- Multiple gestations

Table 11.3 Predictors of adverse maternal outcomes

Risk factors (ZAHARA)	Risk factors (CARPREG II)
History of arrhythmias (1.5 points)	Prior cardiovascular event or arrhythmias (3 points)
Cardiac medications before pregnancy (1.5 points)	NYHA class > II or cyanosis (3 points)
NYHA class > II (0.5 points)	Resting oxygen saturation < 90% (3 points)
LVOT with peak gradient >50 mm Hg or AVA < 1 cm^2 (2.5 points)	Mechanical valve (3 points)
Moderate or severe systemic AV valve regurgitation (0.75 points)	Systemic ventricular dysfunction with LVEF <49% (2 points)
Pulmonary AV valve regurgitation (0.75 points)	High left side obstruction, peak LVOT >30%, AVA < 1.5 cm^2 (2 points)
Mechanical valve prosthesis (4.25 points)	Pulmonary hypertension (2 points)
Cyanotic heart disease (1 points)	Coronary artery disease (2 points)
	High risk aortopathy (2 points)
	No prior cardiac intervention (1 points)
	Later pregnancy assessment (2 points)
Score CV risk	Score CV risk
0–0.5:2.9%	0–1:5%
0.51–1.50:7.5%	2:10%
1.51–2.50:17.5%	3:15%
2.52–3.50:43.1%	4:22%
≥3.51:70.0%	≥4:41%

- Use of anticoagulants throughout pregnancy
- Cardiac medication before pregnancy
- At birth cyanotic heart disease
- Mechanical valve prosthesis
- Maternal cardiac event during pregnancy
- Maternal decline in cardiac output during pregnancy
- Abnormal uteroplacental Doppler flow

11.5 General Management Approach in Pregnancy with Heart Disease

11.5.1 Preconception Counseling

It should be offered to everyone with preexisting heart disease. In the case of CHD, it should be started before the transition from the pediatric to adult cardiac service.

Should include:

1. Both males and females need to be informed about short- and long-term prognosis and chance of inheritance of condition
2. Optimum timing of pregnancy
3. Contraindications to pregnancy along with full discussion to attain motherhood, which include surrogacy and adoption
4. CHD along with single gene defect or a genetic syndrome such as Di George's syndrome can consider preimplantation genetic diagnosis
5. How pregnancy impact their condition and how their condition affect the pregnancy should be considered
6. Importance of optimal weight, physical exercise, smoking cessation, effects of alcohol and drugs, folic acid for supplementation prepregnancy, cervical screening, choice of contraception, medication history, and importance of vaccination (covid and influenza)
7. Review of medications to optimize cardiac function and/or avoid fetal exposure to known teratogens, for example, angiotensin converting enzyme (ACE) inhibitors, angiotensin receptor blockers, amiodarone, warfarin, and spironolactone
8. Women with CHD requiring cardiac intervention generally are advised to proceed with intervention prior to pregnancy (e.g., percutaneous aortic balloon valvuloplasty for asymptomatic severe aortic stenosis (AS) to reduce maternal and fetal risks)
9. Women needing valve replacement should be counseled about the risks and benefits of autografts/homografts; bioprosthetic and metallic heart valves (conflicting maternal and fetal risk and benefits of anticoagulation) must be discussed with the patient
10. Cardiac surgery during pregnancy should be minimized or avoided. Maternal risks are same as those in nonpregnant women, but cardiopulmonary bypass during pregnancy incurs risk for the fetus

11. In case of subfertility, if requirement of ART or diagnostic laparoscopy-associated pneumoperitoneum or hysteroscopy (needing fluid distension of uterine cavity) can cause life-threatening compromise to a woman with a uni-ventricular circulation or pulmonary hypertension, it is important to discuss with the gynecologist who will be undertaking this care and should have clear guidance regarding the cardiac tolerance of the patient
12. Prepregnancy risk assessment should be done using the modified WHO classification (mWHO) and include risk to both mother and baby (Table 11.1)
13. Preconception evaluation should include a detailed history, baseline investigations including a full blood count, liver, thyroid and renal function, information on prior interventions (surgical and percutaneous), symptom status, a complete physical exam, a 12-lead electrocardiogram, a transthoracic echocardiogram, and an assessment of functional status
14. For women who have not had preconception counseling, a complete risk evaluation should be done at first prenatal visit
15. An inter-pregnancy interval of at least 18 months is recommended for women classified as mWHO class II-IV
16. Advice regarding effective and safe contraception should be given, counseling should be provided in a joint clinic by an obstetrician with expertise in heart disease, and a cardiologist with specialized training in adult congenital heart disease

11.5.2 Contraception

Patients with congenital heart disease should be made aware of the risks associated with getting pregnant as well as contraception.

The efficacy of various techniques, patient-specific traits that affect adherence, medical conditions that affect the risk–benefit profile of various methods, and the preference for sterilization or a reversible form of contraception are among the factors taken into account.

It is vital to have efficient contraception in order to optimize the clinical state, change medication, and prepare ready for pregnancy.

Patients with preexisting heart disease or hypertension should avoid taking the combination oral contraceptive pill (OCP) due to its potential to increase the risk of venous thromboembolism (VTE) and elevate blood pressure.

The typical dosage of ethinyl estradiol ranges from 20 to 35 mcg. A 20 mcg dose might result in reduced thromboembolic consequences.

Progestin-only contraception can be administered through many methods such as the levonorgestrel-releasing IUD, depot medroxyprogesterone injections (e.g., Depo-Provera), progestin-only pills (e.g., Micronor tablets, Nor-QD, or generics), or the etonogestrel implant (Nexplanon).

Patients with congestive heart failure (CHF) can safely utilize progesterone only pills (POP), especially the higher dose (Desogestrel 75 mg), which is more dependable because it prevents ovulation.

Depo-Provera is contraindicated in people with heart failure due to its propensity to induce fluid retention.

Barrier methods include condoms for males and diaphragms with spermicide for ladies. While these treatments are usually less efficient than other techniques, they carry almost little risk of problems. Women with heart conditions should avoid using these methods due to their high failure rates (18% for male condoms).

An intrauterine device (IUD) is suitable for women with low risk of sexually transmitted infections who desire a reversible contraceptive technique and have mild or no cyanosis. A copper intrauterine device (IUD) can endure for a minimum of 10 years, reducing the frequency of replacements and lowering the risk of infection. It does not impact medication metabolism, does not induce hormonal side effects, and has minimal contraindications associated with medical disorders.

Women who are anemic or cyanotic with hematocrit levels above 55% should avoid using copper-containing IUDs due to the higher risk of excessive monthly bleeding caused by intrinsic hemostatic abnormalities, which is more common with copper IUDs than levonorgestrel-releasing IUDs.

Infective endocarditis prophylaxis is not needed for insertion of these devices.

IUD implantation, however, may result in a vasovagal reaction, necessitating hospitalization, particularly for patients with Eisenmenger syndrome and Fontan syndrome.

Tubal occlusion is not reversible but can be accomplished safely, even in relatively high risk women.

Vasectomy for the male is an equally efficacious option that incurs no maternal risk.

Copper IUD, LNG, and ulipristal acetate (UPA) are safe choices for emergency contraception that do not elevate the risk of thrombosis.

11.5.3 Termination of Pregnancy

A candid conversation about the necessity of considering therapeutic termination is crucial for patients with complicated congenital heart disease (CHD) who face a significant risk of maternal morbidity or mortality if they continue the pregnancy. Termination has higher maternal risks as pregnancy progresses, regardless of the procedure used, hence it is crucial for patients to make decisions promptly.

The therapeutic advantage of ending pregnancies at ≥20 weeks is debated due to the established physiological changes in the mother's body, which may not be improved by terminating the pregnancy.

First Trimester Surgical dilation and suction curettage is the most often used way for terminating a pregnancy up to 12 weeks of gestation. Choice of anesthetic method may be determined by the mother's condition. The procedure should be conducted in a hospital setting with readily available meticulous monitoring. Medical abortion using mifepristone and misoprostol is as effective as suction curettage if done within the first 7 weeks of pregnancy. However, due to the unpredictable nature of the process and the potential for hemorrhage in an unmonitored outpatient setting, it may not be suitable for patients who are hemodynamically fragile.

Second Trimester Mid-trimester medical termination can be performed using transvaginal misoprostol to initiate labor while the patient is hospitalized. Drawbacks of this method include extended duration (>24 h), discomfort during labor, and the need for uterine curettage in case of placental retention. Surgical dilatation and evacuation are commonly performed, providing the main benefit of allowing termination in a controlled environment in a surgical setting [32].

11.5.4 Antenatal Care with CHD

Women with CHD should be cared for by a MDT, including a cardiologist, obstetrician, anesthetist, specialist nurse, and midwife.

High risk of complications: Miscarriage, fetal growth restriction (FGR), pre-eclampsia, preterm labor, postpartum hemorrhage (PPH), and neonatal death; and cardiological: HF, arrythmias, aortic dissection, VTE, and maternal cardiovascular collapse and death.

To minimize these risks, the MDT must pay close attention to both the routine and patient-specific aspects of antenatal care.

Vaccination for covid and influenza should be recommended, and for pertussis in later pregnancy.

Requirement of anticoagulation:

Indication—Congenital heart disease
Pulmonary hypertension
Atrial fibrillation
Mitral stenosis with left atrial thrombus
Mechanical heart valve

Anticoagulants used—oral: warfarin, INR monitoring required

Injectable—Unfractionated heparin, aPPT monitoring required
Low molecular weight heparin, Anti-Xa monitoring required

According to AHA and ACA there are four types of regimen

- Adjusted dose LMWH given twice daily with peak anti-Xa level drawn 4 h after injection.
- Adjusted dose of IV unfractionated heparin (UFH) given iv infusion to keep mid interval aPTT more than equal to twice of control.
- LMWH or UFH till 13 weeks then switch to warfarin till 36 weeks then switch to LMWH or UFH.

- Patients with high risk of thrombosis efficacy and safety of heparin, warfarin is suggested throughout pregnancy. Heparin substituted close to delivery with aspirin 75–100 mg daily.

11.5.4.1 First Trimester (0–14 Weeks)

Cardiology Care

The first appointment should involve examining the patient's cardiac history and preconception diagnostic tests to identify any new symptoms including palpitations, shortness of breath, or edema.

The physician should conduct a thorough cardiovascular examination, including the typical physiological changes that occur at 12 weeks of pregnancy.

Special focus should be placed on monitoring for the emergence of arrhythmias, new murmurs, or signs of heart failure.

Review the existing prescription regimen for proper indications, potential dangers, and the necessity for dose modifications or cessation.

The first trimester nuchal fold thickness can detect certain significant congenital cardiac abnormalities in fetuses.

After antepartum treatment is initiated, the frequency of cardiology visits is determined based on estimated risk, symptoms, and problems.

Obstetric Care CHD guidelines advise that these individuals should be treated by an obstetrician specialized in maternal–fetal medicine or with expertise in managing patients with CHD.

However, patients living far from a specialist care center may find it difficult to attend planned prenatal checkups. It is crucial to have clear and constant communication between local and tertiary center clinicians regarding the clinical state of both the mother and fetus.

Having a plan that ensures quick transportation in case of a sudden complication and also involves the patient moving closer to the tertiary care center during the early or mid-third trimester (34–36 weeks) will increase the chances of a well-monitored delivery.

Prenatal care appointments are often arranged chronologically. For straightforward pregnancies, appointments are usually planned every 4 weeks up to 28 weeks, every 2 weeks up to 36 weeks, and then weekly until delivery. Some individuals with congenital heart disease may need more frequent prenatal checkups to monitor how their body responds to the increasing blood volume as pregnancy progresses. The frequency of these visits can be adjusted based on each person's specific needs.

Lifestyle Issues

- Physical activity: The amount of physical activity varies based on the patient's prepregnancy functional capacity. Most patients can maintain a normal exercise routine like walking or swimming, but they should avoid activities that could reduce their heart's ability to pump blood effectively. Prolonged exposure to high temperatures can lead to peripheral vasodilation, resulting in reduced cardiac output causing harm to fetus. Patients should refrain from strenuous exertion on hot days and lengthy hot baths; the use of saunas or hot tubs should be avoided.

- Hydration: Adequate maternal hydration is generally suggested for all pregnancies but may be more important for pregnancies in the CHD group. Restricting salt intake is advisable for those with reduced ventricular function who are at risk of heart failure.
- Thromboembolism prevention: Pregnancy indicates an increased tendency for blood clotting. Graduated compression stockings for the lower extremities can alleviate orthostatic symptoms and lower extremity edema, but they may not decrease the likelihood of thrombosis [33].
- Job: Several patients can safely maintain their employment during pregnancy. Providers should evaluate the specific work circumstances of each patient and talk about potential adjustments that could be needed, especially as the pregnancy progresses.
- Intercourse: Cardiovascular responses (heart rate, blood pressure, oxygen consumption) varied significantly among individuals, but overall, sexual activity is comparable to moderate physical exercise. Just like with physical activity and job, sexual activity should be regulated by symptoms and may need to be restricted for obstetric reasons such as placenta previa, cervical incompetence, or a history of preterm labor. While not explicitly researched in individuals with congenital heart disease (CHD), there is no indication that engaging in sexual activity during pregnancy raises the likelihood of negative pregnancy outcomes [34].

11.5.4.2 Second Trimester (14–28 Weeks)

The second trimester is characterized by the most significant hemodynamic alterations.

The examination frequency must be tailored to each individual. A follow-up echocardiography may be necessary to assess the impact of pregnancy on heart and valvular function.

Fetal echocardiogram is typically conducted between 18 and 22 weeks of gestation and can be repeated if a fetal abnormalities is found.

By the end of the second trimester, a detailed and organized plan for labor, delivery, and postpartum care should be created and shared with all members of the multidisciplinary team, including labor and delivery professionals, in case of a spontaneous or indicated premature delivery.

A multidisciplinary planning meeting should be arranged for high-risk patients, such as those with pulmonary hypertension or severe AS, with all relevant healthcare providers after confirming fetal viability, typically around week 23–24 of pregnancy.

A detailed delivery schedule is provided with provisions for early hospitalization and the need for immediate birth. If ventricular assist devices are needed or if cardiac surgery is being planned during pregnancy or at the time of delivery, the cardiothoracic team should be involved. In high-risk circumstances, it is important to consider involving social services and potentially an institutional ethics team.

11.5.4.3 Third Trimester (28–42 Weeks)

Cardiac assessment frequency throughout late pregnancy should be tailored to each individual.

It is advised to have routine fetal growth screenings at 28, 32, and 36 weeks of gestation to detect FGR and determine the appropriate timing and method of delivery.

As pregnancy progresses and reaches its peak hemodynamic load, common pregnancy symptoms like swelling and difficulty breathing during physical activity may develop. It is important to constantly monitor patients to differentiate between typical pregnant symptoms and signals that may indicate hemodynamic compromise.

Engaging in physical exercise, work, and sexual activity may become challenging as the pregnancy advances; all activities should be restricted based on symptoms or obstetric issues. Delivery plans and contingencies should be completed throughout the third trimester.

The Multidisciplinary Team (MDT) should create a birth plan between 20 and 32 weeks of pregnancy.

Admission to patient:

Elective—Grade 1: 2 weeks prior to estimated due date (EDD)
- Grade 2: At 28 weeks especially in case of unfavorable surrounding
- Grade 3 and 4: As soon as pregnancy is diagnosed

Emergency——Deterioration of functional grading
- Appearance of symptoms of dyspnea, cough, basal crepitations, or tachyarrythmias
- Apperance of any pregnancy related complication like anemia

11.5.5 Intrapartum Care

Women and her attendants should be explained about all the risks in labor and a high risk consent must be obtained followed by arrangement of ICU and emergency medications.

Preterm labor is a significant worry, particularly in cyanotic pregnant women with fetuses that are likely to be underdeveloped.

Tocolytic therapy, which aims to inhibit uterine contractions, can be achieved through pharmacological means such as indomethacin, nifedipine, a beta-adrenergic agonist, or atosiban, an oxytocin receptor antagonist.

Possible consequences of beta adrenergic agonist treatment may involve volume expansion and elevated maternal heart rate, potentially leading to heart failure [35]. Nifedipine or indomethacin are typically the recommended choices. Nifedipine could be detrimental in patients with substantial aortic stenosis or cyanotic congenital heart disease.

For women with minor unrepaired congenital heart disease or those who have had successful cardiac surgery without substantial issues, the approach to labor and delivery is similar to that of typical pregnant women, with the exception of a possible higher risk of infective endocarditis.

Pregnant women with unrepaired or postoperative congenital heart disease who are deemed to be functionally normal can proceed to experience spontaneous labor.

If there are doubts regarding the heart and circulation's functional sufficiency, labor should be induced in a controlled environment unless there are obstetrical reasons against vaginal birth.

Induction timing is personalized based on the gravida's heart health, cervical readiness for induction, and likelihood of fetal lung maturity indicated by gestational age and/or amniocentesis.

Avoid prolonged inductions in women with an unfavorable cervix. Inducing labor in pregnant women with a favorable cervix typically involves administering oxytocin and artificially breaking the membranes.

Various procedures can be used to ripen an unfavorable cervix. A softened and dilated cervix is more receptive to labor induction.

Techniques such as Cook's balloon, prostaglandin E1 mimic, slow-release formulation of 10 mg prostaglandin E2, and artificial rupture of membranes with oxytocin are considered safe methods for labor induction.

After the amniotic sac breaks during labor, it is essential to rapidly start labor augmentation to reduce the risk of infection. Oxytocin ought to be employed for this objective in order to reduce the frequency of vaginal examinations.

Mechanical approaches are favored for patients with cyanosis to avoid any negative effects from a decrease in systemic vascular resistance and/or blood pressure.

If a mechanical approach is not feasible, we prefer using misoprostol.

A mechanical approach, like a Foley catheter, is preferred over pharmaceutical treatments for cervical ripening to avoid potential negative effects. Nevertheless, there is a potential possibility of infection due to the insertion of a foreign object.

Although there are no absolute contraindications to using misoprostol or dinoprostone, there is a potential risk of coronary vasospasm and a minimal risk of arrhythmias. Dinoprostone has significant effects on blood pressure and should not be used in those with cardiovascular disease.

11.5.5.1 First stage

- The gravida should lie on her side during labor to reduce pressure on the abdominal aorta and inferior vena cava, which helps to lessen the changes in blood flow caused by strong uterine contractions when lying on her back.
- Continuous electronic fetal heart rate monitoring is advised for labor. Uterine contractions normally lead to decreased uterine blood flow and placental oxygen supply, but the fetus is able to extract sufficient oxygen to fulfill its requirements. Fetal hypoxemia can result from issues such abruptio placentae, cord compression, maternal hemodynamic instability, or fetal growth restriction.
- Continuous monitoring of maternal blood pressure, heart rate, oxygen saturation, intermittent chest auscultation, and ECG is recommended during labor. An arterial line may be deemed appropriate for high-risk patients.

- In-between contraction if pulse rate is more than 110/min or respiratory rate of more than 24/min associated with dyspnea is suggestive of impending ventricular failure. Immediately give medical management and then take appropriate decision after assessing both maternal and fetal condition.
- It is crucial to maintain systemic pressures in pregnant women to ensure the equilibrium of systemic and pulmonary blood flow.
- If systemic vascular resistance (SVR) decreases or pulmonary vascular resistance (PVR) increases, it causes more right-to-left shunting, leading to higher levels of hypoxemia and an elevated risk of maternal and fetal mortality.
- An arterial line is useful for monitoring changes in fluid distribution and blood volume. Hemodynamic monitoring should be maintained for 24 h postpartum if initiated.
- Oxygen treatment is frequently used during labor, particularly in women with cyanosis. Transcutaneous fingertip oximetry is adequate for monitoring maternal oxygen levels.
- Desaturation not corrected during labor with oxygen is indicative of pulmonary edema.
- Fluid equilibrium must be closely observed restricted to 75 ml/h. Generally, right-sided heart lesions rely more on sufficient filling pressure to sustain cardiac output, while excessive fluid is more prone to causing pulmonary edema in the case of a left-sided lesion. Following childbirth, the transfer of blood from the placenta to the mother's bloodstream can lead to a temporary increase in blood volume and may contribute to the rise in heart failure observed during this time [36].
- Administer intravenous crystalloid as needed for hydration while closely monitoring fluid balance.
- Regional epidural anesthetic is the recommended choice for cesarean section unless contraindicated by recent anticoagulation, past spinal surgery, or clinically required in the context of pulmonary hypertension at certain medical facilities. During vaginal delivery, it is advisable to use an epidural to reduce cardiovascular strain. Other options include patient-controlled remifentanil, especially if the patient has just received LMWH or have life-threatening complications Severe AS, multiple sclerosis (MS), pulmonary artery hypertension, hypertrophic obstructive cardiomyopathy (HOCM):, CoA, Marfan syndrome with dilated aortic root.
- According to AHA/ACA antimicrobial prophylaxis for bacterial endocarditis is not typically advised for most women with congenital heart disease throughout pregnancy and delivery but recommend specific care for high-risk adults with congenital heart disease.
    1. Structural heart disease
    2. Rheumatic heart disease
    3. Cyanotic congenital heart disease
    4. Presence of dental/respiratory infections
    5. Hypertrophic obstructive cardiomyopathy
    6. Prosthetic heart valve
    7. Prior h/o IE

8. I.V drug abusers
9. Valvulopathy after cardiac transplant

- Antibiotic of choice —Ampicillin 2 gm IV stat + gentamicin 1.5 mg/kg (not exceeding 80 mg) IV stat at the onset labor followed by TDS.
- Per vaginal examination should be done under aseptic precautions and when indicated.

11.5.5.2 Second Stage

- The fetal head should drop to the perineum naturally during labor without mother pushing to prevent the negative circulation effects of the Valsalva maneuver.
- Delivery can be facilitated using low forceps or vacuum extraction.
- Cesarean delivery's role—Anticipation and control of labor, delivery, and the postpartum period are critical for pregnant women with a major congenital heart defect, independent of prior surgical correction, in order to minimize risks. Cesarean delivery should only be performed for obstetrical reasons, such as breech presentation, failure to progress, placenta previa, or aberrant fetal heart rate patterns and for some specific cardiac lesions: Dilated aortic root >4 cm, acute severe CHF, recent MI, severe symptomatic AS, warfarin administration within 2 weeks of delivery, need for emergency valve replacement immediately after delivery, and severe pulmonary hypertension
- The potential hazards of cesarean delivery in these women encompass:
  1. General anesthesia carries the risk of hemodynamic instability due to intubation and the anesthetic drug
  2. Blood loss amounting to at least double that of a typical vaginal delivery
  3. Elevated risks of wound and uterine infections and surgical thrombophlebitis
  4. Incisional bleeding may occur in people using anticoagulants and in pregnant women with cyanosis who have underlying coagulation abnormalities
- IV Ergometrine following delivery of anterior shoulder should be withheld to prevent sudden overloading of heart.
- Intermittent chest auscultation.

11.5.5.3 Third Stage

- Intermittent chest auscultation.
- Following placental expulsion, bleeding is minimized with uterine massage and the gradual intravenous delivery of oxytocin, at a rate of less than 2 U/min, to prevent low blood pressure.
- Following childbirth, there is an increase in intravascular volume due to a process called "autotransfusion," where 500 mL of blood from the shrinking uterus is transferred back into the bloodstream.

11.5.5.4 Puerperium

During uncomplicated pregnancies, stroke volume and cardiac output rise by 71% and 60–80%, respectively. The alterations start to reverse shortly after birth and gradually decrease over the following 24 h, resolving throughout the next 6–8 weeks [4, 37, 39, 40]. But may last for up to 6 months [41].

Monitor blood pressure, pulse rate, respiratory rate hourly and intermittent chest auscultation.

The extravascular fluid buildup that happens during pregnancy usually resolves within a comparable timeframe.

Due to the simultaneous occurrence of various hemodynamic alterations, cardiopulmonary problems may arise shortly after delivery, depending on the mother's ability to compensate hemodynamically.

If volume overload then diuretics can be usedMisoprostol, a prostaglandin E1 analogue at a dose of 1000 mcg is deemed safe for managing postpartum hemorrhage. However, ergometrine and prostaglandin F analogues should be avoided.

Metoprolol, nadolol, enalapril, captopril, amlodipine, furosemide, and warfarin are safe to use while breastfeeding.

Women with intricate congenital heart disease should be monitored collaboratively by their cardiologist and obstetrician, 6–12 weeks after giving birth [42, 43].

Risk of thromboembolism in postpartum period is likely due to relative immobilization, pooling of blood in lower extremity, peripartum alteration in coagulation, and fibrinolysis.

Thorough leg hygiene, elastic support stockings, LMWH prophylaxis, and early ambulation are crucial preventive steps that lower the risk of thromboembolism following childbirth. Heparin can exacerbate the inherent blood clotting abnormalities in pregnant women with cyanosis, potentially leading to severe and life-threatening bleeding. Anticoagulation should be resumed 6 h after vaginal delivery and 12 h after cesarean section if the patient was on anticoagulation during the prenatal period. Administer heparin for up to 7 days postpartum, then transition to warfarin. Therefore, postpartum monitoring recommendations are mostly based on the patient's congenital cardiac abnormalities, tendency for arrhythmias, existence of heart failure signs or symptoms, and clinical progression during pregnancy and delivery. Cardiac telemetry monitoring should be maintained for a minimum of 24 h for patients displaying symptoms or signs of notable arrhythmias throughout pregnancy or labor. Patients at highest risk or showing signs of decompensation during pregnancy or delivery should be managed in an intensive care unit or critical care unit for the initial 24–48 h post-birth for hemodynamic monitoring. Patients who have maintained clinical stability during pregnancy and childbirth can be quickly transferred to postpartum units with guidance to watch for cardiopulmonary symptoms. Discharge planning should incorporate scheduled follow-up appointments for standard postpartum and cardiac assessment, along with thorough patient guidance on recognizing signs and symptoms requiring medical attention. Feeding a newborn through breastfeeding can be tiring and has a modest risk of mastitis with bacteremia. Therefore, some women with symptomatic congenital cardiac disease opt for bottle-feeding instead of breastfeeding (Fig. 11.2).

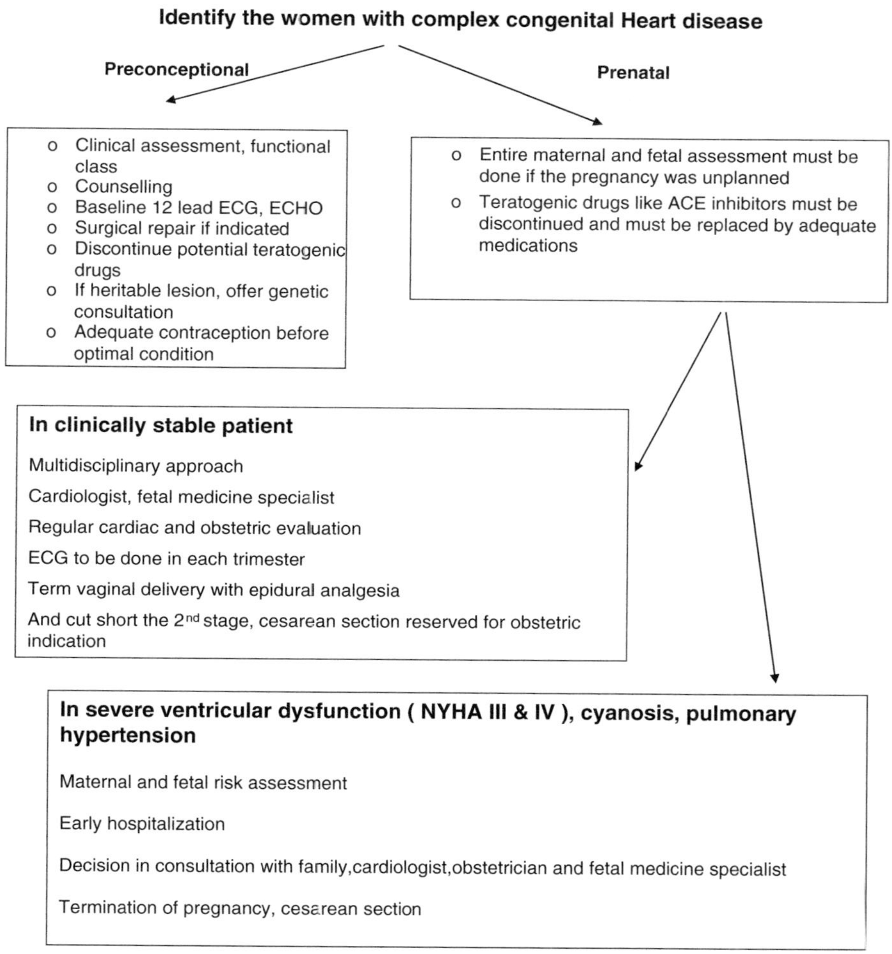

Fig. 11.2 Flow chart

Key Points

1. Congenital heart disease is a condition that affects around 0.8% of newborn infants worldwide. Due to recent medical and surgical improvements, more than 85% of these infants now survive into adulthood.
2. Pregnancy induces diverse physiological alterations in the cardiovascular system and these alterations in blood circulation impact the heart's functionality.
3. In a woman with known heart disease it is important to ensure the nature of lesion and physical status of the patient.
4. Before getting pregnant, proper counseling regarding prognosis, inheritance, appropriate timing of pregnancy, contraception, contraindications of pregnancy,

other methods of attaining motherhood of the women, partner, and family members is essential.

5. A pregnant women with congenital heart disease should be properly worked up, regularly followed up till at least 6 months after delivery by multidisciplinary approach both cardiology and maternal unit.
6. Depending upon the severity of disease, decision of mode, timing, and center of delivery should be decided.

References

1. Nieminen HP, Jokinen EV, Sairanen HI. Late results of pediatric cardiac surgery in Finland: a population-based study with 96% follow-up. Circulation. 2001;104:570–5.
2. Thorne S, Deanfield J. Long-term outlook in treated congenital heart disease. Arch Dis Child. 1996;75:6–8.
3. Hunter S, Robson SC. Adaptation of the maternal heart in pregnancy. Br Heart J. 1992;68:540–3.
4. Robson SC, Dunlop W, Moore M, et al. Combined Doppler and echocardiographic measurement of cardiac output: theory and application in pregnancy. Br J Obstet Gynaecol. 1987;94:1014–27.
5. Robson SC, Hunter S, Boys RJ, et al. Serial study of factors influencing changes in cardiac output during human pregnancy. AmJ Physiol. 1989;256:H1060–5.
6. Melchiorre K, Sharma R, Thilaganathan B. Cardiac structure and function in normal pregnancy. Curr Opin Obstet Gynecol. 2012;24:413–21.
7. Thorne SA. Pregnancy in heart disease. Heart. 2004;90:450–6.
8. Galie N, Humbert M, Vachiery JL, Gibbs S, Lang I, Torbicki A, Simonneau G, Peacock A, Vonk Noordegraaf A, Beghetti M, Ghofrani A, Gomez Sanchez MA, Hansmann G, Klepetko, et al. ESC/ERS guidelines for the diagnosis and treatment of pulmonary hypertension. Eur Heart J. 2016;37:67–119.
9. Peacock AJ, Murphy NF, McMurray JJ, Caballero L, Stewart S. An epidemiological study of pulmonary arterial hypertension. Eur Respir J. 2007;30:104–9.
10. Mandalenakis Z, Rosengren A, Skoglund K, Lappas G, Eriksson P, Dellborg M. Survivorship in children and young adults with congenital heart disease in Sweden. JAMA Intern Med. 2017;177:224–30.
11. Sliwa K, van Hagen IM, Budts W, Swan L, Sinagra G, Caruana M, Blanco MV, et al. Pulmonary hypertension and pregnancy outcomes: Data from the Registry of Pregnancy and Cardiac Disease (ROPAC) of the European Society of Cardiology. Eur J Heart Fail. 2016;18:1119–28.
12. Hemnes AR, Kiely DG, Cockrill BA, Safdar Z, Wilson VJ, Al Hazmi M, Preston IR, MacLean MR, Lahm T. Statement on pregnancy in pulmonary hypertension from the pulmonary vascular research institute. Pulm Circ. 2015;5:435–65.
13. Duan R, Xu X, Wang X, Yu H, You Y, Liu X, Xing A, Zhou R, Xi M. Pregnancy outcome in women with Eisenmenger's syndrome: A case series from west China. BMC Pregnancy Childbirth. 2016;16:356.
14. Cha KS, Cho KI, Seo JS, Choi JH, Park YH, Yang DH, Hong GR, Kim DS. Effects of inhaled iloprost on exercise capacity, quality of life, and cardiac function in patients with pulmonary arterial hypertension secondary to congenital heart disease (the Eisenmenger syndrome) (from the EIGER Study). Am J Cardiol. 2013;112:1834–9.
15. Ladouceur M, Benoit L, Basquin A, Radojevic J, Hauet Q, Hascoet S, Moceri P, Le Gloan L, Amedro P, Lucron H, Richard A, Gouton M, Nizard J. How pregnancy impacts adult cyanotic congenital heart disease: A multicenter observational study. Circulation. 2017;135:2444–7.

16. Regitz-Zagrosek V, Roos-Hesselink JW, Bauersachs J, Blomstrom-Lundqvist C, Cıfkova R, De Bonis M, Iung B. ESC Guidelines for the management of cardiovascular diseases during pregnancy. Eur Heart J. 2018;2018(39):3165–241.
17. Yap SC, Drenthen W, Meijboom FJ, Moons P, Mulder BJ, Vliegen HW, van Dijk AP, Jaddoe VW, Steegers EA, Roos-Hesselink JW, Pieper PG. Comparison of pregnancy outcomes in women with repaired versus unrepaired atrial septal defect. BJOG. 2009;116:1593–601.
18. Balci A, Drenthen W, Mulder BJ, Roos-Hesselink JW, Voors AA, Vliegen HW, Moons P, Sollie KM, van Dijk AP, van Veldhuisen DJ, Pieper PG. Pregnancy in women with corrected tetralogy of fallot: Occurrence and predictors of adverse events. Am Heart J. 2011;161:307–13.
19. Lima FV, Koutrolou-Sotiropoulou P, Yen TY, Stergiopoulos K. Clinical characteristics and outcomes in pregnant women with Ebstein anomaly at the time of delivery in the USA: 2003–2012. Arch Cardiovasc Dis. 2016;109:390–8.
20. Bowater SE, Selman TJ, Hudsmith LE, Clift PF, Thompson PJ, Thorne SA. Longterm outcome following pregnancy in women with a systemic right ventricle: Is the deterioration due to pregnancy or a consequence of time? Congenit Heart Dis. 2013;8:302–7.
21. Cataldo S, Doohan M, Rice K, Trinder J, Stuart AG, Curtis SL. Pregnancy following Mustard or Senning correction of transposition of the great arteries: a retrospective study. BJOG. 2016;123:807–13.
22. Hornung TS, Bernard EJ, Celermajer DS, Jaeggi E, Howman-Giles RB, Chard RB, Hawker RE. Right ventricular dysfunction in congenitally corrected transposition of the great arteries. Am J Cardiol. 1999;84(1116–1119):A1110.
23. Gouton M, Nizard J, Patel M, Sassolas F, Jimenez M, Radojevic J, Mathiron A, Amedro P, Barre E, Labombarda F, Vaksmann G, Chantepie A, Le Gloan L, Ladouceur M. Maternal and fetal outcomes of pregnancy with Fontan circulation: a multicentric observational study. Int J Cardiol. 2015;187:84–9.
24. Cauldwell M, Von Klemperer K, Uebing A, Swan L, Steer PJ, Gatzoulis M, Johnson MR. Why is post-partum haemorrhage more common in women with congenital heart disease? Int J Cardiol. 2016;218:285–90.
25. Nora JJ. From generational studies to a multilevel genetic-environmental interaction. J Am Coll Cardiol. 1994;23:1468–71.
26. Siu SC, Colman JM, Sorensen S, Smallhorn JF, Farine D, Amankwah KS, et al. Adverse neonatal and cardiac outcomes are more common in pregnant women with cardiac disease. Circulation. 2002;105:2179–84.
27. Siu SC, Sermer M, Harrison DA, Grigoriadis E, Liu G, Sorensen S, et al. Risk and predictors for pregnancy-related complications in women with heart disease. Circulation. 1997;96:2789–94.
28. Siu SC, Sermer M, Colman JM, Alvarez AN, Mercier LA, Morton BC, et al. Prospective multicenter study of pregnancy outcomes in women with heart disease. Circulation. 2001;104:515–21.
29. Silversides CK, Grewal J, Mason J, et al. Pregnancy outcomes in women with heart disease: the CARPREG II study. J Am Coll Cardiol. 2018;71(21):2419–30.
30. Drenthen W, Boersma E, Balci A, et al. Predictors of pregnancy complications in women with congenital heart disease. Eur Heart J. 2010;31(17):2124–32.
31. Lu CW, Shih JC, Chen SY, et al. Comparison of 3 Risk estimation methods for predicting cardiac outcomes in pregnant women with Expert Review of Cardiovascular Therapy 597 congenital heart disease. Circ J. 2015;79(7):1609–17.
32. Bryant AG, Grimes DA, Garrett JM, Stuart GS. Second-trimester abortion for fetal anomalies or fetal death: labor induction compared with dilation and evacuation. Obstet Gynecol. 2011;117:788–92.
33. Kahn SR, Lim W, Dunn AS, Cushman M, Dentali F, Akl EA, Cook DJ, Balekian AA, Klein RC, Le H, Schulman S, Murad MH. American College of Chest Physicians. Prevention of VTE in nonsurgical patients: Antithrombotic Therapy and Prevention of Thrombosis, 9th ed: American College of Chest Physicians Evidence-Based Clinical Practice Guidelines. Chest. 2012;141(suppl):e195S–226S.

34. Sayle AE, Savitz DA, Thorp JM, Hertz-Picciotta I, Wilcox AJ. Sexual activity during late pregnancy and risk of preterm delivery. Obstet Gynecol. 2011;283–289:283.
35. Armson BA, Samuels P, Miller F, et al. Evaluation of maternal fluid dynamics during tocolytic therapy with ritodrine hydrochloride and magnesium sulfate. Am J Obstet Gynecol. 1992;167:758.
36. San-Frutos L, Engels V, Zapardiel I, et al. Hemodynamic changes during pregnancy and postpartum: a prospective study using thoracic electrical bioimpedance. J Matern Fetal Neonatal Med. 2011;24(11):1333–40.
37. Robson SC, Dunlop W, Boys RJ, Hunter S. Cardiac output during labour. Br Med J (Clin Res Ed). 1987;295:1169–72.
38. Ueland K, Hansen JM. Maternal cardiovascular dynamics, 3: labor and delivery under local and caudal analgesia. Am J Obstet Gynecol. 1969;103:8–18.
39. Adams JQ, Alexander AM Jr. Alterations in cardiovascular physiology during labor. Obstet Gynecol. 1958;12:542–54.
40. Kjeldsen J. Hemodynamic investigations during labour and delivery. Acta Obstet Gynecol Scand Suppl. 1979;89:1–252.
41. Capeless EL, Clapp JF. When do cardiovascular parameters return to their preconception values? Am J Obstet Gynecol. 1991;165(pt 1):883–6.
42. Davis Melinda B, Arendt K, Bello NA, et al. Team-based care of women with cardiovascular disease from pre-conception through pregnancy and postpartum. J Am Coll Cardiol. 2021;77(14):1763–77.
43. Lima F, Nie L, Yang J, et al. Postpartum cardiovascular outcomes among women with heart disease from a nationwide study. Am J Cardiol. 2019;123(12):2006–14. https://doi.org/10.1016/j.amjcard.2019.03.01.
44. Canobbio MM, Warnes CA, Aboulhosn J, Connolly HM, Khanna A, Koos BJ, Mital S, Rose C, Silversides C, Stout K, American Heart Association Council on Cardiovascular and Stroke Nursing; Council on Clinical Cardiology; Council on Cardiovascular Disease in the Young; Council on Functional Genomics and Translational Biology; and Council on Quality of Care and Outcomes Research. Management of pregnancy in patients with complex congenital heart disease: a scientific statement for healthcare professionals from the American Heart Association. Circulation. 2017;135(8):e50–87.

Peripartum Cardiomyopathy

12

Rachna Chaudhary and Komal Rastogi

Peripartum cardiomyopathy (PPCM) is a form of systolic heart failure (HF) with reduced left ventricular ejection fraction affecting women during last trimester of pregnancy or in the first 5 to 6 months of the postpartum period. Delays in diagnosis may occur as signs, and symptoms of PPCM can mimic normal findings of late pregnancy and peripartum period. Although some women may have mild disease and complete recovery, others experience significant morbidity and mortality [1–5].

PPCM diagnosis is made after ruling out other cardiac conditions (Fig. 12.1).

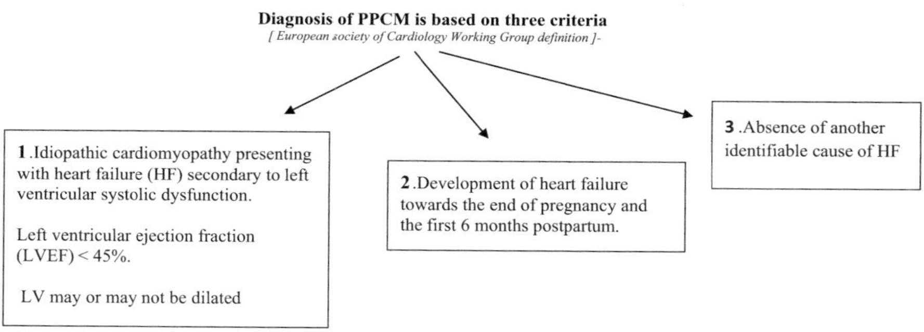

Fig. 12.1 Diagnosis of PPCM [4–6]

R. Chaudhary · K. Rastogi (✉)
Department of Obstetrics and Gynaecology LLRM Medical College, Meerut, India

R. Sharma, A. Kumar (eds.), *Systemic Disorders in Pregnancy*,
https://doi.org/10.1007/978-981-96-4876-4_12

Table 12.1 Risk factors [10–15]

Higher incidence of PPCM is seen in:
Multiparous women
Maternal age >30 years
Hypertensive women, women with history of eclampsia/preeclampsia
Those conceived with in vitro fertilization
Multifetal gestation
Women of African descent
Use of tocolytic agents

12.1 Epidemiology

Incidence of PPCM vary according to the racial and geographical background and it has been found that risk is more among Africans and African Americans [7].

12.1.1 Pathophysiology

PPCM is multifactorial condition, including nutritional deficiencies (selenium), genetic factors, hormonal abnormalities, myocarditis (viral or antigen induced), hemodynamic changes of pregnancy, or any underlying genetic predisposition (Table 12.1) [8, 9].

12.2 Genetic Predisposition

A hereditary or genetic component to PPCM has been identified in several studies. A family history of heart failure has been reported in approximately 16% of the patients [16] and therefore screening such families with genetic testing is helpful, e.g., sarcomeric protein titin (TTN), a mutation near the vascular homeostasis parathyroid hormone-like hormone (PTHLH) gene, dystrophic gene, beta-myosin heavy chain (MYH7), sodium voltage-gated channel alpha subunit 5 (SCN5A), and myosin-binding protein C (MYBPC3) [17, 18] etc.

12.3 Oxidative Stress and Prolactin

Oxidative stress plays a very important role in the pathogenesis of the disease. Kleiner et al. [19] tried to explain the increased oxidative stress in PPCM patients based on a genetic mouse model. This theory was further confirmed by the beneficial effect of blockade of prolactin cleavage with bromocriptine in some studies [19, 20].

12.3.1 Inflammation

A pro-inflammatory state may also play an important role in the pathophysiology of PPCM. Various studies have found significant circulating levels of pro-inflammatory cytokines (interleukin-6, tumor necrosis factor-α, C-reactive protein, interferon-ϒ, and soluble death receptor sFas/Apo1). This observation is further emphasized by the benefit of pentoxifylline, anti-inflammatory agent in a nonrandomized trial of 58 patients with PPCM [21, 22].

12.3.2 Myocarditis (Viral Myocarditis and Antigen-Induced Autoimmune Myocarditis)

Viral cardiomyopathy as a cause of PPCM was first reported by Goulet et al. [23]. Viruses include Epstein–Barr virus, human cytomegalovirus, human herpes virus 6, and parvovirus B19.

12.4 Diagnosis

12.4.1 Clinical Presentation

Women with PPCM typically develop symptoms in the first month postpartum, but it can occur in the third trimester or up to 6 months postpartum [24]. While most patients present with typical heart failure signs and symptoms, patients can also present with thromboembolic complications, life-threatening arrhythmias, and even cardiac death (Table 12.2).

Rarely, patients can also present with severe arrhythmias, cardiogenic shock, and neurological deficits secondary to cardiac thrombus embolization [24].

Table 12.2 Clinical features of PPCM

Symptoms	Physical examination
Dyspnea on exertion	Raised JVP
Orthopnea	Displaced apical impulse
Paroxysmal nocturnal dyspnea	Presence of S3
Dry cough	Pan systolic murmur consistent with functional MR
Pedal edema	Pulmonary rales
Nonspecific symptoms: Fatigue, malaise, palpitations, lightheadedness, abdominal discomfort	Peripheral edema

12.4.2 Diagnostic Testing

The diagnostic criteria for PPCM include development of an unclear cause of HF in the last month of pregnancy up until 6 months postpartum in the absence of known preexisting heart disease, with an eft ventricular ejection fraction (LVEF) of <45% and often (but not required) LV dilatation. Echocardiography should be performed in any suspected case and remains at the central point of diagnosis.

Rule out anemia, infection, thyroid disorders, electrolyte imbalance, kidney or liver function impairments [24]. BNP and NT-proBNP levels correlate with clinical outcomes and recovery of LVEF.

Electrocardiographic (ECG) may show nonspecific findings. Sinus tachycardia and arrhythmia, ventricular tachycardia, and atrial fibrillation/flutter have been reported. QRS prolongation in ECG of more than 120 ms is related to increased mortality. Chest radiography may show cardiomegaly or signs of congestion (vascular redistribution, interstitial edema, pleural effusions.

Echocardiography is the mainstay of diagnosis and should be performed in every suspected case of PPCM (Table 12.3).

Echocardiographic ECHO findings—LVEF <45%, left ventricular dilatation, enlarged fourth chamber, raised pulmonary artery pressures, mitral or tricuspid regurgitation, and right ventricular enlargement. A left-ventricular end-systolic diameter of <5.5 cm is associated with better cure rates and shorter recovery times [25]. Intracardiac thrombus, leading to an increased risk of thromboembolism may occur in 10–17% of women with PPCM [25].

Endomyocardial biopsy is indicated only if giant cell myocarditis, is suspected (Table 12.4).

Table 12.3 Echocardiographic feature of PPCM

Diagnostic features
Left ventricular ejection fraction (LVEF) <45% and/or
Fractional shortening <30%
Additional features
LV and right ventricular dilatation and/or dysfunction
Functional mitral and/or tricuspid regurgitation
Pulmonary hypertension
Left atrial or biatrial enlargement

Table 12.4 Differential diagnosis

Preexisting cardiomyopathy	Most of these patients present during second trimester in comparison to PPCM patients, who present in the early postpartum period
Preexisting congenital or acquired valvular heart disease, undetected congenital heart disease, patent ductus arteriosus, atrial septal defects, and ventricular septal defects	Should be excluded on the basis of clinical presentation and echocardiography
Hypertrophic cardiomyopathy and noncompaction cardiomyopathy	Can also be excluded by echo or cardiac MRI
Myocarditis	Should be considered if there is a viral prodrome or fulminant presentation
Ischemia due to thromboembolic disease or coronary artery dissection	Can be excluded on the basis of presentation with anginal chest pain, cardiac biomarker and ECG changes, and echocardiogram showing regional wall motion abnormalities

12.5 Management

A multidisciplinary approach involving cardiologist, obstetrician, intensivist, and pediatrician is crucial for management of PPCM patients (Table 12.5).

Diuretics, like furosemide and hydrochlorothiazide, should be given to treat peripheral edema or pulmonary edema. Vasodilators like amlodipine, hydralazine, and nitroglycerin can be given during pregnancy, but nitroprusside is contraindicated due to risk of cyanide toxicity.

Beta-1 selective blockers (metoprolol, carvedilol, bisoprolol) are safe during pregnancy. Angiotensin-converting enzyme (ACE) inhibitors, angiotensin II receptor blockers (ARBs), neprilysin inhibitors, and mineralocorticoid receptor antagonists are contraindicated due to teratogenicity.

Anticoagulation Pregnancy and heart failure both are hypercoagulable states; anticoagulation has been proposed in PPCM patients with LVEF <35%. Anticoagulation is recommended if a documented left ventricular thrombus is pres-

Table 12.5 Management during pregnancy based on grades [26–28]

Grades	Clinical scenario	Treatment	Level of care
Mild PPCM	Subacute heart failure	Oral HF medications Oral diuretics	General ward Ambulatory treatment in selected cases
Moderate PPCM	Acute heart failure Respiratory failure	Oral HF medications Diuretics Consider bromocriptine and anticoagulation Oxygenation	Intermediate care
Severe PPCM	Cardiogenic shock Respiratory failure	Diuretics Vasodilators Inotropes/pressors Bromocriptine and anticoagulation Oxygenation	Cardiac ICU

ent or if bromocriptine is used. Bromocriptine is associated with increased thromboembolic events but is however considered investigational at this time. Warfarin is the preferred anticoagulant if the dose is less than 5 mg. Unfractionated and low molecular heparin are alternate agents. In the second and third trimesters, the preferred agent is warfarin. Warfarin should be switched over to adjusted dose continuous infusion of unfractionated heparin, prior to planned vaginal delivery.

Intra-aortic balloon counter pulsation (IABP), venoarterial extracorporeal membrane oxygenation (ECMO), LV assist device (LVAD), and Impella heart pump devices can be used if mechanical circulatory support is needed in cardiogenic shock.

Bromocriptine inhibits prolactin secretion and prevents the formation of 16 kDA N terminal. Although clinical benefit of bromocriptine is seen in several studies, there are no definite guidelines [28, 29].

12.5.1 Intrapartum

Consider expectant management if both mother and fetus are stable. Prompt delivery must be considered for maternal cardiovascular indications or hemodynamic instability. Planned cesarean delivery is preferred for women with advanced heart failure requiring inotropic therapy or mechanical circulatory support [30].

12.5.2 Postpartum

For women with PPCM who have delivered and are not breastfeeding, acute and chronic heart failure should be managed using standard GDMT therapy. Clinically stable women can breastfeed the baby.

Table 12.6 Maternal risks based on residual LVEF [30–33]

LVEF	≥ 50%	LVEF <50%
Maternal risks	20% have a relapse	Higher risk of relapse
	Severe deterioration is rare	50% show further deterioration in LV dysfunction
	Mortality unlikely	Increased morbidity and mortality
	Rate of subsequent recovery is high	Premature delivery and abortion more common

Beta blockers, enalapril, and spironolactone are compatible with breast feeding and can be given. Neprilysin inhibitors, ARBs, and Ivabradine should be avoided during pregnancy and lactation.

12.5.3 Role of Defibrillators

Thirty percent of demises have been reported due to sudden cardiac death at 6 months, suggesting the potential role of defibrillators. Defibrillators can be an acceptable option to prevent sudden cardiac death while either monitoring for LVEF recovery or for patients awaiting heart transplantation [31]. Thus, it is reasonable to wait for 6 months of optimal medical therapy when considering the timing of implantable defibrillators or Cardiac Resynchronization Therapy.

12.5.4 PPCM Recurrence in Subsequent Pregnancy

- Recurrence depends upon the extent of recovery of the myocardial function.
- In case of persistent myocardial dysfunction (LVEF <50%) women should be counseled about high risk of heart failure, deterioration of cardiac function, and mortality including discussions of alternative ways like surrogacy and adoption.
- Risk of abortion, stillbirth, and preterm birth is more among women with persistent LV dysfunction. 2018 guidelines from European Society of Cardiology discouraged subsequent pregnancy if LVEF is <50–55%.
- Women with LVEF >50% have lower risk of complications during a subsequent pregnancy, however, there is possibility of recurrent HF (Table 12.6).

12.6 Prognosis

12.6.1 Predictors for Poor Outcomes and Less Probability of Full Recovery

- Increased LV end-diastolic diameters (LVEDD ≥6 cm)
- LVEF <35% at time of diagnosis
- Right ventricular dysfunction

- Older age
- Later diagnosis
- African ancestry
- Elevated inflammatory markers

Subsequent pregnancy is discouraged when the LVEF has not returned to the values from before pregnancy. Continuation of guideline-directed medical therapy (GDMT) is recommended for the long term in these patients. Women with PPCM with persistent left ventricular (LV) dysfunction or LV ejection fraction (LVEF) $\leq$25% at diagnosis are at high risk of recurrent PPCM and should avoid future pregnancy [33].

Key Points

1. PPCM is a cardiomyopathy of unknown etiology occurring in the last trimester or the first 6 months postpartum.
2. Multidisciplinary care, with a focus on maternal and fetal well-being, is needed for the appropriate management of these patients.
3. Patients with PPCM with recovered LVEF have a better prognosis but a high rate of recurrence with future pregnancies.

Bibliography

1. Ritchie C. Clinical contributions to the pathology, diagnosis, and treatment of certain chronic diseases of the heart. Edinb Med Surg J. 1849;72(181):325–39.
2. Hull EHF. Toxic postpartum heart disease. New Orleans Med Surg J. 1937;89:550–7.
3. Bauersachs J, König T, van der Meer P, et al. Pathophysiology, diagnosis and management of peripartum cardiomyopathy: a position statement from the heart failure Association of the European Society of Cardiology Study Group on peripartum cardiomyopathy. Eur J Heart Fail. 2019;21(7):827–43. https://doi.org/10.1002/ejhf.1493.
4. Sliwa K, Hilfiker-Kleiner D, Petrie MC, et al. Current state of knowledge on aetiology, diagnosis, management, and therapy of peripartum cardiomyopathy: a position statement from the heart failure Association of the European Society of Cardiology Working Group on peripartum cardiomyopathy. Eur J Heart Fail. 2010;12(8):767–78. https://doi.org/10.1093/eurjhf/hfq120.
5. Stergiopoulos K, Lima FV. Peripartum cardiomyopathy-diagnosis, management, and long term implications. Trends Cardiovasc Med. 2019;29(3):164–73. https://doi.org/10.1016/j.tcm.2018.07.012.
6. Irizarry OC, Levine LD, Lewey J, et al. Comparison of clinical characteristics and outcomes of peripartum cardiomyopathy between African American and non-African American Women. JAMA Cardiol. 2017;2(11):1256–60. https://doi.org/10.1001/jamacardio.2017.3574.
7. Kolte D, Khera S, Aronow WS, et al. Temporal trends in incidence and outcomes of peripartum cardiomyopathy in the United States: a nationwide population-based study. J Am Heart Assoc. 2014;3(3):e001056. https://doi.org/10.1161/JAHA.114.001056.
8. Pearson GD, Veille JC, Rahimtoola S, et al. Peripartum cardiomyopathy: National Heart, Lung, and Blood Institute and Office of Rare Diseases (National Institutes of Health) workshop recommendations and review. JAMA. 2000;283(9):1183–8. https://doi.org/10.1001/jama.283.9.1183.
9. Anderson JL, Horne BD. Birthing the genetics of peripartum cardiomyopathy. Circulation. 2010;121(20):2157–9. https://doi.org/10.1161/CIRCULATIONAHA.110.956169.

10. Fett JD, Sundstrom BJ, Etta KM, Ansari AA. Mother-daughter peripartum cardiomyopathy. Int J Cardiol. 2002;86(2–3):331–2.
11. Goli R, Li J, Brandimarto J, et al. Genetic and phenotypic landscape of peripartum cardiomyopathy. Circulation. 2021;143(19):1852–62. https://doi.org/10.1161/CIRCULATIONAHA.120.052395.
12. Hilfiker-Kleiner D, Kaminski K, Podewski E, et al. A cathepsin D-cleaved 16 kDa form of prolactin mediates postpartum cardiomyopathy. Cell. 2007;128(3):589–600. https://doi.org/10.1016/j.cell.2006.12.036.
13. Damp J, Givertz MM, Semigran M, et al. Relaxin-2 and soluble Flt1 levels in peripartum cardiomyopathy: results of the multicenter IPAC study. JACC Heart Fail. 2016;4(5):380–8. https://doi.org/10.1016/j.jchf.2016.01.004.
14. Bhattacharyya A, Basra SS, Sen P, Kar B. Peripartum cardiomyopathy: a review. Tex Heart Inst J. 2012;39(1):8–16.
15. Zagelbaum NK, Bhinder J, Gupta CA, Frishman WH, Aronow WS. Peripartum cardiomyopathy incidence, risk factors, diagnostic criteria, pathophysiology, and treatment options. Cardiol Rev. 2020;28(3):148–55.
16. Ware JS, Li J, Mazaika E, et al. Shared genetic predisposition in peripartum and dilated cardiomyopathies. N Engl J Med. 2016;374(3):233–41. https://doi.org/10.1056/NEJMoa1505517.
17. Koziol KJ, Aronow WS, Giuliani E, Nunziata A. Peripartum cardiomyopathy: current understanding of pathophysiology, diagnostic workup, management, and outcomes. Curr Probl Cardiol. 2023;48(8):101716.
18. Toescu V, Nuttall SL, Martin U, Kendall MJ, Dunne F. Oxidative stress and normal pregnancy. Clin Endocrinol. 2002;57(5):609–13. https://doi.org/10.1046/j.1365-2265.2002.01638.x.
19. Hilfiker-Kleiner D, Sliwa K. Pathophysiology and epidemiology of peripartum cardiomyopathy. Nat Rev Cardiol. 2014;11(6):364–70. https://doi.org/10.1038/nrcardio.2014.37.
20. Ballo P, Betti I, Mangialavori G, Chiodi L, Rapisardi G, Zuppiroli A. Peripartum cardiomyopathy presenting with predominant left ventricular diastolic dysfunction: efficacy of bromocriptine. Case Rep Med. 2012;2012:476903. https://doi.org/10.1155/2012/476903.
21. Ekizler FA, Cay S. A novel marker of persistent left ventricular systolic dysfunction in patients with peripartum cardiomyopathy: monocyte count- to- HDL cholesterol ratio. BMC Cardiovasc Disord. 2019;19(1):114. https://doi.org/10.1186/s12872-019-1100-9.
22. Sliwa K, Skudicky D, Candy G, Bergemann A, Hopley M, Sareli P. The addition of pentoxifylline to conventional therapy improves outcome in patients with peripartum cardiomyopathy. Eur J Heart Fail. 2002;4(3):305–9. https://doi.org/10.1016/S1388-9842(02)00008-9.
23. Goulet B, McMillan T, Bellet S. Idiopathic myocardial degeneration associated with pregnancy and especially the puerpernium. Am J Med Sci. 1937;194(2):185–99. https://doi.org/10.1097/00000441-193708000-00005.
24. Patel PA, Roy A, Javid R, Dalton JA. A contemporary review of peripartum cardiomyopathy. Clin Med (Lond). 2017;17(4):316–21. https://doi.org/10.7861/clinmedicine.17-4-316.
25. Felker M, Mann D. A companion to Braunwald's heart disease. Heart failure Vol Fourth Volume Elsevier Inc.; 2020.
26. Rodriguez Ziccardi M, Siddique MS. Peripartum cardiomyopathy, StatPearls Publishing, 2020 drugs AAoPCo. Transfer of drugs and other chemicals into human milk. Pediatrics. 2001;108:776–89.
27. Halpern DG, Weinberg CR, Pinnelas R, Mehta-Lee S, Economy KE, Valente AM. Use of medication for cardiovascular disease during pregnancy: JACC state-of-the-art review. J Am Coll Cardiol. 2019;73:457–76. https://doi.org/10.1016/j.jacc.2018.10.075.
28. Regitz-Zagrosek V, Blomstrom Lundqvist C, Borghi C, et al. ESC guidelines on the management of cardiovascular diseases during pregnancy: the task force on the Management of Cardiovascular Diseases during pregnancy of the European Society of Cardiology (ESC). Eur Heart J. 2011;32(24):3147–97. https://doi.org/10.1093/eurheartj/ehr272.
29. Lindley K, Verma V, Blauwet L. Peripartum cardiomyopathy. Heart Fail Clin. 2019;15(1):29–39. https://doi.org/10.1016/j.hfc.2018.08.004.

30. Drugs AAoPCo. Transfer of drugs and other chemicals into human milk. Pediatrics. 2001;108(3):776–89.
31. Sliwa K, Petrie MC, van der Meer P, et al. Clinical presentation, management, and 6-month outcomes in women with peripartum cardiomyopathy: an ESC EORP registry. Eur Heart J. 2020;41(39):3787–97.
32. McNamara DM, Elkayam U, Alharethi R, et al. Clinical outcomes for peripartum cardiomyopathy in North America: results of the IPAC Study (Investigations of Pregnancy-Associated Cardiomyopathy). J Am Coll Cardiol. 2015;66(8):905–14. https://doi.org/10.1016/j.jacc.2015.06.1309.
33. Habli M, O'Brien T, Nowack E, Khoury S, Barton JR, Sibai B. Peripartum cardiomyopathy: prognostic factors for long-term maternal outcome. Am J Obstet Gynecol. 2008;199(4):415.e411–5.

Rheumatic Heart Disease in Pregnancy 13

Richa Sharma and Bharti Singh

Nearly 1–3% of all pregnancies are complicated by heart diseases and in India Rheumatic heart disease (RHD) is a major challenge and accounts for 70% in pregnancy. Although the attack rate for rheumatic fever is roughly equal among genders, mitral stenosis is two to three times more common in women and is generally believed that the M protein antigen held in common between the heart and group A hemolytic *Streptococcus* results in an autoimmune attack of the heart in response to streptococcal infection [1].

Women with cardiac disease face a greater risk of mortality and morbidity during pregnancy in comparison to women without it. In patients with RHD, mitral stenosis is the most common heart lesion. Physiological changes of pregnancy (Table 13.1) are tolerated poorly by women with severe heart abnormality.

Rheumatic fever is the leading cause of acquired valvular heart disease. Although incidence of RF has declined, it still remains a prevalent cause of maternal cardiovascular morbidity and mortality in nonindustrialized countries.

Mitral stenosis is the most common rheumatic heart lesion. In general, regurgitant lesions are better tolerated than stenotic lesions because increase in intravascular volume and decrease in SVR improves forward flow through the valve in regurgitant lesion.

R. Sharma (✉)
Department of Obstetrics and Gynecology, UCMS–GTB Hospital, New Delhi, Delhi, India
e-mail: gautamdrricha1@gmail.com

B. Singh
Consultant OBCGY, Gorukhpur, UP, India

R. Sharma, A. Kumar (eds.), *Systemic Disorders in Pregnancy*,
https://doi.org/10.1007/978-981-96-4876-4_13

Table 13.1 Normal physiological changes in pregnancy and labor

Parameters	First trimester	Second trimester	Third trimester	Labor
Cardiac output (CO)	+ 5–10%	+ 35–45%	+ 35–45%	+ 30–50%
Heart rate (HR)	+ 3–5%	+ 10–15%	+ 15–20%	During uterinecontractions:+40–50%
Systemic vascular resistance (SVR)	−30%	Nadir at 24 weeks	After 24 weeks starts increasing reaching prepregnancy at term	
Blood pressure (BP)	−10%	−5%	+5%	During uterinecontractions: +SBP 15–25% +DBP 10–15%
Plasma volume	Increase by 45–55% by 32 weeks			
RBC volume	Increase by 20–30% by 32 weeks			

Discrepancy between plasma volume and RBC volume leads to physiological anemia of pregnancy.

13.1 Pathophysiology

The normal diameter of mitral valve orifice is 4–5 cm^2, which maintains equal pressures in both left atrium and left ventricle during diastole. *If* mitral valve gets narrowed then a pressure gradient develops between both the chambers and causes increase in left atrial pressure, left atrial enlargement, and pulmonary congestion (Table 13.2).

During pregnancy, the pathophysiology is often exacerbated by the physiological demands of pregnancy. During the second trimester, cardiac output increases by ≈70%. Prepregnancy resting transmitral gradient of 4 mm Hg might become 12 mm Hg during pregnancy, resulting in a left atrial pressure of 25 mm Hg, in turn causing cardiac symptoms.

Rule of 1 class is valid: that is, during pregnancy, the patient's symptomatic status will increase by 1 New York Heart Association class.

Table 13.2 Grades of mitral stenosis severity

Severity	Mitral valve area MVA,cm^2	Gradient, mmHg	Pulmonary artery pressure PAP	Symptoms	Signs	Therapy
Mild	>1.8	2–4	Normal	Usually absent	S2-OS > 120 ms, normal P2	Infective endocarditis (IE) prophylaxis
Moderate	1.2–1.6	4–9		Class II	S2-OS, 100–120 ms,normal P2	IE prophylaxis, diuretics
Moderate-severe	1.0–1.2	10–15	Mild pulmonary HTN	Class II-III	S2-OS,80–120 ms, increased P2	IE prophylaxis, BMV if required or surgery if symptoms
Severe	<1.0	>15	Mild–severe pulmonary HTN	Class II-IV	S2-OS < 80 ms, increased P2	IE prophylaxis, BMV

13.2 Management of Valvular Heart Disease in Pregnancy

Management of cardiac disease in pregnancy must include a multidisciplinary team: the pregnancy heart team.

13.3 Diagnostic Evaluation and Risk Stratification

The initial diagnostic evaluation should include the following:

- Detailed history, including family history
- Review of medications
- Arterial oxygen saturation
- Baseline laboratory studies, including complete blood count, electrolytes, thyroid and liver function tests
- ECG
- Exercise stress test
- Echocardiogram
- Genetic counseling (to discuss the risk of inheritance of cardiac disease in fetus)
- Fetal Echocardiography

13.3.1 Echocardiogram (ECG)

Left axis shift corresponding to elevation of diaphragm is seen normally in pregnancy. PR, QRS, and QT intervals are shortened due to raised heart rate. ST segment depression or inverted T waves in lead III also occurs.

13.3.2 Echocardiography (ECHO)

Transthoracic echocardiography is the imaging of choice. Mild dilatation of the chambers, a change in LV wall thickness, and an increase in pressure gradient across valves may be found in normal pregnancy. If needed transesophageal echocardiography can also be performed for added information and is relatively safe [2].

13.3.3 Brain Natriuretic Peptide (BNP)

Brain natriuretic peptide (BNP) and N-terminal pro-BNP, which do not change significantly during normal pregnancy and may be mildly elevated in the setting of pre-eclampsia, are associated with adverse maternal cardiac events in high concentrations. A BNP level of greater than 100 pg/mL and an NT-proBNP level > 450 pg/ml is associated with adverse cardiac events [3].

13.3.4 Magnetic Resonance Imaging (MRI)

MRI is helpful in the assessment of extracardiac vascular structures, including the aorta and left ventricular myocardium.

13.3.5 Exercise Testing

In asymptomatic women with severe valve disease who are considering pregnancy, exercisetesting is reasonable before pregnancy for risk assessment [4]. ESC 2018 guidelines recommend submaximal exercise testing (80% of predicted maximal heart rate) in asymptomatic patients with suspected heart disease if already pregnant. There is no evidence that it increases the risk of spontaneous miscarriage [2].

13.3.6 Risk Scoring

CARPREG (CARdiac disease in PREGnancy), ZAHARA (translated in English as "Pregnancy and Congenital Heart Disease"). Modified WHO (mWHO) classification are the accurate risk scoring systems [2].

13.4 Interventions

13.4.1 Choice of Prosthetic Valve Before Pregnancy

If a woman is planning pregnancy then she should be counseled about benefits and risks of both mechanical and bioprosthetic valves. Generally, in young patients, mechanical valve is preferred because of long life of the mechanical valve. In case of pregnancy, however, the risk of anticoagulation with the mechanical valve should be weighed against the risk of valve resurgery with bioprosthetic valve.

American College of Cardiology (ACC) and American Heart association (AHA) (2020) guidelines on intervention in valvular heart disease in pregnancy have suggested following recommendations [4]

- In women who require a valve intervention before pregnancy, the choice of prosthetic valve should be based on a shared decision-making process that accounts for the patient's values and preferences, including discussion of the risks of anticoagulation with mechanical valves during pregnancy and the reduced durability of bioprosthetic valves in young women.

- In women of childbearing age who require valve replacement, bioprosthetic valves are preferred over mechanical valves because of the increased maternal and fetal risks of mechanical heart valves in pregnancy.

13.5 Management of Cardiac Disease in Pregnancy (Fig. 13.2)

13.5.1 Antepartum Management

- Risk assessment is done by a multidisciplinary team and plan of follow-up frequency, place of care and delivery, risks to the fetus (Fig. 13.1), modes and risks of anticoagulation should be clearly discussed with the patient [5].
- In patients with a known genetic defect, prenatal echocardiography, prenatal invasive diagnostic testing including chorionic villus sampling and amniocentesis to detect known mutations in fetus can be offered. Preimplantation diagnostic testing is also available.

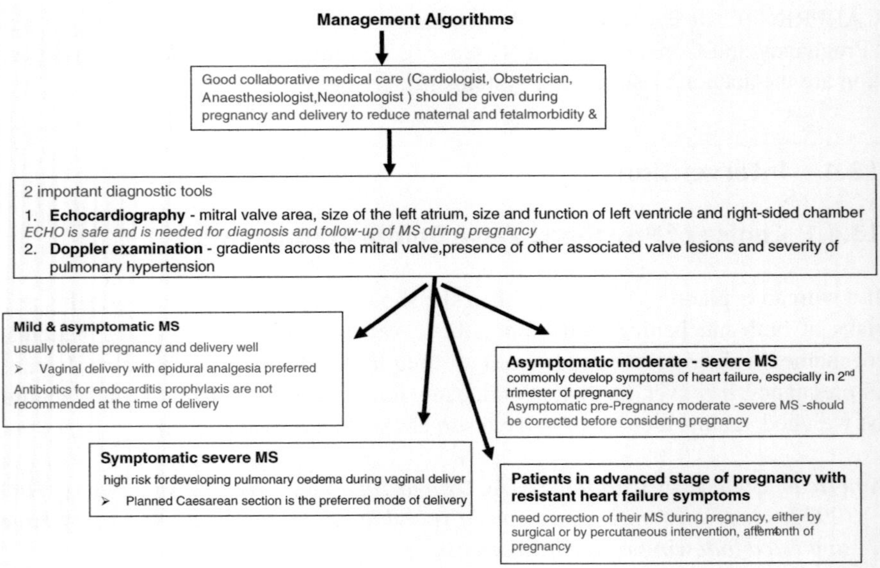

Fig. 13.1 Management algorithms

13.5.2 Management of Heart Failure

- Risk of heart failure increases toward the end of the second trimester of pregnancy, when the cardiovascular demands reach their peak and then again at peri and early postpartum [6].
- Diagnosis of heart failure is difficult in pregnancy as its signs and symptoms (shortness of breath on exertion, peripheral edema, and sinus tachycardia) may be difficult to distinguish from normal findings of pregnancy.
- Index of suspicion should be kept high and evaluation should be done by the above-mentioned investigations.
- Patients should be managed at a tertiary care center by a pregnancy heart team.
- Precipitating factors should be sought and treated.
- Inotropes may be needed to improve contractility.
- Diuretics should be used carefully to treat pulmonary congestion and overdiuresis must be avoided as it may worsen uteroplacental flow.
- Renin-angiotensin-aldosterone inhibitors are contraindicated during pregnancy, but during lactation, they can be restarted.
- In patients with bed rest, thromboembolic prophylaxis is necessary.
- In case of persistent hemodynamic instability, irrespective of the duration of gestation, delivery should be contemplated. Lung maturity induction with corticosteroids may lead to fluid retention and worsening of heart failure.

13.5.3 Management of Arrhythmia

Pregnancy lowers the threshold for isolated rhythm disturbances. Most common arrhythmias during pregnancy are premature atrial beats and supraventricular tachycardia. In women with structural heart disease atrial fibrillation and flutter can occur [3]. Management is individualized.

13.6 Anticoagulation in Women with Mechanical Heart Valve

American College of cardiology, ACC, and American heart association (AHA) (2020) recommendations for anticoagulation for pregnant women with mechanical prosthetic heart valves are as follows [4]:

- Pregnant women with mechanical prostheses should receive therapeutic anticoagulation with frequent monitoring during pregnancy. Patients on warfarin, to be changed to unfractionated heparin (UFH) from 6 to 12 weeks of gestation after detailed counseling regarding risks and benefit of continuing warfarin versus switching over to UFH and taking written informed consent. Warfarin to be restarted after 12 weeks with switchover to UFH 36 weeks of gestation or earlier in patients with threatened preterm labor or any other complication requiring early delivery.
- Women with mechanical heart valves who cannot maintain therapeutic anticoagulation with frequent monitoring should be counseled against pregnancy.
- Women with mechanical heart valves should be informed that vitamin K antagonists (VKA) during pregnancy is
- associated with the lowest likelihood of maternal complications but the highest likelihood of miscarriage, fetal death, and congenital abnormalities, particularly if taken during the first trimester and if the warfarin dose exceeds >5 mg/day.
- Pregnant women with mechanical valve prostheses who are on warfarin should switch to twice-daily low-molecular-weight heparin (LMWH) (with a target anti-Xa level of 0.8 U/mL to 1.2 U/mL at 4 to 6 h after dose) or intravenous UFH (with an activated partial thromboplastin time [aPTT] 2 times control) at least 1 week before planned delivery.
- Pregnant women with mechanical valve prostheses who are on LMWH should switch to UFH (with an aPTT 2 times control) at least 36 h before planned delivery.
- Pregnant women with valve prostheses should stop UFH at least 6 h before planned vaginal delivery.
- If labor begins or urgent delivery is required in a woman therapeutically anticoagulated with a VKA, caesarean section should be performed after reversal of anticoagulation.
- For pregnant women with mechanical prostheses who require a dose of warfarin ≤5 mg/d to maintain a therapeutic INR, continuation of warfarin for all three trimesters is after proper counseling.

- For pregnant women with mechanical prostheses who require >5 mg/d of warfarin to achieve a therapeutic INR, dose-adjusted LMWH (with a target anti-Xa level of 0.8 to 1.2 U/mL at 4 to 6 hours after dose) at least two times per day during the first trimester, followed by warfarin during the second and third trimesters, is reasonable.
- For pregnant women with mechanical prostheses who require a dose of warfarin >5 mg/d to achieve a therapeutic INR, dose adjusted LMWH at least two times per day during the first trimester followed by warfarin in second and third trimesters may be considered. In case of unavailability of LMWH dose adjusted continuous intravenous UFH during the first trimester (with aPTT 2 times control), followed by warfarin in second and third trimesters is reasonable.
- For pregnant women with mechanical prostheses, aspirin 75 to 100 mg daily may be considered, in addition to anticoagulation, if needed for other indications.
- For pregnant women with mechanical prostheses, LMWH should not be administered unless anti-Xa levels are monitored 4 to 6 h after administration and dose is adjusted according to levels.
- Newer anticoagulants like direct thrombin inhibitor dabigatran and anti Xa agents should not be administered.

13.7 Management of Labor and Delivery in Women with Heart Disease

There is increased risk of fetal growth restriction and preterm delivery in these pregnancies attributable both to the disease and the medications used. Figure 13.1 summarizes fetal risks in pregnancies with cardiac diseases.

13.7.1 Labor Induction

- Vaginal delivery is the recommended mode of delivery with some exceptions where cesarian section is preferred (see later).
- In the absence of spontaneous onset of labor or indicated delivery before term, scheduled induction of labor may be considered for pregnant women with cardiac disease between 39 and 40 weeks of gestation with inputs from pregnancy heart team [3].
- Misoprostol, dinoprostone, artificial rupture of membranes, and oxytocin can be used safely.
- Cardiovascular side effects and contraindications of drugs used in obstetric management are discussed in Table 13.3 [3].

Table 13.3 Cardiovascular side effects and contraindications of drugs used in obstetric management

Drug	Cardiovascular side effects	Contraindications
Corticosteroids for fetal lung maturity	Fluid retention Hypertension Electrolyte disturbances	Use with caution in HF/severe hypertension
PGE2	None reported	Considered to be safe
Misoprostol	Rare	Considered to be safe
Oxytocin	Arrhythmias Hypotension	Avoid rapid intravenous bolus Titrate carefully
Magnesium sulfate	Hypotension Vasodilation Syncope	Titrate carefully in hypertrophic obstructive cardiomyopathy and stenotic valvular lesions Caution in heart block
Terbutaline	TachycardiaHypotension-ArrhythmiasMyocardial ischemia	Hypertrophic obstructivecardiomyopathy Patients at risk of arrhythmiasor ischemia Stenotic valvular lesionsespecially mitral stenosis Do not use beyond 48–72 h
Tranexamic Acid	Risk of thrombosis	Uncorrected cardiovascular disease
Ergot alkaloids	Coronary artery vasospasmHypertension Arrhythmia	Coronary artery disease orrisk for ischemia AortopathiesDo not give intravenously
Carboprost	Hypertension Bronchospasm	Pulmonary hypertension

13.7.2 Mode of Delivery

Preferred mode of delivery is always vaginally if the women is clinically stable.

Indications for cesarean section

- Obstetric indications
- Patients presenting in labor on oral anticoagulants (OACs)
- Severe aortic pathology (severe aortic stenosis or ascending aorta diameter > 45 mm)
- Intractable HF
- Severe forms of PH (including Eisenmenger's syndrome)

13.8 Delivery in Women on Anticoagulation [2, 3]

Pregnant women on anticoagulation should be switched from low-molecular-weight heparin (LMWH) regimens to unfractionated heparin (UFH) at or near 36 weeks of gestation.

13.8.1 Recommendations

- For women who are receiving prophylactic LMWH (e.g., enoxaparin 40 mg s.c/ day), discontinuation is recommended at least 12 h before scheduled induction of labor or cesarian delivery.
- For patients on therapeutic LMWH (e.g., enoxaparin 1 mg/kg 12 hourly), this interval should be at least 24 h.
- For Unfractionated heparin UFH dose of 7500 units subcutaneously twice daily or more a 12 h interval as well as evaluation of coagulation status is recommended.
- In moderate and high risk patients, an infusion of UFH is started with regular checks of aPTT and the infusion stopped at least 4–6 h prior to insertion of regional anesthesia or anticipated delivery.
- In high-risk women, therapeutic UFH can be restarted at 6 h postdelivery.
- In women at moderate or low risk, a single prophylactic dose of LMWH can be given at 6 h postdelivery, and therapeutic LMWH is restarted 12 h later.

13.8.2 Reversal of Therapeutic Anticoagulation

- Delivery in a patient on therapeutic anticoagulation carries a high risk of maternal hemorrhage.
- For UFH, protamine sulfate should be given.
- In the case of LMWH, protamine sulfate can be used but dose need to be repeated as the half-life of LMWH is longer and absorption after subcutaneous injection is prolonged.
- If the patient is on oral anticoagulants then to prevent the risk of fetal intracranial hemorrhage, cesarean section must be considered.
- Four-factor prothrombin complex concentrate (given as an individualized dose dependent on maternal weight, initial INR, and target INR than fresh frozen plasma (12–15 mL/kg), should be given prior to cesarean delivery to achieve an INR $\leq$1.5.
- Vitamin K (5–10 mg IV.) may also be given, but may take up to 8–12 h to reverse the INR and has a persistent effect making re-anticoagulation more difficult.
- Fetus may remain anticoagulated for 8–10 days after discontinuation of maternal OACs, and may need to be given fresh frozen plasma as well as vitamin K.

13.8.3 Labor

- Maternal blood pressure, heart rate, oxygen saturation and continuous ECG monitoring should be done to detect early signs of decompensation.
- Labor should be conducted in a right or left lateral tilt position as this reduces compression of the inferior vena by the gravid uterus and maintains cardiac preload. IV fluids need to be given carefully.
- Epidural analgesia reduces pain during labor and can be converted to anesthesia if cesarian is needed. Dose should be carefully titrated because it can cause systemic hypotension.
- To cut short the second stage, forceps or vacuum-assisted delivery must be done.
- American heart association does not consider high risk of bacteremia in either vaginal or cesarian delivery and does not recommend antibiotic prophylaxis; however, in rare settings of endocarditis, consequences could be grave. Therefore, it is reasonable to give antibiotics 30 min before the anticipated delivery [4].
- Patients should be monitored for signs of decompensation for at least 24 h postpartum. Early ambulation and use of support stockings should be encouraged to prevent thromboembolic accidents.

13.8.4 Rheumatic Heart Disease and Pregnancy Outcomes: Findings from the Registry of Pregnancy and Cardiac Disease Registry

The ROPAC registry (Registry of Pregnancy and Cardiac Disease) reports the largest prospective cohort of pregnant women with RHD.

The key features of the study are as follows:

1. Mild and asymptomatic mitral valve disease are well tolerated in pregnancy.
2. MS was less well tolerated than MR, heart failure was highest in severe and moderate MS (49.1%).
3. Women with mixed moderate to severe MS/MR had and stenosis had adverse pregnancy outcomes same as severe MS.
4. Severe MS is an independent risk factor for adverse fetal outcomes, e.g., preterm birth, low birth weight.

13.8.5 Contraception

Intrauterine contraceptive devices are the preferred nonpermanent option in patients with high risk cardiovascular conditions. Progestin-only contraceptives (oral, depot medroxyprogesterone acetate injection, or implant) are potentially effective alternatives for women with cardiac disease.

13.9 Prepregnancy Counseling and Management

Prepregnancy counseling and optimization of pre-existing heart condition must be achieved (Table 13.4).

13.9.1 Goals of Preconception Counseling

- To identify other maternal risk factors, such as obesity, hypertension, and tobacco use that can further aggravate the risk of pregnancy.
- Exercise testing before pregnancy for risk assessment in asymptomatic women with severe valve disease who are considering pregnancy.
- In symptomatic women with severe VHD who are considering pregnancy, intervention is indicated before planning pregnancy.
- Risks of anticoagulation should be discussed and appropriate changes are done.
- Issues regarding health of the baby should be discussed (Fig. 13.2).

Table 13.4 Indications for surgical interventions

Procedure	Indications	Contraindications	Advantages	Disadvantages
BMV	MVA < 1.5 cm^2 with good valve score Pulmonary HTN,MVA < 1.5 cm^2 with good valve score Surgery or pulmonary HTN + high risk surgery and any valve score	MV >1.5 cm^2 Left atrial thrombus More than moderate mitral regurgitation	*Percutaneous*	*Reduced applicability with poor valve morphology*
Open commissurotomy	Surgery, MVA <1.5cm^2, pulmonary HTN with MVA < 1.5 cm^2	MVA > 1.5 cm^2	Avoids prosthetic valve	Limited applicability

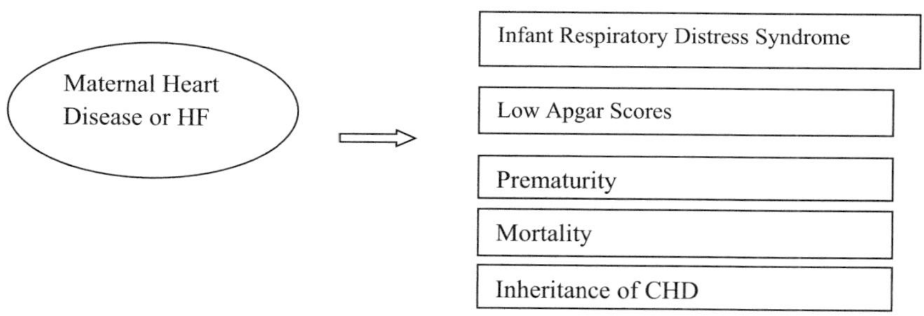

Fig. 13.2 Fetal/neonatal risks of maternal cardiac disease

- The risk of recurrence to the offspring should be discussed. It depends on the heart lesion and increases if heart lesion is associated with any syndrome like Marfan syndrome.
- Prenatal vitamins and folate have been shown to reduce this risk of recurrence [7].
- Medications should be reviewed and change of drugs should be considered if necessary (Table 13.5).

Table 13.5 Safety profile and teratogenic effects of the cardiac drugs [8–10]

Drugs	Can cross placenta	Teratogenic effects	Previous FDA category[a]
Beta blocker	Yes	Not associated with an increased risk of congenital malformations Beta-adrenergic blocking agents are generally safe in pregnancy Risk of FGR and hypoglycemia Beta-1-selective drugs like metoprolol have lower rates of fetal growth retardation Unselective beta-blockers, e.g., atenolol, are contraindicated as have increased risk for FGR	B
Loop diuretic	Yes	Oligohydramnios Inadequate human data Monitoring of fetal growth is recommended	C
CCB	Yes	No increased risk of teratogenicity Verapamil is fairly safe during pregnancy Diltiazem—limited data available	C
Digoxin	Yes	Considered to be safe	C
ACE inhibitors	Yes	Contraindicated due to extreme teratogenicity.	D
ARBs	Unknown	Same as above	D
Warfarin	Yes	Use in the first trimester can result in embryopathy (limb defects and nasal hypoplasia) in 0.6–10% of cases At doses <5 mg/day risk of embryopathy is <1% 0.7–2% risk of fetopathy (e.g., ocular and central nervous system abnormalities and intracranial hemorrhage) when VKAs are used in the second and third trimesters	D
LMWH	No	Prolonged use: less chance of osteoporosis and thrombocytopenia than UFH.	B
UFH	No	Same as above	B
Aspirin	Yes	No teratogenic effects	B
Bromocriptine	Yes	Appears to be safe in fetus	B
Spironolactone	Yes	Oral clefts Inadequate human data	D
Statins	Yes	Statins should not be prescribed in pregnancy or during breastfeeding to treat hyperlipidemia since their harmlessness is not proven	X

[a]The FDA classification has been replaced by the Pregnancy and Lactation Labeling Rule in 2015

13.9.2 Feto–Maternal Morbidity and Mortality

This is greatest during labor and during the immediate postpartum period. Sudden increase in preload immediately after delivery may flood the circulation, resulting in pulmonary edema.

Fetal growth retardation, low birth weight, and preterm delivery increase with increasing severity of MS.

Key Points

- Prepregnancy risk assessment and counseling is indicated in all women with known or suspected congenital or acquired cardiovascular diseases..
- Multidisciplinary unit of obstetricians, neonatologists, cardiologist, intensive care etc.
- ECHO is recommended for unexplained or new cardiac disease suspicion during pregnancy.
- Interventions in symptomatic heart disease should be planned before pregnancy.
- In women considering pregnancy and requiring heart valve surgery, it is recommended to choose the prosthesis in consultation with a pregnancy heart team.
- It is recommended to manage pregnancy in women with mechanical heart valves in a center
- with a pregnancy heart team.
- Peripartum cardiomyopathy is a form of systolic heart failure affecting young women toward the end of pregnancy or in the months following pregnancy.
- Variable outcomes include complete recovery, persistent heart failure, arrhythmias, thromboembolic events, and death. Subsequent pregnancy confers substantial risk of relapse and even death if there is incomplete myocardial recovery.

References

1. Canobbio MM, Warnes CA, et al. Management of pregnancy in patients with complex congenital heart disease: a scientific statement for healthcare professionals from the American Heart Association. Circulation. 2017;135:e50–87. https://doi.org/10.1161/CIR.0000000000000458.
2. Regitz-Zagrosek V, Roos-Hesselink JW, et al. ESC Scientific Document Group, 2018 ESC Guidelines for the management of cardiovascular diseases during pregnancy: The Task Force for the Management of Cardiovascular Diseases during Pregnancy of the European Society of Cardiology (ESC). Eur Heart J. 2018;39(34):3165–241. https://doi.org/10.1093/eurheartj/ehy340.
3. ACOG Practice Bulletin No. 212: Pregnancy and Heart Disease, Obstetrics & Gynecology: 2019;133(5):e320–56. https://doi.org/10.1097/AOG.0000000000003243.
4. Van Hagen IM, Thorne SA, Taha N, Youssef G, Elnagar A, Gabriel H, ElRakshy Y, Iung B, Johnson MR, Hall R, Roos-Hesselink JW, on behalf of the ROPAC Investigators and EORP Team. Pregnancy outcomes in women with rheumatic mitral valve disease: results from the Registry of Pregnancy and Cardiac Disease. Circulation. 2018;137:806–16.

5. Otto CM, Nishimura RA, et al. 2020 ACC/AHA guideline for the management of patients with valvular heart disease: a report of the American College of Cardiology/American Heart Association Joint Committee on Clinical Practice Guidelines. J Am Coll Cardiol. 2021;77:e25–197.
6. Davis MB, Arany Z, et al. Peripartum cardiomyopathy: JACC state-of-the-art review. J Am Coll Cardiol. 2020;75:207–21.
7. Pandit V, Shetty S, Kumar A, Sagir A. Incidence and outcome of peripartum cardiomyopathy from a tertiary hospital in South India. Trop Dr. 2009;39:168–9.
8. Feng Y, Wang S, Chen R, Tong X, Wu Z, Mo X. Maternal folic acid supplementation and the risk of congenital heart defects in offspring: a meta-analysis of epidemiological observational studies. Sci Rep. 2015;5:8506. https://doi.org/10.1038/srep08506. PMID: 25687545; PMCID: PMC4330542.
9. van Hagen IM, Roos-Hesselink JW. Pregnancy in congenital heart disease: risk prediction and counselling. Heart. 2020;106:1853–61.
10. Cowan JR, Ware SM. Genetics and genetic testing in congenital heart disease. Clin Perinatol. 2015;42(2):373–93, ix. https://doi.org/10.1016/j.clp.2015.02.009. Epub 2015 Apr 14. PMID: 26042910.

Acute Fatty Liver in Pregnancy

14

Samta Gupta and Shivangini Sahay

Acute fatty liver of pregnancy (AFLP) is a rare serious life-threatening complication of pregnancy that can lead to fulminant hepatic failure. It carries high risk of maternal and neonatal mortality if not diagnosed and treated promptly. Due to fatty infiltration of liver parenchyma, acute liver dysfunction occurs, which can precipitate coagulopathy, electrolyte imbalance, and multiorgan failure with an onset typically in late pregnancy.

14.1 Background

Williams in 1903 termed this as acute yellow atrophy and cited its rarity in pregnancy. Sheehan in 1940 concluded that most maternal deaths attributed to fatty liver were iatrogenic and related to either hepatic toxins, such as chloroform or fulminant viral hepatitis.

However, Burroughs' observations of widespread microvesicular fat infiltration on liver biopsy of patients with liver failure in pregnancy led to the clinical understanding and significance of this rare, life-threatening condition and disregarded its iatrogenic etiology.

14.2 Epidemiology and Risk factors

The incidence of acute fatty liver of pregnancy varies widely from 1 in 7000 to 1 in 20,000 pregnancies. It does not appear to be significantly affected by geographical or ethnic factors.

S. Gupta (✉) · S. Sahay
School of Medical Sciences and Research Greater, Noida, India

R. Sharma, A. Kumar (eds.), *Systemic Disorders in Pregnancy*,
https://doi.org/10.1007/978-981-96-4876-4_14

Table 14.1 Risk factors for AFLP

Maternal	Fetal
Multifetal gestation Nulliparity Previous episodes of AFLP Diabetes Intrahepatic cholestasis Preeclampsia	Male fetus Disorders of fatty acid oxidation

Risk factors associated with acute fatty liver of pregnancy include multifetal gestation, nulliparity, a male fetus, and past history of acute fatty liver of pregnancy. Some other risk factors are metabolic diseases such as diabetes mellitus, and other hepatic disorders—intrahepatic cholestasis [7]. There is also a well-known association with preeclampsia but the cause and effect are not clear. Usually it presents in the third trimester, but can occur in the second trimester or in puerperium (Table 14.1).

During earlier times between 1940 and 1970, maternal mortality from acute fatty liver of pregnancy was reported to be as high 80%. Since that time, however, maternal and perinatal death rates have diminished significantly; the perinatal mortality rate, which had been correspondingly high, has now reported to be about 15% and maternal mortality recent estimates are dramatically lower—around 2%.

14.3 Etiopathogenesis

During normal pregnancy, placental dehydrogenases in placenta break down triglycerides into free fatty acids, which then enter the fetal compartment where free fatty acids are used for fetal growth and development. Autosomal recessive mutations in various genes that encode enzymes for the fatty acid metabolism pathway lead to defects in the fatty acid oxidation pathway of the fetal placental unit, causing accumulation of intermediate products of fatty acid metabolites, which instead enter the maternal circulation. These fatty acids and their metabolites cause microvesicular fatty infiltration in maternal liver and mitochondrial dysfunction.

Fetal fatty acid oxidation disorders are linked to acute fatty liver in the mother. Other fatty acid oxidation defects that have been reported to be associated with acute fatty liver of pregnancy include medium-chain dehydrogenase, very-long chain dehydrogenase, and carnitine palmitoyl transferase 1 deficiency. If the fetus has fatty acid oxidation disorders, then mothers are carriers due autosomal recessive inheritance, i.e., have heterozygous LCHAD deficiency. *Newborn of mother affected by acute fatty liver of pregnancy should be appropriately screened and monitored for signs, symptoms, and complications of fatty acid oxidation disorder like hypoglycemia and metabolic derangements.*

Preconception carrier screening for fatty acid oxidation defects is recommended, if there is prior history of AFLP.

14.4 Clinical Presentation and Diagnosis

Patients have 1–2 weeks history of symptoms—nausea, vomiting, anorexia, abdominal pain, malaise, headache, or jaundice. Few women may have hypertension and proteinuria, as a sequela of coexisting HELLP syndrome or preeclampsia.

Acute liver failure leads to jaundice, ascites, coagulation disorders, confusion, and rapidly occurring multiorgan failure.

Diagnosing AFLP can be challenging because it has symptoms that are similar to preeclampsia and HELLP syndrome.

14.5 Laboratory Parameters

- Always raised aspartate aminotransferase (AST) and alanine aminotransferase (ALT) found
- Elevated serum bilirubin, ammonia, and WBCs
- Hypoglycemia
- Low platelets
- Prolonged prothrombin time, INR ratio
- Low fibrinogen in AFLP as a result of hepatic dysfunction whereas in preeclampsia it occurs as a result of consumption derangements. As a result, AFLP frequently shows signs suggestive of liver failure, and PE and HELLP syndrome usually show signs suggestive of substantial liver injury with little impact on hepatic synthetic function.

14.6 Radiological Examinations

Radiology is supportive but nondiagnostic. Ultrasound, CT scan, and MRI can reveal fatty infiltration in the liver.

14.7 Liver Biopsy

Usually not recommended but must be considered if the liver function does not improve in postpartum, or in very early stages of AFLP.

"Swansea criteria" have been proposed for the diagnosis of AFLP. The positive predictive value of 85% and negative predictive value is 100% (Table 14.2, Figs. 14.1 and 14.2).

Table 14.2 Swansea criteria

Clinical	Biochemical	Hematological	Radiological	Histological
Vomiting Encephalopathy Polydipsia Polyuria Abdominal pain	Elevated bilirubin (over 0.8 mg/dL or 14 micromol/L) Hypoglycemia (less than 72 mg/dL or 4 mmol/L) Elevated transaminases (AST or ALT) (greater than 42 international unit/L) Elevated ammonia (over 47 micromol/L) Elevated uric acid (above 5.7 mg/dL or 340 micromol/L) Acute kidney injury, or creatinine over 1.7 mg/dL or 150 micromol/L	Leukocytosis (over 11,000 cells/microL) Coagulopathy or prothrombin time greater than 14 s	Ascites or bright liver on ultrasound scan	Microvesicular steatosis on liver biopsy

To establish the diagnosis of AFLP, ≥ 6 criteria to be present, in the absence of another known cause of liver dysfunction

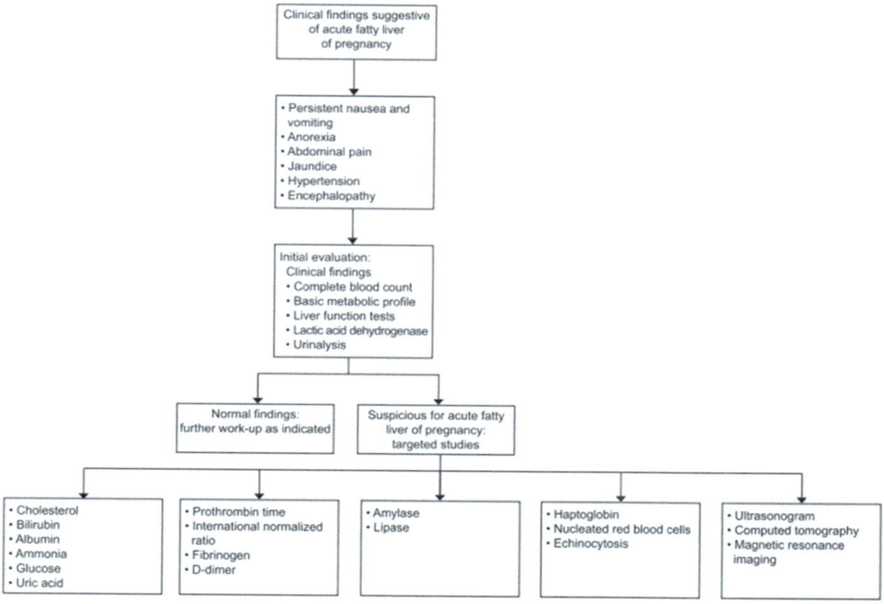

Fig. 14.1 Algorithm for the diagnosis of acute Fatty liver of pregnancy. Nucleated red bllod cells and echinocytes will be reported by complete blood count and peripheral smear. (Nelson Acute Fatty Liver of Pregnancy. Obstet Gynecol 2021)

Fig. 14.2 Section of liver in AFLP—Oil red o stain is picked by triglycerides and other lipids

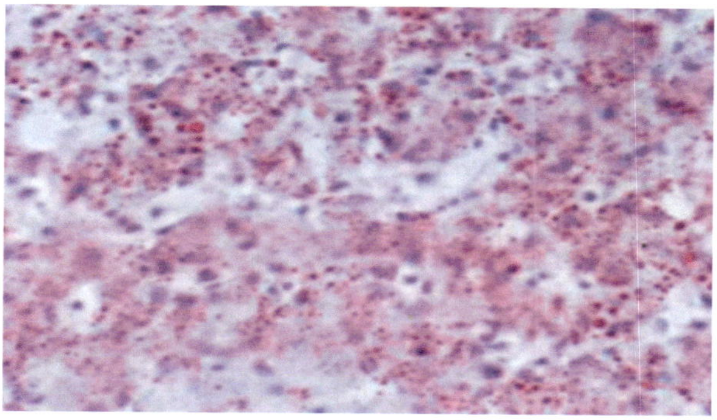

14.7.1 Differential Diagnosis

Characteristics & findings	AFLP	HELLP	Preeclampsia	ICP
Prevalence	0.005–0.010%	0.2–0.6%	5–7%	0.1–0.3%
Maternal age	>20 years	>25 years	<20 years and >45 years	Advanced maternal age
Parity	Nulli-/multiparity, multifetal pregnancy, pregnancies carrying a male fetus	Multiparity	Nulli-/multiparity, multifetal pregnancy	Multiparity, multifetal pregnancy
Family history	Occasionally	No	Often	Often
Onset	3rd trimester or postpartum	Late 2nd/3rd trimester or postpartum	Late 2nd/3rd trimester	3rd trimester
Symptoms	Abdominal pain, vomiting, polydipsia/polyuria, encephalopathy	Abdominal pain, vomiting, proteinuria, headache, peripheral edema	Abdominal pain, hypertension, proteinuria, headache, blurred vision, peripheral edema	Pruritis, jaundice
Sign Laboratory	Ascites ±	No ascites	No ascites	Icteric, no ascites
Thrombocytopenia	± ↓	± ↓	± ↓	± ↓
Bilirubin	<10 mg/dL	<5 mg/dL	<5 mg/dL	<5 mg/dL
Hypoglycemia	±	–	–	–
Aminotransferases	5–10×	1–100×	1–100×	1–5×
Uric acid	↑ (80%)	↑	↑	–
Hemolysis	–	↑	±↑	–
Creatinine	↑	–	↑	–
Proteinuria	±↑	±↑	↑	–

Zein, Ahmad Fariz Malvi Zamzam & Anwar, Irma & Sanityoso, Andri. (2019). The Diagnosis and Management of Acute Fatty Liver of Pregnancy [16]

14.8 Management

Early diagnosis, resuscitation and prompt fetal delivery are the mainstay of management. *Multidisciplinary approach involving ICU, gastroenterology, and perinatology.*

Maternal supportive care and stabilization should be initiated first which includes

- Airway management
- Electrolyte imbalance corrections
- Management of hypoglycemia, coagulopathy,hypertension.
- Frequent maternal and fetal monitoring
- If needed, fluid replacement and blood products transfusion

Anaesthetic management must be tailored according to-

- Hepatic dysfunction of the patient
- Coagulation status
- Degree of neurological involvement in the patient

1. Steroids for lung maturity
2. Magnesium sulfate to be given if gestational age <32 weeks to prevent neonatal cerebral palsy

Inductionof labour
Caesarean deliveryfor maternal or fetal distress and deterioration
Keep the Platelets to a level of 40000 to 50000

After delivery

Monitor for bleeding, hypoglycemia, or renal dysfunction

hepatic transplant, as a life saving procedure can be considered if liver functions does not resolve after delivery.

Maternal follow up outcome

LFTs return to normal by 4 to 8 weeks postdelivery

- Transient diabetic insipidus can occur in 25%
- Acute pancreatitis in 20%
- Recurrence of acute fatty liver of pregnancy in a subsequent pregnancy is unusual.

Follow up of child of AFLD affected mother

1. Molecular testing for LCHAD deficiency,
2. Close monitoring for its manifestations, including hypoglycemia and fatty liver

Key Points

1. AFLP is life-threatening, uncommon, occurring in the third trimester or early postpartum.
2. Coexisting conditions like preeclampsia, viral hepatitis, or cholestasis of pregnancy may cause dilemma in diagnosis.
3. Laboratory and imaging findings with careful history and physical examination helps in clinching the diagnosis.
4. Prompt delivery of the infant and intensive supportive with multidisciplinary team is required to effectively manage these patients.

Bibliography

1. Williams JW. Obstetrics: a textbook for students and practitioners. D Appelton and Company; 1903. p. 444.
2. B Sheehan HL. The pathology of acute yellow atrophy and delayed chloroform poisoning. J Obstet Gynecol. 1940;47:49–62. https://doi.org/10.1111/j.1471-0528.1940.tb14731.x.
3. Burroughs AK, Seong NH, Dojcinov DM. Idiopathic acute fatty liver of pregnancy in 12 patients. Q J Med. 1982;51(481):97.
4. C Sherlock S. Acute fatty liver of pregnancy and the microvesicular fat diseases. Gut. 1983;24:265–9. https://doi.org/10.1136/gut.24.4.265.
5. Zondek B, Bromberg YM. Infectious hepatitis in pregnancy. J Mt Sinai Hosp N Y. 1947;14:222–43.
6. Fesenmeier MF, Coppage KH, Lambers DS, Barton JR, Sibai BM. Acute fatty liver of pregnancy in 3 tertiary care centers. Am J Obstet Gynecol. 2005;192:1416–9. [PubMed: 15902124].
7. Liu J, Ghaziani TT, Wolf JL. Acute fatty liver disease of pregnancy: Updates in pathogenesis, diagnosis, and management. Am J Gastroenterol. 2017;112:838–46. [PubMed: 28291236].
8. Nelson DB, Yost NP, Cunningham FG. Acute fatty liver of pregnancy: clinical outcomes and expected duration of recovery. Am J Obstet Gynecol. 2013;209(456):e1–7. https://doi.org/10.1016/j.ajog.2013.07.006.
9. Castro MA, Fassett MJ, Reynolds TB. Reversible peripartum liver failure: a new perspective on the diagnosis, treatment, and cause of acute fatty liver of pregnancy, based on 28 consecutive cases. Am J Obstet Gynecol. 1999;18:389–95. https://doi.org/10.1016/s0002-9378(99)70567-3.
10. Browning MF, Levy HL, Wilkins-Haug LE. Fetal fatty acid oxidation defects and maternal liver disease in pregnancy. Obstet Gynecol. 2006;107:115–20. https://doi.org/10.1097/01.aog.0000191297.47183.bd.
11. Ko HH, Yoshida E. Acute fatty liver of pregnancy. Can J Gastroenterol. 2006;20(1):25–30.
12. Westbrook RH, Dusheiko G, Williamson C. Pregnancy and liver disease. J Hepatol. 2016;64(4):933–45.
13. Wei Q, Zhang L, Liu X. Clinical diagnosis and treatment of acute fatty liver of pregnancy: a literature review and 11 new cases. J Obstet Gynaecol Res. 2010;36(4):751–6.
14. Knight M, Nelson-Piercy C, Kurinczuk JJ, Spark P, Brocklehurst P. UK Obstetric Surveillance System. A prospective national study of acute fatty liver of pregnancy in the UK. Gut. 2008;57(7):951–6.

15. Goel A, Ramakrishna B, Zachariah U, Ramachandran J, Eapen CE, Kurian G, Chandy G. How accurate are the Swansea criteria to diagnose acute fatty liver of pregnancy in predicting hepatic microvesicular steatosis? Gut. 2011;60(1):138–9; author reply 139–40.
16. Zein AF, Zamzam M, Anwar I, Sanityoso A. The diagnosis and management of acute fatty liver of pregnancy. Indones J Gastroenterol Hepatol Digest Endosc. 2019;20:111–7. https://doi.org/10.24871/2022019111-117.
17. Tran TT, Ahn J, Reau NS. ACG Clinical Guideline: Liver disease and pregnancy. Am J Gastroenterol. 2016;111(2):176–94; quiz 196.
18. Naoum EE, Leffert LR, Chiltilian HV, Gray KJ, Bateman BT. Acute fatty liver of pregnancy: Pathophysiology, anesthetic implications, and obstetrical management. Anesthesiology. 2019;130(3):446–61. https://doi.org/10.1097/ALN.0000000000002597.
19. Ockner SA, Brunt EM, Cohn SM, Krul ES, Hanto DW, Peters MG. Fulminant hepatic failure caused by acute fatty liver of pregnancy treated by orthotopic liver transplantation. Hepatology. 1990;11(1):59–64.
20. Riely CA. Acute fatty liver of pregnancy. Semin Liver Dis. 1987;7(1):47–54.

Systemic Lupus Erythematosus and Pregnancy

15

Vijayata Sangwan

Systemic lupus erythematosus (SLE) is an autoimmune disease, involving multiple organs. It predominantly affects women of childbearing age in a ratio of 10:1 as compared to men [1] with no bearing on fertility but complicates pregnancy. Pregnant women with SLE are highly predisposed to complications like preeclampsia, preterm birth, exacerbation of disease, miscarriages, intrauterine growth restriction, and stillbirths. Active disease, prior lupus nephritis, presence of thrombocytopenia and antiphospholipid antibodies (aPLs) are the predictors of adverse pregnancy outcomes. Primigravida are at higher risk for pregnancy complications. Women desiring conception should be stabilized on drugs for at least 6 months [2]. However, currently, most patients of SLE have successful pregnancies due to preconception counseling, strict monitoring, and improved therapy with minimal complications for mother and fetus [3]. A multidisciplinary team approach, with close rheumatologist, obstetric, dermatologist, and nephrologist monitoring, is essential for optimal outcomes. This chapter will highlight major issues in SLE pregnancy and discuss the recent management strategies to minimize maternal and fetal risks.

Immunophysiology of pregnancy and imunopathology of SLE Pregnancy is an allograft with 50% paternal antigens, with a trophoblast layer inhibiting the contact between fetal and maternal antigens. The founder stone of pregnancy is immune tolerance of maternal immune system toward paternal antigens and T-regulator (Treg) cells that develops immune tolerance. On the other side, SLE results in alterations of immune tolerance to self-antigens only and decreases the number and function of Treg cells resulting a challenge for maternal immune system to how to adapt itself and provide a favorable environment to the embryo. Besides, pregnancy is also associated with high level of estrogen and other immune modulating hor-

V. Sangwan (✉)
BPS Govt Medical College for Women, Khanpur Kalan, Sonepat, Rohtak, Haryana, India

R. Sharma, A. Kumar (eds.), *Systemic Disorders in Pregnancy*,
https://doi.org/10.1007/978-981-96-4876-4_15

mones, which are directly associated with SLE flare. At the same time, maternal immune system also has to maintain the anti-infectious immune capacity of the mother. So, in such pregnancies the immunological monitoring of pregnancy, as well as of the mother's disease, is required. In the postpartum period also because of elevated levels of prolactin and change in neuroendocrine axis and levels of estrogen and progesterone SLE flares occurs. Because of all these immunological, pathophysiological changes, and heterogeneity of disease, the management of pregnancy with SLE is challenging [3, 4].

Diagnosis The typical signs and symptoms of SLE include fatigue, fever, arthritis, photosensitive rash, serositis, glomerulonephritis, vasculitis, and hematological abnormalities (Table 15.1). Usually, pregnancy does not cause flares of SLE, however if flares develop, they occur during the first or second trimester or during the first few months after delivery. Signs and symptoms of pregnancy that must be differentiated from include [2]:

- Chloasma versus malar rash
- Proteinuria secondary to preeclampsia versus proteinuria due to lupus nephritis
- Preeclampsia versus kidney disease
- Thrombocytopenia in pregnancy—HELLP syndrome to thrombocytopenia of lupus exacerbation.
- Pedal edema and fluid accumulation in joints in the late stages of pregnancy versus arthritis of SLE.

The accepted classification criteria for SLE are depicted in Figs. 15.1 and 15.2 below.

Table 15.1 Prepregnancy assessment of patients for risk stratification [2, 3]

Organ system	Complications/manifestations/investigations
Cardiac	Pulmonary hypertension, valvular heart disease, cardiomyopathy assess with echocardiography
Respiratory	Pulmonary fibrosis: Assess with chest X-ray, computed tomography, pulmonary function tests if underlying restrictive respiratory involvement is there
Renal	Renal function tests to assess preexisting renal disease. Urine dipstick and protein creatinine ratio to screen underlying proteinuria. Document and quantify presence of hematuria, hypertension, and renal impairment (lupus nephritis)
Hematology	Complete blood count, liver function tests, coagulation profile for thrombosis assessment
Immunology	Anti-dsDNA, anti-Ro/La antibody, complement C3/C4levels
APLA screening	Lupus anticoagulant (LA), immunoglobulin G(IgG), IgM anticardiolipin (aCL), IgG& IgM anti-beta2-glycoprotein (GP) antibodies
Thyroid function tests	

Entry criterion
Antinuclear antibodies (ANA) at a titer of ≥1:80 on HEp-2 cells or an equivalent positive test (ever)

↓

If absent, do not classify as SLE
If present, apply additive criteria

↓

Additive criteria
Do not count a criterion if there is a more likely explanation than SLE.
Occurrence of a criterion on at least one occasion is sufficient.
SLE classification requires at least one clinical criterion and ≥10 points.
Criteria need not occur simultaneously.
Within each domain, only the highest weighted criterion is counted toward the total score§.

Clinical domains and criteria	Weight	Immunology domains and criteria	Weight
Constitutional		***Antiphospholipid antibodies***	
Fever	2	Anti-cardiolipin antibodies OR	
Hematologic		Anti-β2GP1 antibodies OR	
Leukopenia	3	Lupus anticoagulant	2
Thrombocytopenia	4	***Complement proteins***	
Autoimmune hemolysis	4	Low C3 OR low C4	3
Neuropsychiatric		Low C3 AND low C4	4
Delirium	2	***SLE-specific antibodies***	
Psychosis	3	Anti-dsDNA antibody* OR	
Seizure	5	Anti-Smith antibody	6
Mucocutaneous			
Non-scarring alopecia	2		
Oral ulcers	2		
Subacute cutaneous OR discoid lupus	4		
Acute cutaneous lupus	6		
Serosal			
Pleural or pericardial effusion	5		
Acute pericarditis	6		
Musculoskeletal			
Joint involvement	6		
Renal			
Proteinuria >0.5g/24h	4		
Renal biopsy Class II or V lupus nephritis	8		
Renal biopsy Class III or IV lupus nephritis	10		

Total score:

↓

Classify as Systemic Lupus Erythematosus with a score of 10 or more if entry criterion fulfilled.

Fig. 15.1 Systemic lupus erythematosus classification criteria [ACR, American College of Rheumatology and European Alliance of Associations for Rheumatology]

Prepregnancy counseling and risk stratification EULAR (European League Against Rheumatism 2017,2023) guidelines recommend that women with SLE and planning for pregnancy should be counseled about the effect of the disease on pregnancy and the effect of pregnancy on the disease [5, 6]. In 2020, the American

4 of 17 criteria, with at least 1 clinical and 1 immunologic criterion or biopsy-proven lupus nephritis in the presence of ANA or anti-dsDNA antibodies]

Clinical criteria	Immunologic criteria
Acute cutaneous lupus	ANA
Chronic cutaneous lupus	Anti-dsDNA
Nonscarring alopecia	Anti-Sm
Oral or nasal ulcers	Antiphospholipid antibodies
Synovitis involving _2 joints	Low complement
Serositis	Direct Coombs test in the absence of hemolytic anemia
Renal: proteinuria >500 mg/24 h or red cell casts	
Neurologic: seizures, psychosis, stroke	
Hemolytic anemia	
Leukopenia or lymphopenia	
Thrombocytopenia	

Fig. 15.2 The clinical and immunologic criteria used in Systemic Lupus International Collaborating Clinics classification criteria. (4 of 17 criteria, with at least 1 clinical and 1 immunologic criterion or biopsy-proven lupus nephritis in the presence of ANA or anti-dsDNA antibodies)

College of Rheumatology strongly recommended prepregnancy counseling [5–7]. Pregnancy is not advised in women with active SLE, mainly lupus nephritis. So thorough prepregnancy evaluation by detailed previous obstetric outcome (abortions, IUGR, preeclampsia, preterm, and stillbirth) and investigations (Table 15.1) is required to assess maternofetal risks, severity of disease, and medication adjustment for future conception [8, 9] .

15.1 Prepregnancy Assessment of Patients for Risk Stratification Includes [2, 3]

- Complete blood count, liver function tests, coagulation profile for thrombosis assessment.
- Thyroid function test-TSH, free T3, T4.
- Cardiac evaluation by ECHO to rule out valvular disease, pulmonary hypertension, cardiomyopathy.
- Respiratory system—chest X-ray, CT scan, pulmonary function tests to rule out pulmonary fibrosis and restrictive lung disease.
- Kidney function tests including urine dipstick and protein creatinine ratio to rule out renal diseases, also presence of hematuria, hypertension, and renal impairment (lupus nephritis).
- Immunological tests—Anti-dsDNA, Anti-Ro/La antibody, complement C3/C4levels.

- Antiphospholipid antibody screening—Lupus anticoagulant (LA), immunoglobulin G(IgG), IgM anticardiolipin (aCL), IgG and IgM anti-beta2-glycoprotein (GP) antibodies.

After the analysis of disease status, these women are stratified into three groups to enable an overall management approach, with due adjustment(s) for individual situations [5]:

1. *SLE in remission, or stable low disease activity*: These women are safe to plan a pregnancy, medication should be reviewed and adjusted accordingly.
2. *SLE at an early stage following recent diagnosis, or active disease*: These women should be encouraged to postpone pregnancy; medication should be reviewed according to their disease with follow-up. The pregnancy can be planned after 6 months of SLE remission.
3. *Severe impairment of organ function and/or preexisting severe organ damage (lupus nephritis, APLA positive, anti-Ro/La positivity, cardiac/lung involvement)*: In view of the serious anticipated health and pregnancy-related risks, the pregnancy should be discouraged; alternatives, including adoption and surrogacy (own or donor eggs), should be discussed.

15.1.1 Impact of Lupus on Mother and Fetus

Medical Complications Studies reports significant high risk of stroke, pulmonary embolism (PE), pneumonia, and deep vein thrombosis (DVT). The risk of sepsis and hematological complications like anemia, thrombocytopenia, and increased need of blood transfusion happens in pregnancy with SLE [2, 8]. Pregnancy exacerbates disease flares in 25–45% of cases. Renal and hematologic flares are more common than musculoskeletal flares with mild to moderate intensity. The maternal mortality is also found 20-fold higher in pregnancy with SLE [8].

Preeclampsia It occurs in 16–30% of women with SLE, compared to 4.6 percent of pregnancies in the general obstetric population [2]. The precipitating factors for preeclampsia specific to SLE include an active or prior history of lupus nephritis, declining complement levels, thrombocytopenia, and presence of APLA [2]. Lagana A.S. et al. [9] labeled the presence of Natural killer cells and endothelial progenitor cells in the bloodstream can be employed as marker in the early stages of preeclampsia. These cells play a crucial role in orchestrating the endometrial environment for implantation and growth [9].

APLA and SLE Antiphospholipid (aPL) antibodies may be present in 40% of patients with SLE compared to 8–10% incidence in normal population. When aPL is associated with thrombotic and obstetric complications it is called antiphospholipid syndrome (APS). The APS may result to fourfold higher rate of preeclampsia fivefold higher rate of pregnancy loss and a significant rise of Intrauterine growth restriction/fetal growth restriction (IUGR). SLE patients with positive APS are further more prone to have obstetric complications. These patients need to be individualized for administration of aspirin, low molecular weight heparin (LMWH), and unfractionated heparin [1, 2, 4].

Preeclampsia versus lupus nephritis The flaring of lupus nephritis flares during pregnancy can mimic the picture of preeclampsia. Therefore the differentiation of (Table 15.2) preeclampsia and lupus nephritis is important as management varies [5–7].

Prematurity Clinical or subclinical inflammation, presence of autoantibodies, hormonal dysfunction, immune alterations of lupus make the environment suboptimal for fetal growth [8]. The common complication is fetal prematurity with a mean pregnancy duration of 29.6 weeks. In women with SLE, the indication for preterm births is preeclampsia, maternal SLE activity, or premature rupture of membranes secondary to use of steroids [2, 10, 11].

Fetal Growth Restriction and Fetal Loss The incidence of IUGR and fetal demise is high in pregnant female with SLE. The reported incidence of IUGR is 10–30% and fetal loss rates up to 25–52% have been reported in patients with active SLE at conception and up to 53% in patients with lupus nephritis [2, 10, 12]. A 6 month preconceptional quiescent phase of SLE is a good predictor for better fetal outcome.

Table 15.2 Differentiating features between Lupus nephritis & preeclampsia

Sr. no	Lupus nephritis	Preeclampsia
1	Proteinuria with active urine sediment (red and white cells and cellular casts)	Proteinuria alone
2	Flares are associated with low complement level and Anti-dsDNA titer increases	Complement level remains normal or increased
3	Thrombocytopenia and elevation of LFT and uric acid are less prominent	Thrombocytopenia and elevation of LFT and uric acid are prominent
4	Multiorgan involvement is more common	Multiorgan involvement is more common
5	Onset of symptoms usually before 20 weeks	Onset of symptoms usually before 20 weeks
6	Biochemical markers: High levels of soluble fms-like tyrosinkinase1(sFlt-1) and soluble endoglin(sEng)	High levels of VEGF and PIGF in active SLE/LN
	Renal biopsy can differentiate the two but pregnancy limits its use	

Evidence of lupus activity in other organs can also help in distinguishing SLE from preeclampsia [1, 2, 10]

Neonatal Lupus Syndrome Babies born to mothers with anti-Ro/SSA or anti-LA/SSB antibodies, inherit lupus due to passively transferred autoimmune disease. This tends to resolve by 6–8 months with clearance of autoantibodies [2, 8].The level of maternal antibodies in the neonatal circulation determines the manifestations like rashes, hematologic and hepatic [2, 8].

The most serious complication in the neonate is congenital complete heart block (CHB), which affects approximately 2 percent of children born to primigravid women with anti-Ro/SSA antibodies and carries 16 to 18 percent chances of recurrence in subsequent pregnancies. Women who have antibodies to Ro/SSA and/or La/SSB need increased fetal surveillance for heart block from 16–26 weeks [2, 8] by fetal doppler echocardiography and fetal kinetocardiogram. Detection of an early conduction defect such as prolonged PR interval should be considered a danger sign [2]. The use of hydroxychloroquine (HCQ) in pregnancy is linked to reduced rates of congenital heart block [1, 2, 8]. The fetal survival benefits of fluorinated corticosteroids, beta adrenergic drugs, and IV Ig have also been reported [1, 5].

Medications for SLE during pregnancy The ACR guidelines recommends intake of hydroxycholoroquine by all pregnant women with SLE and dexamethasone 4 mg is recommended for all women with positive anti-Ro/SSA and /or anti La/ SSB antibodies and first or second degree heart blocks on fetal echo. The ACR also conditionally recommend treating SLE patients with low dose aspirin daily beginning in the first trimester.

15.2 Medications Commonly Used to Treat Patients with SLE [1, 5] (Table 15.3)

15.2.1 Safe to Use

- Hydroxychloroquine—Safe to continue antenatally and postnatally, although it crosses the placenta in small amounts. Decreased incidence of flare may reduce risk of congenital heart block (CHB) in fetus of antiRo/La-positive mothers.
- Low-dose Aspirin (75-81 mg/day)—Reduce risk of preeclampsia and fetal growth restriction, if started around 12 weeks gestation and continued antenatally.

15.2.2 Selective Use During Pregnancy

- *Corticosteroids*—(prednisolone, methylprednisolone, hydrocortisone) Safe (benefits outweigh risks). They have anti-inflammatory and immunosuppressive property, betamethasone and dexamethasone (are used for fetal lung maturity, beta and dexamethasone cross placenta readily) and prednisolone and hydrocortisone cross less well, Potential risks include diabetes, hypertension, preeclamp-

Table 15.3 Pharmacological agents used in the treatment of SLE [1, 5]

Drug	Mechanism of action	Placental transfer	Maternofetal effects	Safety in pregnancy and breastfeeding
Safe during pregnancy				
Hydroxychloroquine Safe	Disrupts lysosome presentation and the processing of antigen	Does cross placenta	Decreases incidence of flare. May reduce risk of CHB in fetus of antiRo/La-positive mothers	Safe to continue antenatally and postnatally
Low dose Aspirin (75–81 mg/day) Safe	Irreversibly acetylate serine 530 of cyclo-oxygenase-1 and inhibits platelet generation of thromboxane 2, resulting in an antithrombotic effect	No	Reduce risk of preeclampsia and fetal growth restriction	Started usually around 12 weeks gestation and continued during pregnancy
Selective use during pregnancy				
Corticosteroids (prednisolone, methylprednisolone, hydrocortisone) Safe (benefits outweigh risks)	Anti-inflammatory and immunosuppressive betamethasone and dexamethasone are used for fetal lung maturity	Beta and dexamethasone cross placenta readily. Prednisolone and hydrocortisone cross less well	Potential risks include diabetes, hypertension, preeclampsia, and infections	Consider a 4-h delay before breastfeeding after prednisolone dose >50 mg and monitor neonate for adrenal suppression

(continued)

Table 15.3 (continued)

Drug	Mechanism of action	Placental transfer	Maternofetal effects	Safety in pregnancy and breastfeeding
Nonsteroidal anti-inflammatory drugs ideally, discontinue prior to conception	Inhibit cyclooxygenase	Yes	Premature closure of ductus arteriosus if taken beyond 30 weeks	Use with caution in first and second trimester Avoid after 30 weeks of gestation. Safe postdelivery provided no renal involvement
Cyclosporin Probably safe, do not stop without guidance from rheumatology staff	It binds to cyclophilin A of T cells, inhibits calcium-dependent events, and suppress immune response	Crosses placenta	Associated with preterm delivery and low birth weight	Used extremely in transplant patients and lupus nephritis
Azathioprine Safe	Immunosuppressive agent, prevents cell proliferation, and inhibits lymphocyte function	Crosses placenta but fetal liver lacks enzyme to convert to active metabolite	No case of congenital abnormalities	Safe in pregnancy and breastfeeding but use at minimum effective dose
Tacrolimus: Safe	It bonds to an immunophilin, FK506-binding protein and inhibits calcium-dependent events like IL-2 gene transcription, NO synthase activation cell degranulation, and apoptosis	Yes	Preterm delivery and low birth weight. Congenital malformations are reported	Used for lupus nephritis flares
Antihypertensives	Methyldopa, labetalol, nifedipine, and hydralazine are used during pregnancy. ACE inhibitors and angiotensin II receptor blockers are contraindicated in pregnancy. Diuretics should be used with caution			
Selective use with caution during pregnancy				
Biologic medications	Rituximab(B-cell depleting antibody), Belimumab (BAFF inhibitor) are last resort for SLE flare			
Contraindicated in pregnancy				
Cyclophosphamide, Mycophenolate mofetil, Methotrexate, Leflunomide: Used as anticancer drugs, are contraindicated during pregnancy as well as breastfeeding, should be stopped at least 3 months prior to conception1,5				

sia and infections. Consider a 4-h delay before breastfeeding after prednisolone dose >50 mg and monitor neonate for adrenal suppression.

- *Nonsteroidal anti-inflammatory drugs*—Should be discontinued prior to conception, causes premature closure of ductus arteriosus if taken after 36 weeks gestation.
- *Cyclosporin*—Probably safe, do not stop without guidance from rheumatology staff, it crosses placenta and is associated with preterm delivery and low birth weight. It should be cautiously used in transplant and lupus nephritis patients.
- *Azathioprine*—Safe in pregnancy and breastfeeding but use at minimum effective dose. It is an immunosuppressive agent, prevents cell proliferation, and inhibits lymphocyte function. It crosses placenta but fetal liver lacks enzyme to convert to active metabolite, so no case of congenital abnormalities.
- *Tacrolimus*—Safe to be used for lupus nephritis flares. It bonds to an immunophilin, FK506 binding protein, and inhibits calcium-dependent events like IL-2 gene transcription, NO synthase activation cell degranulation, and apoptosis. Adverse effects are preterm delivery and low birth weight. Few congenital malformations are reported.
- *Antihypertensives*—Methyldopa, labetalol, nifedipine, and hydralazine are used during pregnancy. ACE inhibitors and angiotensin II receptor blockers are contraindicated in pregnancy. Diuretics should be used with caution.

15.3 Selective Use with Caution During Pregnancy

- *Biologic medications*—Rituximab (B-cell depleting antibody) and belimumab (BAFF inhibitor) are the last resort for SLE flare.

15.4 Contraindicated in Pregnancy

Cyclophosphamide, mycophenolate mofetil, methotrexate, leflunomide used as anticancer drugs are contraindicated during pregnancy as well as breastfeeding and should be stopped at least 3 months prior to conception [1, 5]

15.4.1 Management During Pregnancy

A tailored management approach with a multidisciplinary surveillance during the pregnancy and puerperium is required for an optimal maternofetal outcome. At first visit the women should be assessed by a team of rheumatologist, obstetrician, and nephrologist to ascertain the disease status and pregnancy risk. After thorough medical, obstetrical history, and physical examination, the women should have routine pregnancy booking blood tests, baseline tests for renal and hepatic function and complete blood counts. The serological tests are Anti-Ro/SSA and anti-La/SSB antibodies, lupus anticoagulant (LA) and anticardiolipin antibody (aCL) assays,

Anti-double-stranded DNA (dsDNA) antibodies, Complement (CH50, or C3 and C4) and thyroid levels [2, 5–7]. The monitoring should be more frequent and treatment and investigations needs to be tailored according to disease flares, presence of specific antibodies, and risk profile of the patient [2, 5].

During the first two trimesters, a monthly platelet count or CBC is recommended and at the end of each trimester.

Following investigations must be done:

(a) GFR and urine protein to urine creatinine ratio.
(b) Anticardiolipin antibody
(c) Complement (CH 50 or C3 and C4)
(d) Anti-dsDNA antibody

Lupus nephritis needs to be differentiated from preeclampsia; flares may be secondary to hypocomplementemia and increased titers of anti-DNA antibodies. In the PROMISSE study (Predictors of Pregnancy Outcome Biomarkers in Antiphospholipid Antibody Syndrome and Systemic Lupus Erythematosus) two angiogenic factors, fms-like tyrosine kinase1(sFlt1) and placental growth factors (PIGF), measured during early pregnancy proved to have high negative predictive value for development of severe adverse outcomes in patients with SLE and/or APLA syndrome [13].

Women should be offered routine pregnancy scans at first trimester and trisomy scan (11–13 weeks) and a fetal anomaly scan (18–22 weeks). Fetal echocardiography is indicated if there is suspected fetal dysrhythmia or myocarditis, especially in the context of positive maternal anti-Ro/SSA or anti-La/SSB antibodies [5–7]. These patients also need supplemental medication like aspirin/LMWH, calcium, folic acid, vitamin D for prevention of certain complications [5–7]. Fetal surveillance during the third trimester using biometric and Doppler findings help to distinguish early and late IUGR. It helps to plan the time of delivery and reduce perinatal morbidity and mortality. The mode (vaginal vs. cesarean section) and timing of delivery are influenced by maternal (hypertensive disorders, anticoagulation status) as well as fetal conditions during pregnancy.

Postpartum care & breast feeding Some women who have had active disease at conception and those with significant end-organ damage are at greater risk of disease flares in the postpartum period. The periodic assessment of disease activity with urinalysis, renal function test, CBC, Anti-dsDNA, and Complement levels (CH50, or C3 and C4) are warranted at the month of delivery [5–7]. A slightly high incidence of postpartum infection have been reported among these women. All postpartum women with active SLE will require thoughtful discussion regarding breastfeeding. Patients can breastfeed if they are not taking azathioprine, methotrexate, cyclophosphamide, or mycophenolate. Long-acting NSAIDS and HCQ are also inadvisable, as they may cause kernicterus in newborn; prednisolone up to 15–20 mg can be given safely to breastfeeding mothers.

Contraception Contraception is imperative for sexually active patients who have severe organ damage that precludes pregnancy due to high maternal risk [10]. The most significant issues affecting contraceptive choice are concern for flare of underlying disease, increased risk of thrombosis, and potential medication interactions. Long-acting reversible contraceptives like IUCD and subdermal contraceptive implants are most effective and are recommended for such women. Estrogen progestin oral contraceptives (COCP) are contraindicated in active SLE or those at increased risk for thrombosis, such as those with positive aPL, history of thrombosis, nephrotic syndrome, or active vasculitis; however women with low active/quiescent may use COCP if they wish. Progestin-only methods are good alternatives for patients who are unable to take estrogen and may decrease menstrual blood loss in patients on anticoagulation [10].

Updated consensus on the management of lupus with pregnancy toward best clinical practice [14, 15]

Preconception Counselling

- Assessment of Clinical and laboratory indices for disease status, organ damage and disease related comorbidities.
- Individualized Risk stratification.
- A minimum of 6 months of disease quiescence (remission or at least low disease activity in absence of severe major organ affection) prior to conception.
- Improve cardiovascular health (dyslipidemia- hypertension- thromboembolic risk- obesity).
- Consider safe discontinuation of potentially teratogenic drugs.
- Design patient tailored therapeutic strategies to sustain remsission using drugs with a proven benefit (hydroxychloroquine with without azathioprine).
- Avoid Pregnancy in patients with severe end organ disease e.g. severe pulmonary hypertension, severe restrictive lung disease, advanced or active renal failure, advanced congestive heart failure, recent cerebrovascular events, prior pregnancy with severe preeclampsia, eclampsia or HELLP syndrome (hemolysis, elevated liver enzymes, low platelets).

Natal Management

- A multidisciplinary team for monitoring including rheumatologist-obstetrician for high risk pregnancy and a neonatologist amongst other subspeciality consultanat according to patients' individual risk and end organ disease.
- Monitor Disease activity using relevant clinical and laboratory indices.
- For patients with positive antiphospholipid profile: maintain on low dose aspirin during pregnancy± low molecular weight heparin prophylaxis (history of repeated abortions and thromboembolic manifestations).
- Management of hypertension in accordance to obstetric guidelines during pregnancy.

- Follow up for predictors or signs of maternal adverse pregnancy outcome (hypertension- thromboembolic manifestations- worsening renal function- preeclampsia- eclampsia- HELLP syndrome- rising autoantiby titer).
- Follow up for predicotrs or signs of adverse fetal outcome (IUGR- Fetal heart block-Still birth) via fetal ultrasound monthly and fetal echocardiography starting 16 weeks and after.
- Monitor and sssess for severity of flare.
- Treat mild flares using safe therapeutic options including low dose corticosteroids, hydroxychloroquine, azathioprine.
- Management of moderate to severe flares with or without major organ affection (calcineurin inhbitors is safe- conditional use of methylprednisolone pulse therapy, cyclophosphamide or mycophenolate mofetil in the second and the third trimester)
- Manage fetal heart block during pregnancy (Flourinated steroids- IVIG and Beta agonists)
- The decision to terminate pregnancy is highly dependable on severity of flares and the response to implemented therapeutic stratgies.

Postnatal Management

- Avoid postnatal maternal complications (bleeding- sepsis- thromboembolism-flares- progression of organ disease).
- Assess for postnatal fetal complications including fetal heart block- neonatal lupus)
- Address fetal complications (observe for neoonatal lupus- pacemaker for heart block)
- Follow up for disease activity and worsening of end organ disease using recommended clinical and ilaboratory indices.
- Breast feeding is an available option.

References

1. Cauldwell M, Nelson-Piercy C. Maternal and fetal complications of systemic lupus erythematosus. Obstetr Gynaecol. 2012;14(3):167–74. https://doi.org/10.1111/j.1744-4667.2012.00113.
2. https://www.uptodate.com/contents/pregnancy-in-women-with-systemic-lupus-erythematosus/contributors. Revised and updated in 2024.
3. Tan Y, Yang S, Liu Q, Li Z, Mu R, Qiao J, Cui L. Pregnancy-related complications in systemic lupus erythematosus. J Autoimmun. 2022;132:102864. https://doi.org/10.1016/j.jaut.2022.102864. Epub 2022 Jul 21.
4. Gluhovschi C, Gluhovschi G, Petrica L, Velciov S, Gluhovschi A. Pregnancy associated with Systemic Lupus Erythematosus: Immune tolerance in pregnancy and its deficiency in Systemic Lupus Erythematosus—An immunological dilemma. J Immunol Res 2015;2015:241547.
5. Andreoli L, Bertsias GK, Agmon-Levin N, et al. EULAR recommendations for women's health and the management of family planning, assisted reproduction, pregnancy and meno-

pause in patients with systemic lupus erythematosus and/or antiphospholipid syndrome. Ann Rheum Dis. 2017;76(3):476–85.
6. Fanouriakis A, Kostopoulou M, Andersen J, et al. Ann Rheum Dis. 2024;83:15–29.
7. Sammaritano LR, Bermas BL, Chakravarty EE, et al. 2020 American College of Rheumatology Guideline for the Management of Reproductive Health in Rheumatic and Musculoskeletal Diseases. Arthritis Rheumatol. 2020;
8. Sangah AB, Jabeen S, Hunde MZ, Devi S, Mumtaz H, Shaikh SS. Maternal and fetal outcomes of SLE in pregnancy: a literature review. J Obstet Gynaecol. 2023;43(1):2205513. https://doi.org/10.1080/01443615.2023.2205513.
9. Laganà AS, et al. Decreased endothelial progenitor cells (EPCs) and increased natural killer (NK) cells in peripheral blood as possible early markers of preeclampsia: a case-control analysis. Arch Gynecol Obstet. 2017;295(4):867–72.
10. Dao KH, Bermas BL. Systemic lupus erythematosus management in pregnancy. Int J Women's Health. 2022;14:199–211. https://doi.org/10.2147/IJWH.S282604.
11. Eudy AM, Jayasundara M, Haroun T, et al. Reasons for cesarean and medically indicated deliveries in pregnancies in women with systemic lupus erythematosus. Lupus. 2018;27:351.
12. Strouse J, Donovan BM, Fatima M, et al. Impact of autoimmune rheumatic diseases on birth outcomes: a population-based study. RMD Open. 2019;5(1):e000878. https://doi.org/10.1136/rmdopen-2018-000878. PMID: 31168407; PMCID: PMC6525602.
13. Kim MY, Buyon JP, Guerra MM, Rana S, Zhang D, Laskin CA, et al. Angiogenic factor imbalance early in pregnancy predicts adverse outcomes in patients with lupus and antiphospholipid antibodies: results of the PROMISSE study. Am J Obstet Gynecol. 2016 Jan;214(1):108.e1–108.e14.
14. Mohammed RHA, Mumtaz H, Sangah AB, et al. Pregnancy in lupus: an updated consensus to guide best practice strategies. Egypt Rheumatol Rehabil. 2022;49:67. https://doi.org/10.1186/s43166-022-00167-5.
15. Society for Maternal-Fetal Medicine. Systemic lupus erythematosus in pregnancy. Am J Obstet Gynecol. 2023;

Antiphospholipid Antibody Syndrome 16

Aruna Verma and Anupam Rani

16.1 Introduction

Antiphospholipid syndrome (APS) is a systemic autoimmune disease that is characterized by arterial or venous thrombosis. It is also associated with pregnancy loss in the presence of persistent expression of antiphospholipid (aPL) antibodies. There are three main types of aPL antibodies: Lupus anticoagulant (LA), anticardiolipin (aCL) antibodies, and anti-beta-2-glycoprotein 1 antibodies (aB2GP1).

Pregnancy-associated adverse events are reduced if treatment of APS is started within a stipulated time period, which improves pregnancy outcome. APS-positive pregnant patients are also at risk of adverse events, including fetal loss, preeclampsia, autoimmune thrombocytopenia, thrombosis, and fetal growth restriction (FGR).

Classification of APS (Fig. 16.1): It is classified as primary or secondary, based on the absence or presence of *other autoimmune disorders:*

1. *Primary APS*—When clinical and laboratory criteria for the disease are present without other autoimmune disorders.
2. *Secondary APS*—It is diagnosed in patients with other important autoimmune diseases such as systemic lupus erythematosus (SLE).

A. Verma (✉) · A. Rani
Department of Obstetrics and Gynecology, LLRM Medical College Meerut (UP), Meerut, UP, India

R. Sharma, A. Kumar (eds.), *Systemic Disorders in Pregnancy*,
https://doi.org/10.1007/978-981-96-4876-4_16

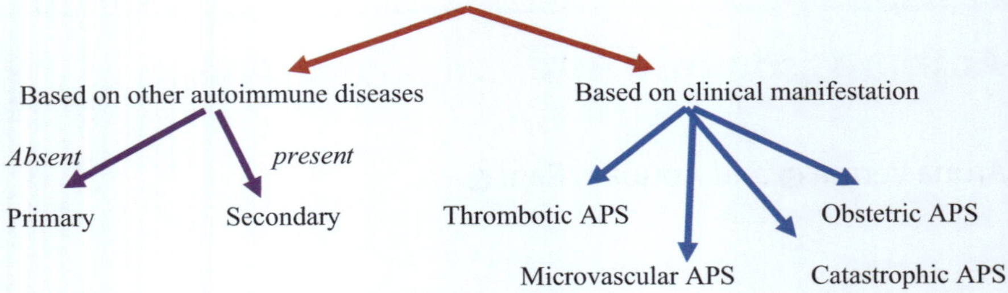

Fig. 16.1 Classification

Classification based on *clinical manifestation* (some cases overlap) with persistent laboratory criteria for aPL:

1. *Thrombotic APS*—is based on venous and /or arterial thrombosis.
2. *Obstetric APS*—based on certain adverse pregnancy outcomes (e.g., fetal death after 10 weeks gestation, premature birth due to severe preeclampsia or placental insufficiency, or multiple embryonic losses [before 10 weeks gestation]).
3. *Microvascular APS*—has small vessel involvement, such as diffuse alveolar hemorrhage or aPL nephropathy, without moderate- to large-vessel thrombosis.
4. *Catastrophic APS*—is a rare, life-threatening form of APS characterized by thrombotic complications (macrovascular and microvascular) affecting multiple organs that develop simultaneously or over a short period.

APS is characterized by the presence of three types of antibodies, namely, lupus anticoagulant (LAC), anticardiolipin (aCL) antibodies, and anti-beta-2 glycoprotein 1(aB2GP1) antibodies. These antibodies cause clotting in vivo, mainly by interfering with the antithrombotic activity of phospholipids. Thus, by initiating the treatment during pregnancy, adverse pregnancy events can be reduced.

16.2 Diagnostic Criteria

Previously Sapporo criteria were used to make the diagnosis, which was modified (Sydney criteria) in 2006.

Revised Sapporo classification criteria for the APS

16.2.1 Clinical Criteria

1. *Vascular thrombosis*

   One or more clinical episodes of arterial, venous, or small vessel thrombosis, except superficial venous thrombosis. For histopathologic confirmation, thrombosis should be present without any significant evidence of inflammation in the vessel wall.

2. *Pregnancy morbidity*
   - One or more unexplained fetal loss at or beyond the 10 weeks of gestation, with normal morphology, documented by ultrasound or by direct examination, or
   - One or more premature births of a morphologically normal neonate before the 34 weeks of gestation because of: (i) eclampsia or severe preeclampsia defined according to standard definitions, or (ii) recognized features of placental insufficiency, or
   - Three or more unexplained consecutive spontaneous abortions before the 10 weeks of gestation, with maternal anatomic or hormonal abnormalities and paternal and maternal chromosomal causes excluded.

16.2.2 Laboratory Criteria

1. aCL antibodies (IgG and/or IgM in serum/ plasma) present in medium or high titer (i.e., >40 IgG phospholipid units (GPL) or IgM phospholipid units (MPL), or > the 99th percentile, or > mean + 3SD of 40 healthy controls), on two or more occasions, at least 12 weeks apart, measured by a standardized enzyme-linked immunosorbent assay (ELISA).
2. Presence of LAC in plasma, on two or more occasions at least 12 weeks apart, detected as per guidelines of the International Society on Thrombosis and Hemostasis (Scientific Subcommittee on Lupus Anticoagulants/Phospholipid-Dependent Antibodies).
3. Anti-B2GP1 antibody (IgG and/or IgM in serum/ plasma), present on two or more occasions, at least 12 weeks apart, measured by a standardized enzyme-linked immunosorbent assay.

Definite APS is present if at least one of the clinical criteria and one out of three laboratory criteria are met, with the first measurement of the laboratory test performed at least 12 weeks from the clinical manifestation (Table 16.1).

American College of Rheumatology 2023 (ACR) and European Alliance of Associations for Rheumatology (EULAR), APS classification includes definitions

Table 16.1 Comparison of laboratory of APS

	Sapporo criteria(1999)	Sydney criteria(2006)
LAC	Screening, mixing, and confirmation tests. Two or more occasions at least 6 weeks apart	Screening, mixing, and confirmation tests. Two or more occasions at least 12 weeks apart
aCL ab	Detected by standardized ELISA IgG and/or IgM Two or more occasions at least 6 weeks apart	Detected by standardized ELISA IgG and/or IgM Medium or high titer (>40 units titer or 99th percentile) Two or more occasions at least 12 weeks apart
Anti-B2GP1 ab		IgG and/or IgM titer >99th percentile Two or more occasions at least 12 weeks apart

of clinical or laboratory criteria, high risk profiles for venous thromboembolism (VTE) and a newer one have higher specificity (99% versus 86%) and lower sensitivity (84% versus 99%) [1].

Patients who fulfill the entry criteria and also have at least three weighted criteria in clinical as well as in laboratory domain (Fig. 16.2) will be diagnosed as APS.

At least one documented clinical criteria mentioned below (D1-D6)

Plus

A positive antiphospholipid(aPL) test, within 3 years of the clinical criteria

↓

If present, apply additive criteria otherwise not diagnose as APS

↓

Additive clinical and laboratory criteria (only count the highest weighted feature toward the total score

↓

Clinical domain and criteria	weight
D1. Macro vascular (venous thromboembolism[VTE])	
• VTE with high risk VTE profile	1
• VTE without high risk VTE profile	3
D2. Macro vascular (Arterial thrombosis [AT])	
• AT with high risk CVD profile	2
• AT without high risk CVD profile	4
D2. Microvascular	
Suspected (one / more of the below mentioned features)	2
o Livedo racemose (examination)	
o Livedo vasculopathy lesion (examination)	
o Acute/chronic aPL nephropathy (examination or laboratory)	
o Pulmonary haemorrhage (symptoms and imaging)	
Established (one / more of the below mentioned features)	5
o Livedo vasculopathy lesion (pathology)	
o Acute/chronic aPL nephropathy (pathology)	
o Pulmonary haemorrhage (Broncho-alveolar lavage or pathology)	
o Myocardial disease (imaging/pathology)	
o Adrenal haemorrhage (imaging/pathology)	
D4. Obstetrics	
• ≥3 consecutive pre-natal (<10 weeks) and/or early fetal (10-15w6d) deaths.	1
• Fetal death (16- 33w6d) in the absence of preeclampsia(PEC) with severe features or placental insufficiency (PI) with severe features.	1

Fig. 16.2 American college of Radiology (ACR) and European Alliance of Associations for Rheumatology (EULAR) classification criteria

• PEC with severe features (<34w 0d) or PI with severe features (<34w 0d) with/without fetal death. • PEC with severe features (<34w 0d) and PI with severe features (<34w 0d) with/without fetal death.	3 4
D5. Cardiac valve • Thickening • Vegetation	2 4
D6. Hematology • Thrombocytopenia	2
Laboratory domain and criteria	**weight**
D7. aPL test by coagulation-based functional assay (lupus anticoagulant[LAC]) • Positive LAC (single-one time) • Persistent LAC (persistent)	**1** **5**
D8. aPL test by solid phase assay (anticardiolipin antibody [aCL] ELISA and/or anti-beta2-glycoprotein1 antibody[aB2GP1] ELISA) {persistent} • Moderate or high positive(IgM) (aCL and/or aB2GP1) • Moderate positive (IgG) (aCL and/or aB2GP1) • High positive (IgG) (aCL **or** aB2GP1) • High positive (IgG) (aCL **and** aB2GP1)	**1** **4** **5** **7**

Fig. 16.2 (continued)

16.3 Adverse Pregnancy Outcomes Defining APS

The new ACR and EULAR classification system defines pregnancy morbidity more explicitly for gestational age and placental insufficiency rather than pregnancy losses. Again, Ig M positivity for aCL and aB2GP1 was given less weightage rather than Ig G positivity.

Obstetric criteria includes:

- Pregnancy morbidity
- Positive aPL test within 3 years of pregnancy morbidity
- Findings not because of other four APS domain (hemolytic, cardiac valve, microvascular, macro vascular)

16.3.1 Pregnancy Morbidity Associated with APS

≥3 consecutive, unexplained prefetal losses at <10 weeks and/or early fetal deaths at (10–16 weeks gestation)

Or

≥1 fetal death (16 weeks 0 days to 34 weeks 0 days) alone (i.e., no preeclampsia with severe features or placental insufficiency with severe features)

Or

Preeclampsia with severe features (<34 weeks 0 days) with or without fetal death

Or

Placental insufficiency with severe features (<34 weeks 0 days) with or without fetal death

Placental insufficiency with severe features is defined by intrauterine fetal growth restriction (FGR) without fetal syndromes or genetic causes of growth restriction *and* at least one of the mentioned features:

- Abnormal or nonreasoning fetal surveillance test(s) suggestive of fetal hypoxemia (e.g., nonreactive nonstress test, low biophysical profile score [0 to 4 out of 10]).
- Abnormal Doppler examination suggestive of fetal hypoxemia (e.g., absent or reversed end-diastolic flow in the umbilical artery).
- Severe fetal/new-born growth restriction (e.g., estimated fetal or postnatal birth weight < 3 percentile for gestational age).
- Oligohydramnios (e.g., amniotic fluid index ≤5 cm, deepest vertical pocket <2 cm).
- Placental histology showing maternal vascular malperfusion (e.g., placental thrombosis/infarction, inadequate remodeling of the uterine spiral arteries [decidual vasculopathy], decreased vasculo-syncytial membranes, increased syncytial knots, or decidual inflammation).

16.4 Factors for Adverse Obstetric Outcome

- Lupus anticoagulant: It appears to be an important major predictor for adverse outcome, especially when it is persistently positive
- Triple positivity: When all three tests (LA, aCL, and aB2GP1) are positive, indicates poor prognosis
- History of thrombosis: Patients with thrombotic APS have high chances of pregnancy complications than those with only obstetric APS

A new biomarker, i.e., C4 complement (low levels) has gained importance, to predict the adverse outcome in APS, but need more data for its clinical significance.

16.5 Etiopathogenesis

Phospholipids are the basic components of all cell membranes. In certain conditions like tissue ischemia, cell injury, or auto immunity, the negatively charged inner layer PLs are exteriorized and act as an antigenic stimulus for production of aPL. In genetically predisposed individuals, alteration of microbes (dysbiosis) may induce APS [15]. Toxoplasma, Rubella, CMV, Varicella, HIV, Parvovirus B19, Streptococci, Staphylococci, and Mycoplasma pneumonia are the most common organisms associated with APS, and molecular mimicry between β_2GP1 viral and bacterial epitomes may be the principal mechanism.

16.6 Management

To start with the antithrombotic therapy, patients are categorized on the basis of prior history of thrombosis versus APS pregnancy morbidity.

(a) APS with prior history of thrombosis (with/without APS pregnancy morbidity)

Therapeutic anticoagulation: Pregnant patients are treated with therapeutic dose of heparin. Both low molecular weight heparin (LMWH) and unfractionated heparin can be used, but LMWH is more preferred because of greater safety and efficacy. Fixed dosing schedule of LMWH is similar to weight adjusted dose of LMWH, so both can be used (Table 16.2).

Table 16.2 Dose of heparin during pregnancy

Indication	Type	Dose
Prevention	LMWH	*Low dose(prophylactic)*:
		Enoxaparin Weight < 100 kg: 40 mg S/C once daily Weight < 100 kg: 60 mg S/C once daily Or *Dalteparin* Weight < 100 kg: 5000 units' S/C once daily Weight < 100 kg: 7500 units S/C once daily
		Intermediate dose: *Enoxaparin* 40 mg S/C once daily, to be increased as per increase in weight during pregnancy (1 mg/kg once daily) Or *Dalteparin* 5000 units S/C once daily, to be increased as per increase in weight during pregnancy (100 units/kg once daily)
	UFH	*According to trimester* First trimester: 5000—7500 units S/C 12 hourly Second trimester: 7500–10,000 units S/C 12 hourly Third trimester: 10,000 units S/C 12 hourly
Therapeutic	LMWH	*Enoxaparin* 1 mg/kg S/C 12 hourly Or *Dalteparin* 100 units/kg S/C 12 hourly
	UFH	Either IV infusion or S/C dose repeated every 12 h. Titration should be done to maintain the aPTT in therapeutic range

LMWH Low Molecular Weight Heparin; *UFH* Unfractionated Heparin

It was observed that chances of thromboses is very low in treated versus non-treated patients (<1% versus >10%) [16].

Low dose aspirin (LDA): Recommended dose is 81 mg (one/two tablets daily) and preferably to be started before pregnancy, or as soon as pregnancy is diagnosed.

(b) APS with pregnancy morbidity alone

Patient with history of embryonic or fetal death In patients with history of prior fetal or embryonic demise prophylactic dose of LMWH (upon confirmation of pregnancy) plus LDA (one or two doses of 81 mg tablet) either before conception or as soon as pregnancy is diagnosed.

Patients with history of Preeclampsia with severe features/placental insufficiency with severe feature In such type of scenario only LDA is recommended. Some clinicians also prefer to give LMWH, but available evidence does not support this approach.

The combination of heparin and LDA significantly reduced pregnancy loss [18] or 1st trimester pregnancy loss [19] and increased live births [21]. These findings were reported in meta-analyses of randomized trials in patients with APS.

16.6.1 Antepartum Feto–Maternal Surveillance

In addition to normal antenatal care, the following recommendations are supported by reproductive health guidelines given by ACR:

1. Baseline levels of aPL [LA, aCL (IgG and IgM), AB2GP1), platelets, serum creatinine, urinary protein to creatinine ratio, liver enzymes, complements (C3 and C4) to compare various manifestation and complications in pregnancy.
2. Screening for anti-LA/SSB and anti-Ro/SSA antibodies. It was observed that these antibodies are associated with higher risk for congenital heart block.
3. Dating ultrasound is mandatory in the first trimester, as these patients are at higher risk of developing fetal growth restriction. Repeat scan should also be done at every 4 weeks to evaluate the fetal growth and amniotic fluid.
4. Once or twice a week nonstress test(NST)/Biophysical profile (BPP) from 32 weeks onward is also recommended.
5. Maternal APS monitoring and management according to the present criteria.
6. If any complication develops during pregnancy, should be managed as per guidelines.

16.6.2 Timings and Mode of Delivery

As there is need to control the timing of discontinuation of anticoagulant medication, delivery is to be done at 39 + 0 weeks of gestation in uncomplicated pregnancy. Early delivery is done only for medical or obstetrical indications.

1. *Anticoagulation*: LMWH should be switched to unfractionated heparin at 36–37 weeks of gestation, which allows regional anesthesia or analgesia and decrease the chances of bleeding if labor starts. According to anesthesia guidelines, there should be at least 24 h gap from the last dose of therapeutic and 12 h gap from the last dose of prophylactic LMWH for the placement of epidural catheter.
2. *Low-dose anticoagulant LDA*: When there is no history of thrombosis, it should be stopped any time after 36 + 0 weeks of gestation, which avoids the minor perioperative bleeding. If there is past history of arterial thrombosis, it can be continued through labor and delivery because continuation outweighs the smaller risk of incisional bleeding.

16.6.3 Postpartum Care

Patients of APS with prior history of thromboses are at risk of recurrence and should be kept on lifetime anticoagulation (started 4–6 h after delivery and 6–12 h after birth) with warfarin. Patients of APS with obstetric morbidity only (no personal or family history of thromboses) should not be prescribed with postpartum anticoagulation. Summary of management is shown in the algorithm (Algorithm 16.1).

16.6.4 Treatment of Pregnant Patients with Adverse Outcome Despite Anticoagulation Therapy

- *Role of hydroxychloroquine (HCQ)*: HCQ appears to decrease the levels of aCL (IgG and IgM). Keeping this fact in mind it is considered that HCQ might be helpful in APS obstetric morbidity. Still no proved data are available, but some retrospective human and animal experimental data has shown some benefit of HCQ in APS or SLE-related obstetric morbidity [7]
- *Role of prednisone and/or intravenous immunoglobulin (IVIG)*: A network meta-analysis of RCTs showed reduction of adverse pregnancy outcomes in patients who received LDA plus LMWH plus IVIG (or LDA plus LMWH plus IVIG plus prednisone) in comparison to LDA plus LMWH [28]·dose prednisone (1–30 mg/day) is preferable to high-dose formulations.

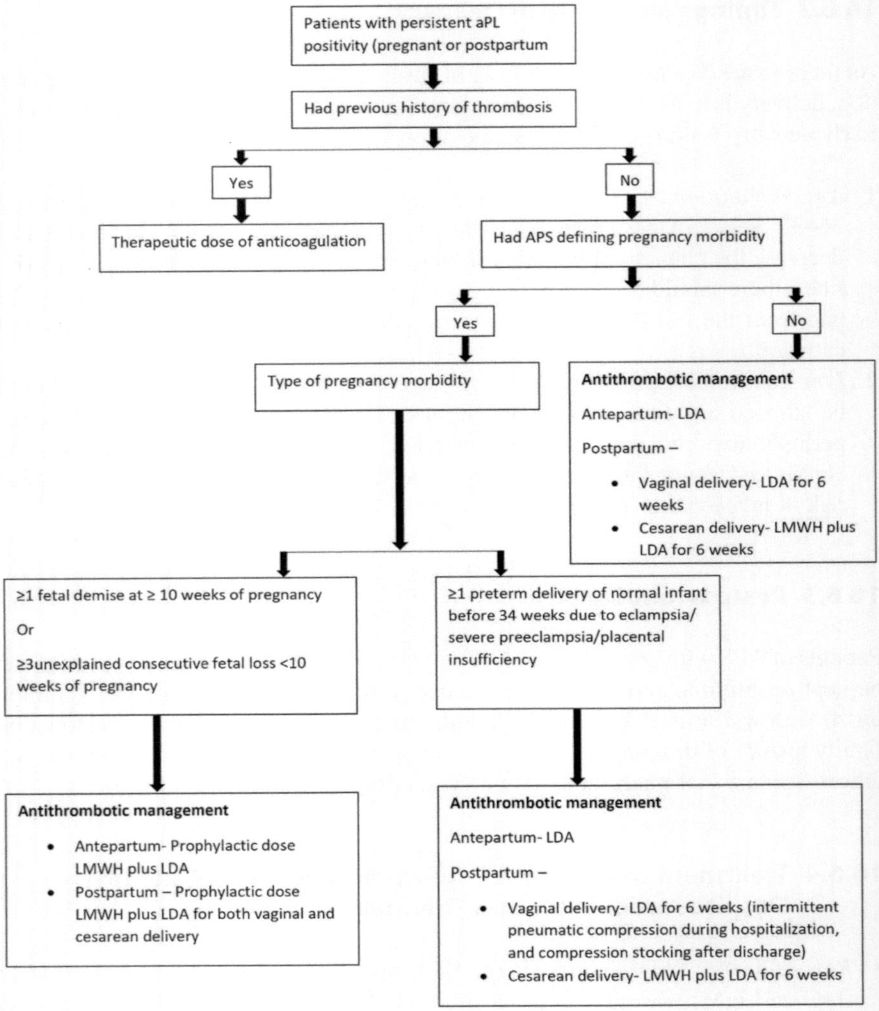

Algorithm 16.1 Management

16.6.5 Special Circumstances

- *Pregnancy with aPL without APS*
- Prevalence of aCL in uncomplicated pregnancy ranged from 0–11% [29–37]. It is difficult to prove the relationship between these antibodies and pregnancy outcome in normal asymptomatic individual. There is lack of information to guide the management of incidental persistent aPL positivity without clinical symptoms. More than 50% of such cases have successful pregnancy outcome without

treatment, but here pregnancy should be monitored to note any evidence of placental insufficiency. Advisory Board of 10th International Congress on aPL has recommended LDA alone for such type of patients.

- *Patients with APS planning in vitro fertilization (IVF)*
- IVF in patients with aPL: Prophylactic antithrombotic therapy is not prescribed for patients who have aPL without any clinical features of APS.
- IVF in APS: Oral anticoagulants must be shifted to therapeutic dose of unfractionated heparin and after conception, LMWH must be started.
- *Neonatal APS*: A least one type of aPL antibodies is present in serum with at least one clinical feature (venous or arterial thromboses, thrombocytopenia).
- *Catastrophic APS (CAPS)*: Only 1% of APS patients are at risk of developing CAPS, which is a life-threatening variant. It is characterized by its rapid onset, very high titers of aPL, widespread coagulopathy, resulting in multiorgan failure. These patients are at high risk of fetal death, when it occurs early in pregnancy. Treatment of pregnant patients are same as nonpregnant individuals.

Key Points

1. Pregnancy morbidity can be treated in part by treating antiphospholipid syndrome. The idea that aPLs can directly bind the placental tissue of both the mother and the fetus and hinder placentation without necessarily causing prothrombotic events is now widely acknowledged, despite the abundance of evidence in the literature.
2. Preconception low dosage aspirin (LDA, 81 mg/day, oral) and low molecular weight heparin (LMWH) at preventive doses (0.4–0.6 mg/kg/day; 4000–6000 IU/day, subcutaneous) are the standard treatments for obstetrics APS. These treatments begin as soon as a pregnancy test is positive. Typically, LMWH and LDA therapy is continued for the full 6 weeks after delivery and throughout the pregnancy.
3. Patients who have experienced thrombotic events in the past should receive full unfractionated or LMWH dosages for secondary thromboprophylaxis
4. Heparin was first thought to be a helpful treatment for OAPS due to the initial notion that intraplacental thrombotic events caused pregnancy morbidity.
5. New mechanisms of action have been proposed by the identification of additional pathogenic processes of aPL-mediated placental damage and the drug's effectiveness in OAPS.
6. Conventional treatment may not be effective in up to 20–25% of instances. Alternative treatment regimens have been explored in this case, including IVIG or plasma exchange, low-prednisone doses, increasing LMWH doses, and hydroxychloroquine (HCQ).
7. Biological therapies, such as those based on the use of immunomodulatory medications or monoclonal antibodies, can stop the pro-coagulant and pro-abortive effects of aPL as well as the activation of the complement.

Bibliography

1. Barbhaiya M, Zuily S, Naden R, et al. The 2023 ACR/EULAR antiphospholipid syndrome classification criteria. Arthritis Rheumatol. 2023;75:1687.
2. Yelnik CM, Laskin CA, Porter TF, et al. Lupus anticoagulant is the main predictor of adverse pregnancy outcomes in aPL-positive patients: validation of PROMISSE study results. Lupus Sci Med. 2016;3:e000131.
3. Lockshin MD, Kim M, Laskin CA, et al. Prediction of adverse pregnancy outcome by the presence of lupus anticoagulant, but not anticardiolipin antibody, in patients with antiphospholipid antibodies. Arthritis Rheum. 2012;64:2311.
4. Saccone G, Berghella V, Maruotti GM, et al. Antiphospholipid antibody profile based obstetric outcomes of primary antiphospholipid syndrome: the PREGNANTS study. Am J Obstet Gynecol. 2017;216:525.e1.
5. Latino JO, Udry S, Aranda FM, et al. Pregnancy failure in patients with obstetric antiphospholipid syndrome with conventional treatment: the influence of a triple positive antibody profile. Lupus. 2017;26:983.
6. Lazzaroni MG, Fredi M, Andreoli L, et al. Triple antiphospholipid (aPL) antibodies positivity is associated with pregnancy complications in aPL carriers: a multicenter study on 62 pregnancies. Front Immunol. 2019;10:1948.
7. Latino JO, Udry S, Aranda F, et al. Risk factors for early severe preeclampsia in obstetric antiphospholipid syndrome with conventional treatment. The impact of hydroxychloroquine. Lupus. 2020;29:1736.
8. Udry S, Peréz SM, Belizna C, et al. Clinical and therapeutic value of the adjusted Global Antiphospholipid Syndrome Score in primary obstetric antiphospholipid syndrome. Lupus. 2022;31:354.
9. Bramham K, Hunt BJ, Germain S, et al. Pregnancy outcome in different clinical phenotypes of antiphospholipid syndrome. Lupus. 2010;19:58.
10. Yelnik CM, Lambert M, Drumez E, et al. Bleeding complications and antithrombotic treatment in 264 pregnancies in antiphospholipid syndrome. Lupus. 2018;27:1679.
11. Bates SM, Greer IA, Middeldorp S, et al. VTE, thrombophilia, antithrombotic therapy, and pregnancy: Antithrombotic Therapy and Prevention of Thrombosis, 9th ed: American College of Chest Physicians Evidence-Based Clinical Practice Guidelines. Chest. 2012;141:e691S.
12. Chighizola CB, Lonati PA, Trespidi L, et al. The complement system in the pathophysiology of pregnancy and in systemic autoimmune rheumatic diseases during pregnancy. Front Immunol. 2020;11:2084.
13. Alijotas-Reig J, Esteve-Valverde E, Anunciación-Llunell A, et al. Pathogenesis, diagnosis and management of obstetric antiphospholipid syndrome: a comprehensive review. J Clin Med. 2022;11
14. Nalli C, Lini D, Andreoli L, et al. Low preconception complement levels are associated with adverse pregnancy outcomes in a multicenter study of 260 pregnancies in 197 women with antiphospholipid syndrome or carriers of antiphospholipid antibodies. Biomedicines. 2021:9.
15. De Luca F, Shoenfeld Y. The microbiome in autoimmune diseases. Clin Exp Immunol. 2019;195(1):74–85. https://doi.org/10.1111/cei.13158. PMID: 29920643; PMCID: PMC6300652.
16. Bistervels IM, Buchmüller A, Wiegers HMG, et al. Intermediate-dose versus low-dose low-molecular-weight heparin in pregnant and post-partum women with a history of venous thromboembolism (Highlow study): an open-label, multicentre, randomised, controlled trial. Lancet. 2022;400:1777.
17. van Hoorn ME, Hague WM, van Pampus MG, et al. Low-molecular-weight heparin and aspirin in the prevention of recurrent early-onset pre-eclampsia in women with antiphospholipid antibodies: the FRUIT-RCT. Eur J Obstet Gynecol Reprod Biol. 2016;197:168.
18. Empson M, Lassere M, Craig JC, Scott JR. Recurrent pregnancy loss with antiphospholipid antibody: a systematic review of therapeutic trials. Obstet Gynecol. 2002;99:135.

19. Ziakas PD, Pavlou M, Voulgarelis M. Heparin treatment in antiphospholipid syndrome with recurrent pregnancy loss: a systematic review and meta-analysis. Obstet Gynecol. 2010;115:1256.
20. Mak A, Cheung MW, Cheak AA, Ho RC. Combination of heparin and aspirin is superior to aspirin alone in enhancing live births in patients with recurrent pregnancy loss and positive anti-phospholipid antibodies: a meta-analysis of randomized controlled trials and meta-regression. Rheumatology (Oxford). 2010;49:281.
21. Hamulyák EN, Scheres LJJ, Goddijn M, Middeldorp S. Antithrombotic therapy to prevent recurrent pregnancy loss in antiphospholipid Syndrome-What is the evidence? J Thromb Haemost. 2021;19:1174.
22. Brito-Zerón P, Izmirly PM, Ramos-Casals M, et al. The clinical spectrum of autoimmune congenital heart block. Nat Rev Rheumatol. 2015;11:301.
23. Hirsh J, Guyatt G, Albers GW, et al. Executive summary: American College of Chest Physicians evidence-based clinical practice guidelines (8th Edition). Chest. 2008;133:71S.
24. Sciascia S, Hunt BJ, Talavera-Garcia E, et al. The impact of hydroxychloroquine treatment on pregnancy outcome in women with antiphospholipid antibodies. Am J Obstet Gynecol. 2016;214:273.e1.
25. Bertolaccini ML, Contento G, Lennen R, et al. Complement inhibition by hydroxychloroquine prevents placental and fetal brain abnormalities in antiphospholipid syndrome. J Autoimmun. 2016;75:30.
26. Ruffatti A, Tonello M, Hoxha A, et al. Effect of additional treatments combined with conventional therapies in pregnant patients with high-risk antiphospholipid syndrome: a multicentre study. Thromb Haemost. 2018;118:639.
27. Duan J, Ma D, Wen X, et al. Hydroxychloroquine prophylaxis for preeclampsia, hypertension and prematurity in pregnant patients with systemic lupus erythematosus: a meta-analysis. Lupus. 2021;30:1163.
28. Yang Z, Shen X, Zhou C, et al. Prevention of recurrent miscarriage in women with antiphospholipid syndrome: a systematic review and network meta-analysis. Lupus. 2021;30:70.
29. Harris EN, Spinnato JA. Should anticardiolipin tests be performed in otherwise healthy pregnant women? Am J Obstet Gynecol. 1991;165:1272.
30. Infante-Rivard C, David M, Gauthier R, Rivard GE. Lupus anticoagulants, anticardiolipin antibodies, and fetal loss. a case-control study. N Engl J Med. 1991;325:1063.
31. Kutteh WH. Antiphospholipid antibodies and reproduction. J Reprod Immunol. 1997;35:151.
32. Polzin WJ, Kopelman JN, Robinson RD, et al. The association of antiphospholipid antibodies with pregnancies complicated by fetal growth restriction. Obstet Gynecol. 1991;78:1108.
33. Lockwood CJ, Romero R, Feinberg RF, et al. The prevalence and biologic significance of lupus anticoagulant and anticardiolipin antibodies in a general obstetric population. Am J Obstet Gynecol. 1989;161:369.
34. Petri M. Diagnosis of antiphospholipid antibodies. Rheum Dis Clin N Am. 1994;20:443.
35. Parke AL, Wilson D, Maier D. The prevalence of antiphospholipid antibodies in women with recurrent spontaneous abortion, women with successful pregnancies, and women who have never been pregnant. Arthritis Rheum. 1991;34:1231.
36. Petri M, Golbus M, Anderson R, et al. Antinuclear antibody, lupus anticoagulant, and anticardiolipin antibody in women with idiopathic habitual abortion. A controlled, prospective study of forty-four women. Arthritis Rheum. 1987;30:601.
37. Haddow JE, Rote NS, Dostal-Johnson D, et al. Lack of an association between late fetal death and antiphospholipid antibody measurements in the second trimester. Am J Obstet Gynecol. 1991;165:1308.
38. Lockshin MD, Druzin ML, Qamar T. Prednisone does not prevent recurrent fetal death in women with antiphospholipid antibody. Am J Obstet Gynecol. 1989;160:439.
39. Del Ross T, Ruffatti A, Visentin MS, et al. Treatment of 139 pregnancies in antiphospholipid-positive women not fulfilling criteria for antiphospholipid syndrome: a retrospective study. J Rheumatol. 2013;40:425.

Inherited Thrombophilia in Pregnancy 17

Shashi L. Kabra Maheshwari and Shalini V. Singh

Thrombophilia's are the conditions where the inhibitory proteins are deficient, which causes hypercoagulability, and thus venous thrombosis and embolism. Thrombophilias may be inherited (genetic) or acquired. Venous thromboembolism (VTE) [1, 2]. Arterial thrombosis is usually rare. The risk of pregnancy-associated VTE is up to six times that of the general population, with an absolute risk up to 12.2 per 10,000, compared with 2 per 10,000 in nonpregnant women [3]. While this disease is more common in Western countries where pulmonary thromboembolism accounts to 1–5% cause of maternal mortality, this entity is underreported in Indian population. However, one of the Indian studies has reported the incidence of venous thromboembolism disorders in India is as common as in the West. The reported incidence is 17.46/10,000 admissions, and it has been on rise, attributed to an increase in the clinical suspicion among treating physicians [4].

17.1 Pathophysiology

Pregnancy causes physiological changes in all the systems including coagulation cascade that affects the Virchow's triad making pregnancy a hypercoagulable state. Pregnancy and puerperium are the times when the risk of venous thrombosis and pulmonary embolism is highest in an otherwise healthy woman. Sultan et al. [5] in 2011 computed the risk to be 6 times higher in the third trimester and 22 times higher in the puerperium. In 2008, Jacobsen et al. [6] reported that deep vein thrombosis (DVT) was more frequent antepartum whereas pulmonary embolism predominated in puerperal women. Physiological changes associated with

S. L. Kabra Maheshwari (✉)
Department of OBG, DDU Hospital, New Delhi, India

S. V. Singh
Rama Medical College, Kanpur, UP, India

R. Sharma, A. Kumar (eds.), *Systemic Disorders in Pregnancy*,
https://doi.org/10.1007/978-981-96-4876-4_17

pregnancy that predispose a woman to thromboembolism are enlisted below (Table 17.1).

Risk factors: Pregnancy is a thrombophilic state. Other risk factors are (Table 17.2):

Table 17.1 Changes in coagulation factors with pregnancy

Increased	Decreased	No change
Virchow's triad: Venous stasis due to compression of pelvic veins and IVC, which also contributes to endothelial cell injury		
Plasma fibrinogen (factor I)		
Factor VII, VIII, X, XII	Factor XI	Factor II, V
Plasminogen activator inhibitor 1 and 2		Plasminogen activator t-PA
Plasminogen, D Dimer, vWF	Free protein S	Protein C, Antithrombin III

Table 17.2 Risk factors associated with increased thrombogenicity

Preexisting risk factors	Score
Previous VTE except a single event related to major surgery	4
Previous VTE provoked by a major surgery	3
Known high-risk thrombophilia	3
Medical disorders	3
Family history of unprovoked or estrogen-related VTE	1
Known low-risk thrombophilia (no VTE)	1
Age > 35 years	1
Obesity	BMI >/=30:1 40 or more: 2
Parity, 3 or more	1
Smoking	1
Gross varicose veins	1
Obstetric risk factors	
Elective cesarean section, instrumental delivery	1
Cesarean section in labor	2
Preeclampsia in current pregnancy	1
ART/IVF pregnancy	1
Multiple pregnancy	1
Prolonged labor (>24 h),	1
Post partum hemorrhage	1
Preterm birth or still birth in current pregnancy	1
Transient risk factors	
Any surgical procedure in pregnancy except episiotomy repair	3
Hyperemesis	3
OHSS in first trimester	4
Current systemic infection	1
Immobility, dehydration	1
Antenatally >/= 4 thromboprophylaxis from first trimester Antenatally >/=3 thromboprophylaxis from 28 weeks Postnatally >/= 2 thromboprophylaxis for at least 10 days Hospitalization antenatally, prolonged stay >3 days postnatally or readmission in puerperium, consider thromboprophylaxis	

Taken from RCOG Greentop guideline 37a [8]

17.2 Classification

Many potentially thrombophilic mutations are discovered apart from the already known ones. Thrombophilia can be divided into inherited and acquired. Flow Chart 17.1 shows the coagulation cascade and the point where these deficiencies affect the cycle. Clinically relevant inherited thrombophilia is enumerated below (Table 17.3):

1. Antithrombin deficiency
2. Protein C deficiency
3. Protein S deficiency
4. Activated protein C resistance (factor V Leiden mutations)
5. Prothrombin mutation

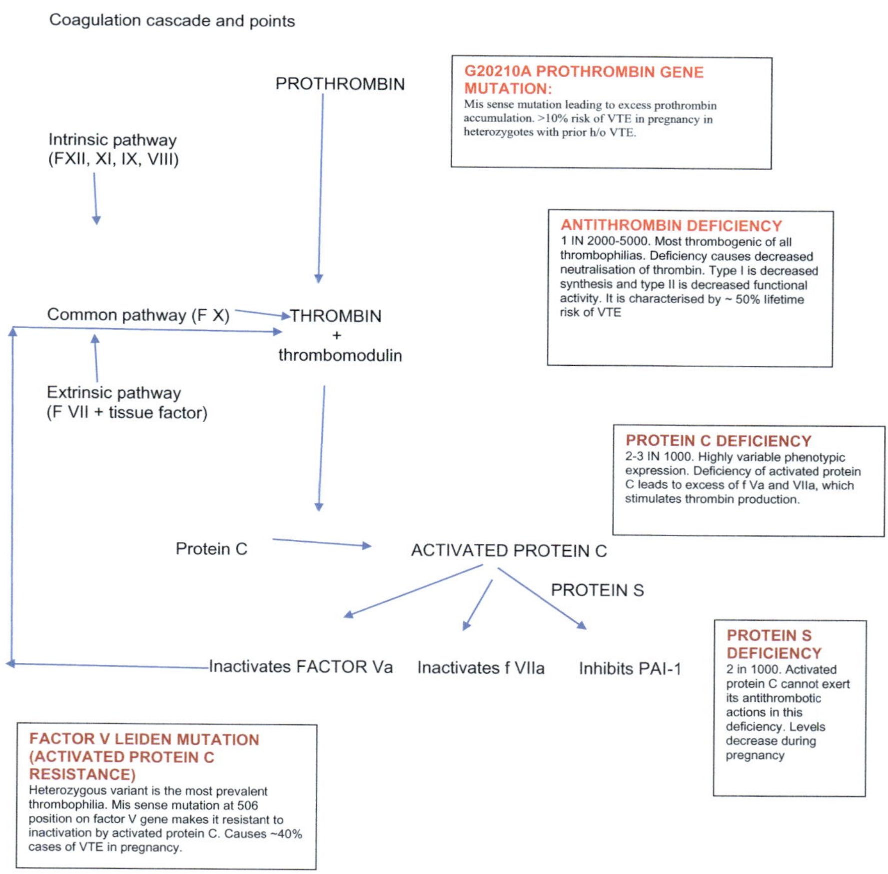

Flow Chart 17.1 Coagulation cascade and points

Table 17.3 Classification of thrombophilia

Inherited		Acquired
High risk	Low risk	
Antithrombin deficiency	Factor V heterozygotes	Lupus anticoagulant
Factor V Leiden homozygotes	PGM heterozygotes	Anticardiolipin antibody
Prothrombin gene mutations	Protein C deficiency	Beta 2 microglobulin
Compound heterozygotes FVL and PGM	Protein S deficiency	
	Hyperhomocysteinemia	

17.3 Clinical Presentation

Women usually present with features of VTE. The odds are increased in the third trimester and puerperium due to compounded risk factors as described above. They may present with features of pulmonary embolism like chest pain, breathlessness, hemoptysis, cough, or with those of DVT such as leg pain, swelling, or pale extremity. High index of suspicion is key to early diagnosis and treatment.

Adverse Pregnancy Outcomes Inherited thrombophilia in pregnancy is less likely to be associated with adverse pregnancy outcomes, which are more correlated to the acquired thrombophilias. A few studies, however, found a modest link, mostly limited to high risk thrombophilia with additional risk factors. Recurrent pregnancy losses, intrauterine fetal death, preeclampsia, abruptio placentae, and fetal growth restriction are the most common pregnancy complications in above condition [7].

17.4 Screening and Diagnosis

Routine screening for inherited thrombophilias in nonselected population is not recommended because of the low frequency of the condition. There is no strong evidence on which recommendations regarding whom to test or the optimal panel of tests could be based [8]. It is appropriate to screen women planning pregnancy when there is

(a) History of VTE associated with a transient risk factor.
(b) History of unprovoked idiopathic VTE, recurrent VTE, or hormone-provoked VTE.
(c) No prior VTE but a first degree relative with a history of high risk thrombophilia.

It is not advocated to advise battery of tests for inherited thrombophilia if a woman presents with a history of recurrent or nonrecurrent early losses, abruption, preeclampsia or fetal growth restriction, or couples with recurrent IVF failures.

However, these women should be thoroughly screened for acquired thrombophilia based on the clinical and laboratory features.

The test panel includes screening for five types of inherited thrombophilias. Timing should ideally be in a nonpregnant state, or 6–8 weeks after pregnancy or any thrombotic event, after ruling out use of oral contraceptives and anticoagulant therapy. If screening in pregnancy is necessary, threshold values for free protein S antigen levels in the second trimester are identified at <30 percent and in third trimester as <24 percent. ACOG does not recommend screening for homocysteine levels, MTHFR polymorphism, PAI-1 polymorphism testing, or factor VIII levels as a part of screening panel [9] (Table 17.4).

A clinical evaluation for thrombophilia should be performed for all patients with previous episode of VTE and those with history of recurrent pregnancy losses, preeclampsia, fetal growth retardation, first trimester abortion, placental abruption, and intrauterine deaths. The evaluation includes accurate family and personal history for thrombosis, past clinical antecedents, associated pathologies and interpretation of existing risk factors, physical examination in particular to skin, lymphatics, peripheral arterial and venous, cardiorespiratory, abdominal, urinary, and neurological system. In a systematic review "The Thrombosis: Risk and Economic assessment of Thrombophilia Screening(TREATS) study shows that selective screening based on prior VTE history is more cost-effective than universal screening [9].

Table 17.4 How to test for inherited thrombophilias

Thrombophilia	Testing method	Is testing reliable during pregnancy?	Is testing reliable during acute thrombosis?	Is testing reliable with anticoagulation?
Factor V Leiden mutation	Activated protein C resistance assay (second generation)	Yes	Yes	No
	If abnormal: DNA analysis	Yes	Yes	Yes
Prothrombin G20210A mutation	DNA analysis	Yes	Yes	Yes
Protein C deficiency	Protein C activity (,65%)	Yes	No	No
Protein S deficiency	Functional assay (55%)	No	No	No
Antithrombin deficiency	Antithrombin activity (60%)	Yes	No	No

ACOG Practice Bulletin 198, 2018 [7]

17.5 Prevention and Preconception Counseling

ACOG and RCOG have published guidelines regarding thromboprophylaxis in various scenarios in pregnant women. The underlying concept however remains that the clinical picture is dynamic, hence documented risk assessment should be done repeatedly as and when the new risk factors come up. Royal College of Obstetrics and Gynaecology (RCOG) has given a comprehensive yet simplified algorithm for scoring. Thromboprophylaxis should be prescribed according to the scoring under a specialist consultation [10]. Routine low-dose aspirin is not recommended in women with inherited thrombophilia, and should be prescribed according to the standard criteria for preeclampsia prophylaxis.

In the context of our topic of interest, some important key points are:

Clinical history remains the most important consideration, hence women with prior history of VTE, recurrent, unprovoked, or hormone related; those who are on long-term anticoagulation; and women with antithrombin deficiency are under very high risk and should be advised high dose LMWH antenatally (after positive urine pregnancy test) and 6 weeks postpartum or till shifted back to oral anticoagulants. Women on long-term anticoagulation should be counseled preconceptionally about the teratogenic effects of oral anticoagulants like warfarin.

Within 2 weeks of the missed period and before 6 week of pregnancy, LMWH should be started. Women should also be told about the conservative measures like avoiding dehydration, graduated compression stockings, mobilization, etc.

Incidence of VTE as per different mutations for inherited thrombophilias is summarized in the Table 17.5

Management of thrombophilia can be simplified and segregated according to the risk category [10] (Table 17.6)

Table 17.5 VTE OR as per different mutation in inherited thrombophilia [14]

Mutation	VTE risk per pregnancy (no prior VTE episode)%	VTE risk per pregnancy (prior VTE episode)%	VTE odds ratio
Factor V Leiden heterozygote	0.5–1.2	10	6.4
Factor V Leiden heterozygote	4	17	35.8
Prothrombin gene heterozygote	<0.5	>10	5.1
Prothrombin gene homozygote	2–4	>17	21.1
Factor V Leiden/ prothrombin gene double heterozygote	4–5	>20	21.2
Antithrombin deficiency	3–7	40	9.5
Protein C deficiency	0.1–0.8	4–17	9.3
Protein S deficiency	0.1	0–22	7.0

Table 17.6 Thrombophilia risk category and management

Risk category	Thromboprophylaxis
Very high risk	
Previous VTE (long-term oral anticoagulants) Antithrombin deficiency, APLA with previous VTE	High dose during pregnancy and up to 6 weeks postpartum low molecular weight heparin or until switched to previous oral anticoagulants. Specialists in hemostasis and high risk pregnancy.
High risk	
Any previous VTE excluding one episode of VTE associated with major surgery	Prophylactic LMWH antenatally and up to 6 weeks postnatally
Intermediate risk	
Asymptomatic high risk thrombophilia, homozygous factor V Leiden mutation, compound heterozygous protein C/S deficiency One episode of previous VTE in major surgery with no risk factors	Prophylactic LMWH antenatally and up to 6 weeks postnatally LMWH to be started from 28 weeks pregnancy and till 6 weeks postnatally
Low risk	
Asymptomatic thrombophilias	Up to 10 days or 6 weeks postnatal

In case of acute event, treatment of choice is unfractionated heparin(UFH), given as intravenous bolus followed by continuous infusion, titrated to achieve an aPTT of 1.5 to 2.5 times control values. Low molecular weight heparins (LMWH) are preferred alternatives in regular use, due to their predictable response, longer half-life, better bioavailability, and fewer bleeding complications [11]. Both the groups act by the same mechanism, i.e., inhibition of factor Xa and thrombin. LMWH shows greater inhibitory activity against factor Xa than thrombin, in contrast to UFH, which has almost equivalent activity against both. Usually, monitoring is not done, though some suggest periodic measurement of anti-factor Xa levels 4 to 6 h after an injection, more so with dose adjustments. LMWH are safe and effective in pregnancy and breastfeeding. Among the complications of anticoagulant treatment, most important is hemorrhage. The dose is calculated on the basis of weight and indication. LMWHs should be cautiously used in women with uncontrolled hypertension, severe renal or liver disease, women at increased obstetric risk of bleeding like placenta previa. Those receiving UFH should be monitored for heparin-induced thrombocytopenia and osteoporosis. Newer anticoagulants like danaparoid and fondaparinux should be reserved in case of intolerance or allergy to heparin and used under strict specialist supervision.

In women on long-term anticoagulation, warfarin can be restarted postpartum after a bridging period. Non-vitamin K antagonist oral anticoagulants (NOACs) should be avoided during pregnancy and lactation.

The thromboprophylactic doses for antenatal and postnatal period is adjusted according to the body weight [10]

- Weight < 50 kgs -Enoxaparin 20 mg daily, Dalteparin 2500 U daily, Tinzaparin 3500 U daily

- Weight 50–90 kgs -Enoxaparin 40 mg daily, Dalteparin 5000 U daily, Tinzaparin 4500 U daily
- High prophylactic dose
- Weight 50–90 kgs- Enoxaparin 40 mg q12h, Dalteparin 5000 U q12h, Tinzaparin 4500 U q12h

17.6 Labor and Delivery

Women should be switched to unfractionated heparin near term, usually in the last month of pregnancy or earlier in case of suspected preterm delivery owing to its shorter half-life and risk of spinal hematoma. Discontinuation is critical with respect to time in planned events. Women on dose adjusted or treatment dosages should discontinue heparin at least 24 h before the planned induction or cesarean [12]. In women who are on prophylactic doses, a gap of 12 h after the last dose is considered as appropriate. If the duration after the last dose is not sufficient, aPTT can be done to verify clearance. Protamine sulfate is an antidote for heparin, however usually not needed at prophylactic doses. After delivery, LMWH should not be given within 4 h of spinal anesthesia or after removal of an epidural catheter, and the catheter should not be removed within 12 h of the most recent injection.

With UFH, an interval of 4 h after the last prophylactic dose is needed. Thromboprophylaxis should be reinstated 4–6 h after uncomplicated delivery once PPH and regional analgesia timings have been considered [10]. Pneumatic compression devices and anti-embolism stockings can be used during the gap and hydration, and mobilization should be adequately taken care of.

17.6.1 Management of Unexpected Delivery on Anticoagulants [15]

1. *If the mother is on warfarin*
   - Check INR
   - If INR < 2.5-cesarean section is safer
   - If INR > 2.5-cesarean section is the mode of delivery, fresh frozen plasma (FFP) to be given, amount will depend upon INR post-FFP
   - If INR > 4.5 vitamin K to be given

Check INR of baby immediately after delivery, Give vitamin K IV into cord. If neonatal bleeding present give 10mg/kg FFP and monitor INR

2. *If the mother is on unfractionated heparin*
   - Check activated partial thromboplastin time

Consider administration of protamine sulfate in case aPTT is prolonged to reduce the risk of bleeding

3. *If the mother is on low molecular weight heparin*
    - If available check anti-factor X levels and testing D-dimers
    - Protamine sulfate may offer limited neutralization in case of bleeding

In case of major bleeding recombinant activated factor VII concentrate to be given

17.7 Biomarkers in Pregnancy

As more women are living with hereditary thrombophilia, nowadays a great deal of research is being done over prognostic biomarkers. Currently, D-dimers is the most used one. Biomarkers provides critical evidence to translate findings from clinical research to clinical practice. In a study conducted in Spain in 2020 over thrombophilic population, microRNA was analyzed by q-PCR in plasma samples and the following results were seen:

1. A total of 752 micro-RNAs were analyzed by qPCR in the genetic analyses of idiopathic thrombophilia population out of which four plasma microRNAs are associated with related intermediate phenotypes (e.g., protein S or factor VII).
2. This microRNA profile is of use for predicting the risk of venous thrombosis, a risk model including the microRNAs, age and sex showed area under ROC of 0.77.

The four microRNAs showed differential expression in patients with VTE: hsa-miR-126-3p, hsa-miR-885-5p, hsa-miR-194-5p, and hsa-miR-192-5p. They displayed a big association with VTE and also proved to be possible predictors of the pathology [13].

miRNA also has a role in the control of gene expression associated with inflammatory response in maternal–fetal immune tolerance, and they are a potential space for research in cases of recurrent pregnancy losses. High quality research is needed to define pathways by which polymorphisms of miRNA machinery genes influence recurrent pregnancy loss.

17.8 Summary and Recommendations

- Pregnancy is a physiological prothrombotic state.
- Heritable thrombophilia is associated with both gestational VTE and, on a slightly modest basis, with high-risk thrombophilia with adverse pregnancy outcomes, like FGR, pregnancy loss, preeclampsia, and placental abruption.
- Screening for inherited thrombophilias is not recommended for women with history of fetal loss or adverse pregnancy outcomes including abruption, preeclampsia, or fetal growth restriction because there is insufficient clinical evidence that

antepartum prophylaxis with unfractionated heparin or low-molecular-weight heparin prevents recurrence in these patients.

- Screening with MTHFR C677T polymorphism and measuring homocysteine levels are not recommended because of the lack of association between it and negative pregnancy outcome.
- LMWH is used on a widespread basis in this condition. Anticoagulants and antiplatelet drugs should be tailored according to the clinical condition of the patient.
- More research is required to have a better understanding of the disease processes, identify possible biomarkers to guide treatment, and explore the possible benefits of better-targeted and newer antithrombotic treatment. Future directions will include mandatory microRNA profiling, which will be a useful tool in both diagnosis and monitoring and prognosis.

References

1. Konstantinides S. 2019 ESC Guidelines for the diagnosis and management of acute pulmonary embolism developed in collaboration with the European Respiratory Society (ERS). Russian J Cardiol. 2020;25(8):3848.
2. Pregnancy Mortality Surveillance System | Maternal and Infant Health | CDC [Internet]. Cdc.gov. 2021 [cited 16 February 2021]. Available from: https://www.cdc.gov/reproductivehealth/maternal-mortality/pregnancy-mortality-surveillance-system.html.
3. Parunov L, Soshitova N, Ovanesov M, Panteleev M, Serebriyskiy I. Epidemiology of venous thromboembolism (VTE) associated with pregnancy. Birth Defects Res C Embryo Today. 2015;105(3):167–84.
4. Edwin S, Vimalin S, Sunil A, Dheepak S, Prabhu P. Deep vein thrombosis is not uncommon in India. Indian J Vasc Endovasc Surg. 2017;4:92–6.
5. Sultan A, West J, Tata L, Fleming K, Nelson-Piercy C, Grainge M. Risk of first venous thromboembolism in and around pregnancy: a population-based cohort study. Br J Haematol. 2011;156(3):366–73.
6. Jacobsen A, Skjeldestad F, Sandset P. Incidence and risk patterns of venous thromboembolism in pregnancy and puerperium—a register-based case-control study. Am J Obstet Gynecol. 2008;198(2):233.e1–7.
7. Rey E, Kahn S, David M, Shrier I. Thrombophilic disorders and fetal loss: a meta-analysis. Lancet. 2003;361(9361):901–8.
8. Torri DM, Neil SS. ACOG Practice Bulletin No. 197: inherited thrombophilias in pregnancy. Obstet Gynecol. 2018;132(1):e18–34.
9. Wu O, Robertson L, Twaddle S, Lowe GD, Clark P, Greaves M, Walker ID, Langhorne P, Brenkel I, Regan L, Greer I. Screening for thrombophilia in high-risk situations: systematic review and cost-effectiveness analysis. The Thrombosis: Risk and Economic Assessment of Thrombophilia Screening (TREATS) study. Health Technol Assess. 2006;10(11):1–110.
10. Royal College of Obstetricians and Gynecologists. Reducing the risk of thrombosis and embolism during pregnancy and the puerperium. Green-top Guideline No. 37a; 2015. www.rcog.org.uk
11. Tapson V. Acute pulmonary embolism. N Engl J Med. 2008;358(10):1037–52.
12. Horlocker T, Wedel D, Rowlingson J, Enneking F. Executive summary: regional anesthesia in the patient receiving antithrombotic or thrombolytic therapy. Reg Anesth Pain Med. 2010;35(1):102–5.

13. Rodriguez-Rius A, Lopez S, Martinez-Perez A, Souto JC, Soria JM. Identification of a plasma microRNA profile associated with venous thrombosis. Arterioscler Thromb Vasc Biol. 2020;40:1392–9.
14. Devis P, Knuttinen MG. Deep venous thrombosis in pregnancy: incidence, pathogenesis and endovascular management. Cardiovasc Diagn Ther. 2017 Dec;7(Suppl 3):S309–19.
15. Habib S, Khuwaja AM, Amjad N. Anticoagulation therapy during pregnancy and puerperium. Anaesth Pain Intens Care. 2014;18(4)

Psychiatric Disorders in Pregnancy 18

Tarun Pal

Perinatal psychiatric disorders constitute a significant clinical concern, bearing implications not only for maternal well-being but also for fetal development and postpartum outcomes. This critical period spans pregnancy and the postpartum.

Incidence of mood and anxiety disorders exhibits notable prevalence throughout the reproductive years [1]. The periods encompassing pregnancy and the postpartum are characterized by increased vulnerability among women with preexisting psychiatric conditions, particularly predisposing them to depressive episodes [2].

Studies have consistently reported the prevalence of depression during pregnancy to range between 10% and 16% [3]. Additionally, women diagnosed with bipolar disorder face escalated risks during these periods, with postpartum relapse rates estimated phase, introduces a unique intersection of physiological, psychological, and social changes, amplifying the vulnerability to psychiatric illness. Despite the societal emphasis on the joyous aspects of pregnancy, it is crucial to recognize the prevalence and complexity of mental health challenges during this time. Studies suggest that about 30–50% of the population experience mental disorders. In the context of obsessive-compulsive disorder (OCD), symptoms typically exacerbate during pregnancy [4]. It is imperative to exercise specialized considerations in managing psychotic disorders during pregnancy.

18.1 Etiology

Mental disorders during the perinatal period stem from a multifactorial etiology. Physiological alterations occurring within the maternal body are recognized as significant contributors, particularly in genetically susceptible women. These changes predominantly involve disruptions in the endocrine and autoimmune systems.

T. Pal (✉)
Department of Psychiatry, L. L. R. M. Medical College, Meerut, India

R. Sharma, A. Kumar (eds.), *Systemic Disorders in Pregnancy*,
https://doi.org/10.1007/978-981-96-4876-4_18

Hence, routine laboratory assessments should be conducted to rule out autoimmune thyroiditis. Additionally, the impact of infectious diseases must not be overlooked. The use of medications by pregnant women, including glucocorticosteroids and sympathomimetics, warrants careful consideration due to potential implications. Conditions associated with cerebral dysfunction, such as eclampsia or preeclampsia-related strokes, as well as neoplastic processes, may also exert considerable influence.

18.2 Risk Factors [5, 6]

- Inadequate social support
- Strained marital relationships
- Single motherhood
- Pessimistic life outlooks
- Unemployment
- Financial instability
- Lack of childcare experience
- Having more than three children
- Maternal age below 20 years

18.2.1 Pregnancy-Related High Factors

- Unwanted or high-risk pregnancies
- Previous traumatic pregnancy experiences (miscarriage, abortion, medical conditions, genetic anomalies)
- Difficult or traumatic childbirths
- Multiple births
- Sleep disturbances
- Sleep deprivation

18.2.2 Others

- History of mental disorders in the mother or family encompassing recurrent depressive disorders, bipolar affective disorder, anxiety disorders, past suicide attempts, and substance use disorders
- Maternal personality traits, characterized by heightened neuroticism, low self-esteem, anxious dispositions, and emotional instability
- Emotional abuse within relationships
- Strained maternal relationships
- Child illnesses
- Inadequate prenatal care
- Childhood experiences of violence

18.3 Classifications

Classifications are key characteristics that describe a specific illness. They help to diagnose conditions more easily by providing a common set of criteria to follow. Their goal is to make the diagnostic process smoother and more efficient. Two classification systems are used worldwide: ICD-11 and DSM-5.

The ICD-11 [7] classification has introduced a new category of mental problems occurring in association with pregnancy, childbirth, and the postpartum period, which includes specific mood disorders and psychotic disorders (block L1-6E2) (Table 18.1).

18.3.1 DSM-5

Specifier is applied to current major depressive episode (or the most recent major depressive episode if major episode is in partial or full remission) if onset of mood symptom occurs during pregnancy or in the 4 weeks following delivery.

18.3.2 Diagnosis

When diagnosing psychosis, it should be determined whether the onset is during pregnancy or within 4 weeks of postpartum. Psychiatric conditions have often been missed, highlighting the importance of including regular screenings for psychiatric disorders during postpartum clinic visits as a crucial aspect of assessment.

Use of a population-specific screening tool such as the "Edinburgh Postnatal Depression Scale," and the "Mood Disorder Questionnaire" can improve awareness of healthcare providers and aid in the early diagnosis of postpartum psychiatric disorders [8].

The Edinburgh Postnatal Depression Scale (EPDS) is a screening tool comprising 10 questions that assess mood over the past week (or 13 during pregnancy). A score exceeding 12 requires clinical evaluation. Typically administered 6 weeks after childbirth, the Beck Depression Inventory (BDI) enables individuals to self-assess depressive symptoms, aiding in determining severity and gauging treatment effectiveness.

Other valuable assessment tools include questionnaires targeting risk factors in pregnancy and postpartum periods, such as the Postpartum Depression Predictors Inventory, Antepartum Questionnaire(APQ), and Bromley Postnatal Depression Scale (BPDS). It is imperative to educate expectant mothers about the complexities of postpartum depression to facilitate early recognition and intervention.

Table 18.1 Classification of Psychiatric illness during pregnancy and childbirth

6E20	Mental or behavioral disorders associated with pregnancy, childbirth, and the puerperium, without psychotic symptoms	A syndrome associated with pregnancy or the puerperium (commencing within about 6 weeks after delivery) that involves significant mental and behavioral features, most commonly depressive symptoms. The syndrome does not include delusions, hallucinations, or other psychotic symptoms. If the symptoms meet the diagnostic requirements for a specific mental disorder, that diagnosis should also be assigned. This designation should not be used to describe mild and transient depressive symptoms that do not meet the diagnostic requirements for a depressive episode, which may occur soon after delivery (the so-called postpartum blues)
6E20.0	Postpartum depression NOS	
6E20.Y	Other specified mental or behavioral disorders associated with pregnancy, childbirth, and thepuerperium, without psychotic symptoms	
6E20.Z	Mental or behavioral disorders associated with pregnancy, childbirth, and the puerperium, without psychotic symptoms, unspecified	
6E21	Mental or behavioral disorders associated with pregnancy, childbirth, or the puerperium, with psychotic symptoms	A syndrome associated with pregnancy or the puerperium (commencing within about 6 weeks after delivery) that involves significant mental and behavioral features, including delusions, hallucinations, or other psychotic symptoms. Mood symptoms (depressive and/ or manic) are also typically present. If the symptoms meet the diagnostic requirements for a specific mental disorder, that diagnosis should also be assigned
6E2Z	Mental or behavioral disorders associated with pregnancy, childbirth, and the puerperium, unspecified	

18.4 Treatment and Its Complications [9]

18.4.1 Recommendations for Psychosis in Pregnancy

- Psychotic women stabilized on antipsychotic drugs should have periconceptional counseling.
- Smoking, alcohol, and drug misuse are aggravating factors and should be avoided.

- Switching medication must be avoided due to the risk of relapse.
- Most reproductive safety data are available for quetiapine, olanzapine, risperidone, and haloperidol with more limited data for clozapine, aripiprazole, and ziprasidone. Quetiapine has low rate of placental passage (Table 18.2).
- Advise pregnant women taking antipsychotic medication about diet and monitor for excessive weight gain.
- Women taking an antipsychotic during pregnancy should be monitored for gestational diabetes. NICE recommends women be offered an oral glucose tolerance test.
- NICE recommends—If a women has noncompliance to oral medication or not responding well then Depot preparations must be considered, otherwise depot should be avoided during periconceptional period, and antenatal and during breastfeeding.
- Class effect—Neonates may present with crying, agitation, increased suckling, etc., if antipsychotic drugs are discontinued.

18.4.2 Recommendations for Depression in Pregnancy

- Antenatal women maintained on any antidepressant should continue it, and if illness progresses then should be further treated with antidepressant drugs (Tables 18.2 and 18.3).
- Sertraline can be considered in previously untreated women.
- Screen for alcohol use and be vigilant for the development of hypertension and preeclampsia.
- Adverse effects of SSRIs include risk of postpartum hemorrhage and persistent pulmonary hypertension of the newborn.
- The neonate may experience discontinuation symptoms, which are usually mild, such as (agitation and irritability, or rarely respiratory distress and convulsions

Table 18.2 Psychotropic drugs in pregnancy

Psychotropic	Recommendations
Antidepressant	Continue same antidepressant during and after pregnancy in women having high risk of relapse When initiating an antidepressant in a woman, consider sertraline
Antipsychotics	Major teratogenic effects are not established, therefore continue antipsychotic drug on which the woman is stabilized and don't switch the drugs Consider OGTT and screen for metabolic disorders Quetiapine has low transplacental passage
Mood stabilizers	Valproate is contraindicated during pregnancy If valproate is the only drug that can work, the woman must be made aware about risks of valproate use in pregnancy Lamotrigine is safe in pregnancy
Sedatives	Benzodiazepines, zopiclone, and promethazine must be avoided during pregnancy although teratogenesis is not established

Table 18.3 Non-pharmacological strategies for the treatment of depression

Mild and moderate postpartum depression	Severe postpartum depression
Computer programs based on assumptions in CBT therapy	CBT or interpersonal psychotherapy
Exercise	Pharmacotherapy if psychotherapy is not sufficient
Psychosocial interventions	
Nondirective counseling (active listening)	
CBT psychotherapy	
Interpersonal psychotherapy	
Pharmacotherapy when others methods fail	

with SSRIs). The risk is assumed to be particularly high with short half-life drugs such as paroxetine and venlafaxine. Continuing to breastfeed and then "weaning" by switching to mixed (breast/bottle) feeding may help reduce the severity of the reactions.

18.4.3 Recommendations for Bipolar Disorder in Pregnancy

- For women who have had a long period without relapse, the possibility of switching the antipsychotic or withdrawing treatment completely before conception and for at least the first trimester should be considered.
- The risk of relapse both pre- and postpartum is very high if medication is discontinued abruptly.
- No mood stabilizer is clearly safe. NICE recommends the use of mood stabilizing antipsychotics as a preferable alternative to continuation with a mood stabilizer.
- Women with severe illness or who are known to relapse quickly after discontinuation of mood stabilizer should be advised to continue their medication following discussion of the risks.

18.5 Prognosis

Research involving women hospitalized due to postpartum illnesses revealed a significant recurrence rate, with 75% experiencing further psychiatric conditions, predominantly non-postpartum-related [10]. Among these, half endured at least three episodes. Diagnostic patterns demonstrated considerable consistency with the initial postpartum episode. Despite this, subjects generally exhibited favorable psychiatric and functional states by the study's conclusion, with reasonable adjustments throughout their lifespan. However, a notable proportion remained reliant on psychotropic medication. These disorders tended to manifest episodically rather than persistently or progressively deteriorating.

A recent study from Denmark (Appleby et al., 1998) highlighted a substantially elevated suicide standardized mortality ratio (SMR) of 1719 among individuals with postpartum disorders.

Severe postpartum illnesses may include typical presentations of mania, depression, or schizophrenia. However, some cases, particularly those with early onset, exhibit atypical features such as fluctuating mood, depressive and elevated states, symptoms resembling schizophrenia, unusual delusions, and cognitive confusion.

Key Points

1. Increased risk of psychiatric illness during pregnancy due to hormonal fluctuations, biological changes, and psychological stressors.
2. Common psychiatric disorders during pregnancy include depression, anxiety disorders, bipolar disorder.
3. Untreated psychiatric illness in pregnancy can have adverse effects on both maternal and fetal health, including increased risk of preterm birth, low birth weight, and developmental issues in the child.
4. Management options in psychiatric illness during pregnancy are psychotherapy, medication, and lifestyle modifications, with careful consideration of potential risks and benefits.
5. Regular screening for psychiatric illness during prenatal care is essential to identify symptoms early and provide appropriate interventions.

References

1. Bie F, Yan X, Xing J, Wang L, Xu Y, Wang G, Wang Q, Guo J, Qiao J, Rao Z. Rising global burden of anxiety disorders among adolescents and young adults: trends, risk factors, and the impact of socioeconomic disparities and COVID-19 from 1990 to 2021. Front Psychiatry. 2024;15:1489427. https://doi.org/10.3389/fpsyt.2024.1489427. PMID: 39691785; PMCID: PMC11651023.
2. Kumarasinghe M, Herath MP, Hills AP, Ahuja KDK. Postpartum versus postnatal period: Do the name and duration matter? PLoS One. 2024;19(4):e0300118. https://doi.org/10.1371/journal.pone.0300118. PMID: 38669219; PMCID: PMC11051636.
3. Răchită AIC, Strete GE, Sălcudean A, Ghiga DV, Rădulescu F, Călinescu M, Nan AG, Sasu AB, Suciu LM, Mărginean C. Prevalence and Risk Factors of Depression and Anxiety among Women in the Last Trimester of Pregnancy: A Cross-Sectional Study. Medicina (Kaunas). 2023;59(6):1009. https://doi.org/10.3390/medicina59061009. PMID: 37374213; PMCID: PMC10303161.
4. Jayasankar P, Manjunatha N, Rao GN, Gururaj G, Varghese M, Benegal V; NMHS India National Collaborator Group. Epidemiology of common mental disorders: Results from National Mental Health Survey of India, 2016. Indian J Psychiatry. 2022;64(1):13–19. https://doi.org/10.4103/indianjpsychiatry.indianjpsychiatry_865_21. Epub 2022 Jan 21. PMID: 35400745; PMCID: PMC8992756.
5. Abdelhafez MA, Ahmed KM, Ahmed NM, Ismail M, Mohd Daud MNB, Ping NPT, Eldiasty A, Amri MFB, Jeffree MS, Kadir F, Pg Baharuddin DM, Bolong MFB, Hayati F, BtAzizan N, Sumpat D, Syed Abdul Rahim SS, Abdel Malek EH. Psychiatric illness and pregnancy: A literature review. Heliyon. 2023;9(11):e20958. https://doi.org/10.1016/j.heliyon.2023.e20958. PMID: 37954333; PMCID: PMC10632674.

6. Ellman LM, Murphy SK, Maxwell SD. Pre- and Perinatal Risk Factors for Serious Mental Disorders: Ethical Considerations in Prevention and Prediction Efforts. J Ethics Ment Health. 2018;10(Spec Iss 4):5. Epub 2018 Jun 15. PMID: 35309950; PMCID: PMC8932439.
7. Seemüller F. ICD-11 and mental disorders: important changes, controversies, and future directions. BMC Psychiatry. 2023;23(1):698. https://doi.org/10.1186/s12888-023-05186-w. PMID: 37749513; PMCID: PMC10521444.
8. Rai S, Pathak A, Sharma I. Postpartum psychiatric disorders: Early diagnosis and management. Indian J Psychiatry. 2015;57(Suppl 2):S216-21. https://doi.org/10.4103/0019-5545.161481. PMID: 26330638; PMCID: PMC4539865.
9. Treatment and Management of Mental Health Conditions During Pregnancy and Postpartum: ACOG Clinical Practice Guideline No. 5. Obstet Gynecol. 2023;141(6):1262–88. https://doi.org/10.1097/AOG.0000000000005202. PMID: 37486661.
10. Shelke A, Chakole S. A Review on Risk Factors of Postpartum Depression in India and Its Management. Cureus. 2022;14(9):e29150. https://doi.org/10.7759/cureus.29150. PMID: 36258936; PMCID: PMC9573019.

Dermatological Conditions During Pregnancy

19

Kavita Bisherwal and Vishal Pal

Pregnancy is a state of immunologic, metabolic, endocrine, and vascular changes, which increases susceptibility to various physiological and pathological changes of the skin and the appendages. These changes can be physiological, alteration of the preexisting skin diseases, or specific dermatoses of pregnancy. Physiological changes include altered pigmentation, changes in the collagen and elastic tissues as well as changes in the skin appendages including hair and nails. Preexisting skin diseases may improve or worsen in pregnancy due to alteration in the immunological profile. Some skin disorders are specifically seen during pregnancy and in the immediate postpartum state.

Pregnancy dermatoses can be broadly classified into the following types:

- Physiological changes of pregnancy
- Dermatoses affected by pregnancy
- Specific dermatoses of pregnancy

19.1 Physiological Changes of Pregnancy

Pregnancy-related skin changes are associated with increased cortisone levels and enhanced production of progesterone and estrogen related to increased maternal adrenal and pituitary gland activity along with an additional contribution from the developing fetal endocrine glands. This hormonal association of skin changes in

K. Bisherwal (✉) · V. Pal
Department of Dermatology & STD, University College of Medical Sciences & GTB Hospital (University of Delhi), New Delhi, India

R. Sharma, A. Kumar (eds.), *Systemic Disorders in Pregnancy*,
https://doi.org/10.1007/978-981-96-4876-4_19

pregnancy is also known as "skin changes of endocrine origin." The physiological skin changes that occur during pregnancy usually resolve or decrease in the postpartum period and do not cause any hazard to the mother and fetus.

Various physiological skin changes seen in pregnancy are enumerated in Table 19.1.

Table 19.1 Physiological changes during pregnancy

Pigmentary	Hyperpigmentation Linea nigra (Fig. 19.1) Melasma Areolar pigmentation Vulvar melanosis Pseudo-acanthotic changes
Hair	Hirsutism Postpartum telogen effluvium Diffuse hair thinning Postpartum male-pattern alopecia
Nails	Subungual hyperkeratosis Distal onycholysis Transverse grooving (Beau's lines) Brittleness
Glandular	Increased eccrine function (Hyperhidrosis) Increased sebaceous gland function (Seborrhea, Acne) Decreased apocrine function (Xerosis)
Connective tissue	Striae (Stretch marks) (Fig. 19.1)
Vascular	Spider angiomas Palmar erythema Pyogenic granuloma (granuloma gravidarum) Gingival hyperemia Varicose veins Hemorrhoids Nonpitting edema Purpura
Mucosa	Jacquemier-Chadwick sign (Erythema of the vestibule and vagina) Goodell's sign (Bluish discoloration of the cervix)

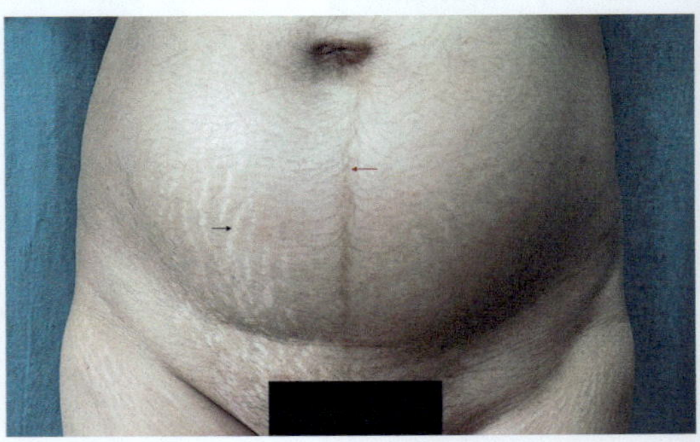

Fig. 19.1 Physiological skin changes of pregnancy seen as striae (black arrow) and linea nigra (red arrow) on the abdomen of a 25-year-old pregnant woman

19.2 Dermatoses Affected by Pregnancy

Pregnancy is an immunosuppressive state attributed to high serum levels of estrogen, which decrease cell-mediated immunity, neutrophil function, natural killer cells activity, and cause impairment of local antibody responses. Another important change is a shift from a predominantly Th1 lymphocyte profile to Th 2 profile leading to reduction in levels of IL 12 and γ-interferon and increased levels of IL- 4 and IL-10. Some drugs may also have to be discontinued during pregnancy due to their teratogenic potential. As a result, many preexisting dermatoses and tumors may remit, exacerbate, or ameliorate during pregnancy. The effect of pregnancy on various dermatoses is listed in Table 19.2.

Table 19.2 Effect of pregnancy on various dermatoses

Dermatoses	Effect of pregnancy
Inflammatory	
Atopic dermatitis Chronic plaque psoriasis Acne vulgaris Hidradenitis suppurativa Fox-Fordyce disease	Likely to worsen, also present for the first time in pregnancy in a person with an atopic diathesis Unaltered or improves. Deterioration likely in postpartum period. Psoriatic arthritis worsens or presents for the first time in pregnancy. Unpredictable, improves in early pregnancy and aggravates in late pregnancy Improves with postpartum disease flare Improves
Infection	
Fungal(candida) Herpes virus (HSV, VZV) Warts HIV Leprosy Trichomonas	Increased susceptibility to frequent and more severe infections
Autoimmune connective tissue	
SLE Systemic sclerosis Dermatomyositis	Flares or worsens if disease is active. Severe if it first presents in pregnancy Usually unaffected, may improve Unaltered, may worsen
Autoimmune vesiculobullous	
Pemphigus vulgaris and foliaceus	Develops or worsen during pregnancy, especially in the first or second trimester
Connective tissue	
Ehlers-Danlos syndrome Pseudoxanthoma elasticum Anetoderma	Likely to have complications such as postpartum bleeding, rupture of major vessels, poor wound healing, uterine lacerations, bladder and uterine prolapse, and abdominal hernia
Metabolic disorders	
Porphyria cutanea tarda Acrodermatitis enteropathica	Exacerbate during pregnancy Worsens and flares during early gestation

(continued)

Table 19.2 (continued)

Dermatoses	Effect of pregnancy
Tumors	
Hemangioma Glomus tumor Dermatofibroma Pyogenic granuloma Leiomyoma Desmoid tumor Keloid Neurofibroma Melanocytic nevus	May appear first time, enlarge, or increase in number
Miscellaneous	
Sarcoidosis	Often decreases during pregnancy
Erythema multiforme Bowenoid papulosis Mycosis fungoides Acanthosis nigricans	Exacerbation or new onset

19.3 Specific Dermatoses of Pregnancy (SDP)

It represents a heterogeneous group of inflammatory dermatoses of unknown etiology associated exclusively with pregnancy and/or the immediate postpartum period. The commonest presenting symptom is severe pruritus. The diagnosis can be sometimes challenging due to their varied clinical presentation and limited tests. Certain specific clinical features might help in distinguishing between various entities. Few SDP are associated with fetal risk and require antenatal surveillance. Early diagnosis and prompt management is therefore imperative.

19.3.1 Classification

Until 1982, no proper classification was present to classify pregnancy dermatoses. In 1982, Holmes et al. proposed a classification that classified pregnancy dermatoses into four major groups: pruritic folliculitis of pregnancy, polymorphic eruption of pregnancy, prurigo of pregnancy and pemphigoid gestationis. Shornick, in 1998, included intrahepatic cholestasis of pregnancy in the group. The most recent rationalized classification has been proposed by Ambros-Rudolph et al. [1] in 2006. They have grouped pruritic folliculitis of pregnancy and prurigo of pregnancy into atopic eruption of pregnancy. Classification of pregnancy dermatoses is given in Table 19.3.

Various pregnancy-specific dermatoses are discussed below.

1. *Pemphigoid Gestationis (PG)* (Herpes gestationis, Gestational pemphigoid)

Table 19.3 Classification of pregnancy dermatoses

Classification of pregnancy dermatoses	
Ambros-Rudolph et al. [1] *2006*	
(a) Pemphigoid gestationis/Herpes gestationis (b) Intrahepatic cholestasis of pregnancy (c) Polymorphic eruption of pregnancy, also known as pruritic urticarial papules and plaques of pregnancy (d) Atopic eruption of pregnancy	
Based on whether dermatosis is associated with fetal risk or not	
(a) Associated with fetal risk	ICP PG
(b) Not associated with fetal risk	AEP PEP

It is a rare autoimmune disorder that presents as an intensely pruritic, vesiculobullous eruption classically in late pregnancy (second and third trimesters) but can develop in any trimester or the immediate postpartum period. Approximately 1 in every 60,000 pregnancies develop PG. [2] Increase risk of other autoimmune diseases like Graves' disease as well as rare association with molar pregnancies and choriocarcinoma have been reported [3].

Pathogenesis PG is characterized by the deposition of autoreactive antibodies directed against BP-180 or bullous pemphigoid antigen 2 located in the hemidesmosomes of the dermo-epidermal junction. The non-collagenous (NC16A) domain of BP-180 is the immunodominant region. BP180 is found in the basement membrane zone (BMZ) of the skin, fetal membranes, and placental tissue suggesting that the disease could be triggered by a placental antigen that causes cross-reaction with the skin antigens. Placental trophoblasts and amniochorionic stromal cells show an abnormal expression of major histocompatibility complex (MHC) class II antigens leading to the presentation of BP180 protein to the antenatal women immune system. The maternal immune system recognizes these specific proteins as foreign, leading to anti-placental IgG antibodies formation, which can cross-react with the same BP180 proteins in the skin. Autoimmune response results due to the binding of these antibodies to the basement membrane. There is activation of complement, immune complexes deposition, and chemoattraction of eosinophils and granulocytes. These eosinophils and granulocytes subsequently degranulate and cause tissue damage and blister formation.

Clinical features It starts with the sudden onset of intense pruritus and inflammatory skin lesions on the abdomen in half of the cases. These skin lesions initially present as urticarial papules and annular plaques, followed by vesicles and finally large tense bullae on an erythematous background (Fig. 19.2). Skin lesions characteristically involve the umbilical region sparing the face and mucous membranes.

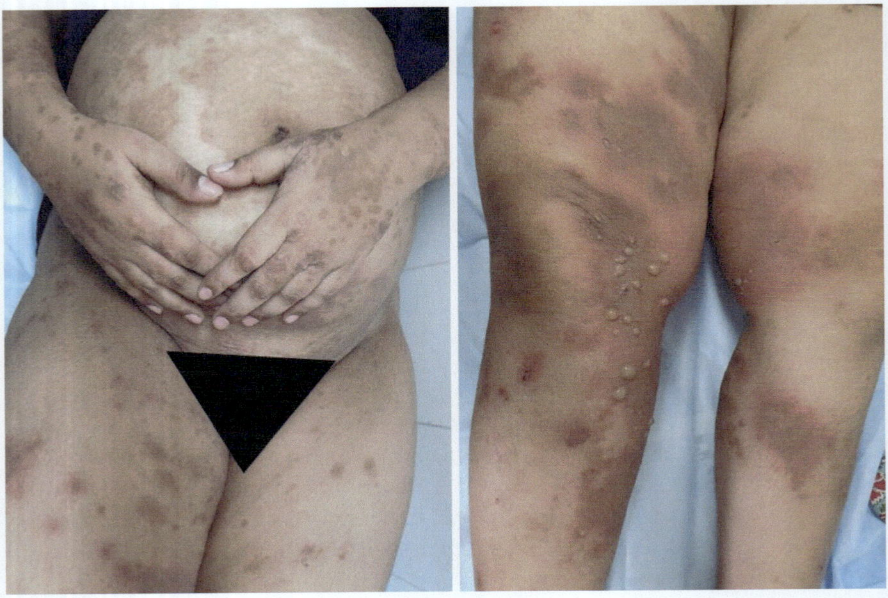

Fig. 19.2 Pemphigoid gestationis in a 27-year-old woman in third trimester, on treatment. Multiple vesicles and tense bullae are present on erythematous background along with urticarial plaques on lower limbs. Post-inflammatory hyperpigmentation of resolved lesions seen on abdomen (with characteristic involvement of umbilical region), distal upper limbs and lower limbs. (Photo courtesy: Dr. Archana Singal, Director Professor & Head, Department of Dermatology & STD, UCMS & GTB Hospital, Delhi)

Differential diagnosis Bullous pemphigoid, polymorphic eruption of pregnancy (in prebullous stage), urticaria (during the urticarial stage).

Diagnosis Histopathology is characterized by the presence of a subepidermal vesicle, spongiosis, and an infiltrate consisting of lymphocytes, histiocytes and eosinophils. Direct immunofluorescence (DIF) shows a linear deposition of C3 (complement 3) in 100% and IgG autoantibodies in 30% cases at the dermo-epidermal junction. Circulating autoantibodies against BP180 can be detected using complement-binding tests such as indirect immunofluorescence (IIF) or ELISA. IIF detects IgG autoantibodies targeting the basement membrane of the skin in 30–100% cases while ELISA reveals circulating IgG antibodies against BP180, particularly against the NC16A domain of BP180.

Course and prognosis Spontaneous resolution is common during late gestation. However, exacerbation at delivery or immediate postpartum occurs in 75% of cases. Recurrences in subsequent pregnancies are also common, seen in approximately one-third to half of the patients and are usually more severe and with an earlier onset [2]. PG is associated with increased risk of premature delivery and low birth weight; the risk of these complications correlates with the maternal disease severity [3, 4].

Around 10% of newborns may develop bullous lesions due to passive placental transfer of the anti–basement membrane zone antibody. These lesions are transient and usually require no therapy.

Treatment The therapy depends on the stage or severity of the disease and aims to diminish pruritus and prevent the development of new blisters. Corticosteroids are the mainstay of management. Topical corticosteroids along with emollients and oral antihistamines are sufficient for the mild cases. For severe cases, oral corticosteroids usually at a dose of 0.5–1 mg/kg are started and gradually tapered to a lower maintenance dose. The dose may have to be increased at delivery to prevent flare. Refractory cases may benefit from systemic immunoadsorption or intravenous immunoglobulin (IVIG). The duration of treatment postpartum is individualized, but the majority of patients are symptom-free after 6 months. In case of persisting (postnatal) symptoms, systemic immunosuppressants should be considered.

2. *Intrahepatic Cholestasis of Pregnancy (ICP)* (cholestasis of pregnancy, obstetric cholestasis, jaundice of pregnancy, prurigo/pruritus gravidarum)

It is a rare, genetically linked, reversible cholestasis that typically occurs in the third trimester of pregnancy in 70% of cases [5]. The incidence varies from 2–24 per 1000 pregnancies [5]. The salient features of ICP include (1) generalized pruritus with or without jaundice, (2) absence of primary skin lesions, (3) biochemical abnormalities consistent with cholestasis, and (4) resolution after delivery.

Pathogenesis Decreased excretion of bile acids results in elevated serum bile acids. This leads to severe pruritus in the mother and may have deleterious effects on the fetus due to passage in the fetal circulation resulting in acute fetal anoxia. The cause is multifactorial. ICP is associated with mutations in the multidrug resistance protein 3 of hepatobiliary transport (MDR3) involved in the biliary secretion of phospholipids, transport protein multidrug resistance-related protein 2 (MRP2), bile salt export pump (BSEP) protein-encoding gene, and cholestatic effects of 17-β-D-estradiol and sulfated metabolites of progesterone leading to changes in the composition of bile. This leads to a progressive increase in the total bile acid levels in the blood. Other contributing factors include cholestatic effects of progesterone, estrogens, and their metabolites, which increase during the pregnancy to reach peak levels in the third trimester and subsequently fall after birth, thus coinciding with the natural history of ICP.

Clinical features ICP is characterized by moderate-to-severe pruritus, either localized to the abdomen, palms, and soles or generalized and occurs in the last trimester of pregnancy. It is the only pregnancy dermatoses that presents without primary skin lesions. Secondary skin lesions in the form of linear excoriations, erosions, and excoriated papules develop due to scratching commonly on the extensor surfaces of the limbs, abdomen, back, and buttocks. Prurigo nodularis is seen in pruritus of longer duration. Mild jaundice may be present in only 10% cases [7].

Differential diagnosis Patients with ICP lack primary skin lesions. Other causes of liver derangement and jaundice, such as viral and nonviral hepatitis, medications, hepatobiliary obstruction, and other intrahepatic diseases (e.g., primary biliary cirrhosis) must be ruled out before making a diagnosis of ICP. Also, in patients presenting with generalized pruritus in pregnancy, other skin dermatoses such as scabies should also be considered.

Diagnosis Histopathologic findings are non-specific and immunofluorescence studies are negative. The most sensitive biochemical marker for the diagnosis is the level of total bile acids (TBA). The cut-off point for diagnosing ICP is defined concentration of TBA exceeding 10 micromoles/L; however, the risk of development of fetal complications occurs at concentrations above 40 micromoles/L. The concentrations of chenodeoxycholic acid (CDCA), cholic acid (CA), and the CA/CDCA ratio are better markers of the disease. The CA/CDCA greater than 1.5 is seen in patients with ICP. A 2–15-fold increase in serum levels of alanine transaminases is observed in 60–85% of patients.

Course and prognosis Pruritus typically persists until delivery. Spontaneous resolution of symptoms within 2–3 weeks of delivery is characteristic. ICP increases the risk of harmful effects to the fetus such as intrauterine asphyxia (up to 44%), premature delivery (20–60%), fetal bradycardia, meconium staining of the amniotic fluid, and stillbirth [6]. Maternal outcomes are generally favorable. Prolonged and severe cases of ICP predispose patients to intra and postpartum hemorrhage secondary to vitamin K depletion. It tends to recur in 45–90% of subsequent pregnancies in a more severe form [6]. Additionally, it also predisposes the affected women toward the development of cholelithiasis or gallbladder disease in later life. Thus, early diagnosis and prompt treatment along with obstetric surveillance is imperative.

Treatment The therapy aims to reduce serum bile acid levels and thereby ameliorate maternal symptoms and reduce fetal risks. The biochemical parameters such as transaminases, total bile acids, and blood coagulation profile should be analyzed on a regular basis. A close obstetric is indicated for the assessment of maternal and fetal well-being. Ursodeoxycholic acid (UDCA) is the treatment of choice administered orally at a dose of 15 mg/kg/day. Topical emollients and oral antihistamines can be added for symptomatic relief. UDCA exerts a hepatoprotective effect through the displacement of hydrophobic bile acids and sulfated progesterone metabolites. UDCA also removes bile acids from the fetus via the transplacental route.

3. *Pruritic Urticarial Papules and Plaques of Pregnancy (PUPPP)* (Polymorphic eruption of pregnancy, Nurse's late onset prurigo of pregnancy, toxic erythema of pregnancy, Toxemic rash of pregnancy)

PUPPP is a benign, intensely pruritic dermatosis that occurs classically in primigravida during the third trimester or immediate postpartum period and does not usually recur in subsequent pregnancies. With a prevalence of 1 in every 130–300 pregnancies, PUPPP is the second most common pregnancy-specific dermatoses [5].

Pathogenesis The exact etiology of PUPPP is still unknown. It has been associated with increased maternal weight gain and multiple gestation. Increased progesterone receptor immunoreactivity has also been suggested. Another possible explanation is rapid abdominal wall distension in primigravidae, which might damage the connective tissue due to over stretching. This leads to conversion of nonantigenic molecules to antigenic ones, thus triggering an inflammatory process.

Clinical features The eruption is polymorphous and occurs late in the third trimester. In the majority, it begins on the abdomen classically within the striae and shows periumbilical sparing. Lesions rapidly spread over a few days to involve the trunk, extremities, and breast. The face, palms, and soles are usually spared. The eruption starts as pruritic erythematous papules, which coalesce to form urticarial plaques. The morphology becomes polymorphic later with development of vesicles, generalized nonurticated erythema, targetoid, and eczematous lesions in approximately half of the patients (Fig. 19.3). Pruritus is usually localized to the involved skin.

Differential diagnosis The most important differential to exclude is pemphigoid gestationis. Contact dermatitis, urticaria, drug eruptions, and viral exanthems should also be considered.

Diagnosis Diagnosis is generally made clinically. Histopathology is nonspecific and shows focal epidermal changes such as parakeratosis, mild acanthosis with spongiotic dermatitis, and a nonspecific perivascular lympho-histiocytic infiltrate and eosinophils in the dermis. DIF studies and laboratory evaluation are routinely negative.

Course and prognosis PUPPP is a benign disorder with a tendency toward spontaneous resolution. The lesions usually resolve within 4–6 weeks, independent of delivery. Recurrence in subsequent pregnancies is uncommon; recurrent condition tends to be less severe than the first episode. It is not associated with fetal or maternal morbidity and mortality.

Treatment Symptomatic treatment is generally sufficient with topical corticosteroids and/or oral antihistamines. Short course of oral corticosteroids is needed in severe and distressing cases.

4. *Atopic eruption of pregnancy(AEP)* (Early-onset prurigo of pregnancy, prurigo of pregnancy, pruritic folliculitis of pregnancy, eczema of pregnancy, prurigo gestationis)

AEP is the most common pregnancy dermatosis accounting for up to 50% (36–49.7%) of all pregnancy dermatoses. The main characteristics include (a) onset

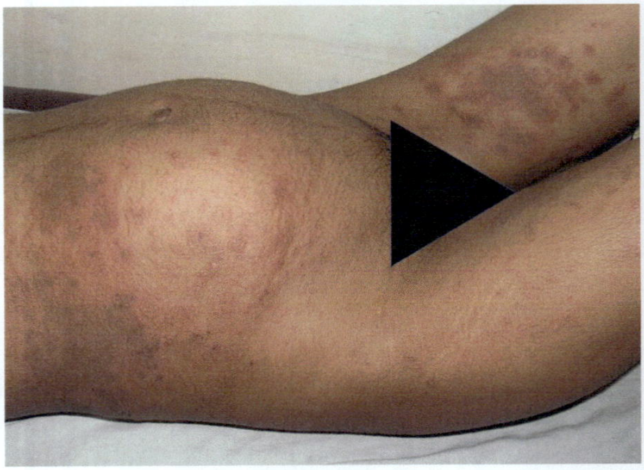

Fig. 19.3 Pruritic urticarial papules and plaques of pregnancy (PUPPP) at 30 weeks gestation in a 29-year-old primigravida. Polymorphic lesions in the form of erythematous papules, plaques, as well as urticarial, targetoid, and eczematous lesions on thighs and abdomen with sparing of the periumbilical region. (Photo courtesy: Dr. Archana Singal, Director Professor & Head, Department of Dermatology & STD, UCMS & GTB Hospital, Delhi)

before the third trimester, (b) presence of an atopic background in the patient or family, (c) recurrence in subsequent pregnancies, and d) elevation of serum total IgE level.

Pathogenesis It has been related to pregnancy-specific immunological changes characterized by low cellular immunity and reduced Th1 cytokines production due to physiological switch from cell-mediated to humoral immunity (Th1 to Th2 shift) occurring during gestation.

Clinical features AEP is characterized by intense pruritus (with the tendency to worsen during the evening or overnight), papular/prurigo lesions, and patchy eczematous skin lesions. Onset is usually early in the first trimester or the second trimester. There are two types of AEP: E-type(eczematous) and P-type (papular/prurigo type). Two-thirds of the patients present with classic eczematous eruption primarily affecting flexural surfaces and the face (E-type). The remaining third presents with discrete, pruritic, excoriated papules with a predilection for extensor surfaces predominantly on the trunk and limbs (P-type) (Fig. 19.4). The coexistence of E and P types can occur. Approximately, 80% of the AEP patients experience an atopic eruption for the first time (or after a long remission) [8]. Minor features of eczema, xerosis, keratosis pilaris, and hyperlinear palms may be noted.

Differential diagnosis PEP, ICP, and other pruritic dermatological conditions like scabies and drug eruptions.

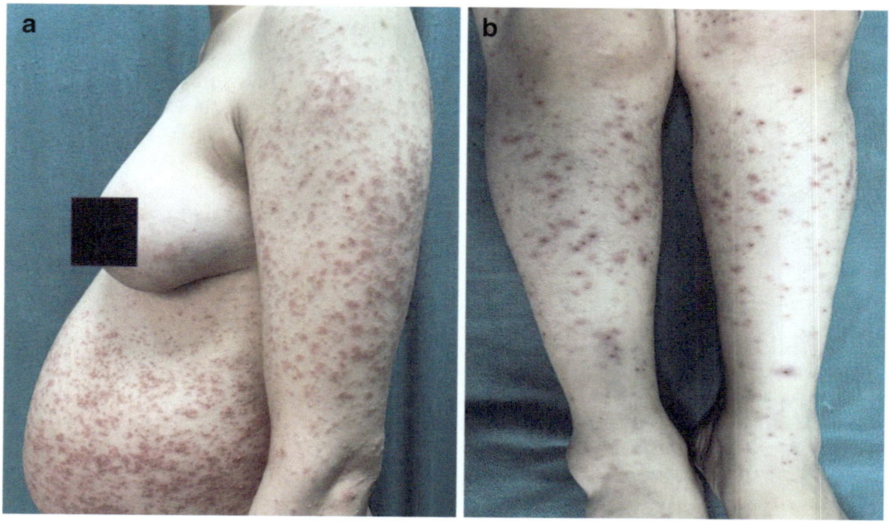

Fig. 19.4 Atopic eruption of pregnancy in a 30-year-old woman presenting as discrete, pruritic, excoriated papules on abdomen and extensor surfaces of arm and legs at second trimester of pregnancy

Diagnosis Diagnosis of AEP is largely clinical and biopsy from the lesions shows nonspecific changes such as hyperkeratosis, parakeratosis, spongiosis, and perivascular lympho-histiocytic infiltrate. Skin immunofluorescence testing (DIF and IIF) is negative. Elevated serum IgE levels are seen in 20–70% of women with AEP.

Course and prognosis Rapid improvement of the skin lesions usually occurs with therapy. Recurrence with subsequent pregnancies is common in patients with atopic diathesis. The maternal and fetal prognosis is excellent. The infant may be at increased risk for atopic dermatitis later on in life.

Treatment Mild to moderate disease shows rapid response with emollients, topical corticosteroids, and antihistamines. For severe recalcitrant cases, a short tapering course of oral corticosteroid may be required.

Pregnancy is a state of altered hormonal and metabolic adaptations, which cause a variety of complex physiological changes in the skin of pregnant patients. These physiological skin changes are benign and self-limiting and do not cause any hazard to the mother and fetus. Many preexisting dermatoses may be modified during pregnancy mainly due to pregnancy-specific immunological changes. Specific dermatoses of pregnancy can be associated with severe fetal outcomes such as fetal distress, premature birth and stillbirth, hence regular follow-up, continuous fetal monitoring, and timely intervention is required.

Salient features of specific dermatoses of pregnancy are listed in Table 19.4.

Table 19.4 Salient features of specific dermatoses of pregnancy

Pemphigoid gestationis	Intensely pruritic, vesiculobullous eruption occurring on abdomen characteristically involving umbilical region. Classically occurs in late pregnancy (second and third trimester). Recurrences in subsequent pregnancies are common with a more severe and an earlier onset. Associated with other autoimmune diseases and an increased risk of premature delivery and low birth weight
Intrahepatic cholestasis of pregnancy	Reversible form of cholestasis occurring in third trimester. Associated with biochemical abnormalities and increased risk of harmful effects to the fetus. Lacks primary cutaneous lesions. Symptoms remit within 2–3 weeks of delivery, but tends to recur in subsequent pregnancies.
Pruritic urticarial papules and plaques of pregnancy	Benign disorder with a tendency toward spontaneous resolution. Classically seen in primigravida during third trimester or immediate postpartum. Eruption is polymorphous and begins on the abdomen classically within the striae with periumbilical sparing and involves trunk, extremities, and breast. Recurrence in subsequent pregnancies is uncommon
Atopic eruption of pregnancy	Most common pregnancy dermatosis usually occurs early in first or second trimester. Resembles classic atopic dermatitis (E-type) or papular/prurigo lesions (p-type). Recurrence with subsequent pregnancies is common in patients with atopic diathesis. The maternal and fetal prognosis is excellent

Brief diagnostic approach for various specific dermatoses of pregnancy is given in Flow Chart 19.1.

Key Points

1. Pregnancy dermatoses are inflammatory skin disorders that occur during pregnancy or immediate postpartum period.
2. The physiological skin changes are benign and self-limiting. The pathological changes cause alteration of the preexisting skin diseases or specific dermatoses of pregnancy.
3. Pregnancy-specific dermatoses include pemphigoid gestationis, intrahepatic cholestasis of pregnancy, pruritic urticarial papules and plaques of pregnancy, and atopic eruption of pregnancy.
4. Correct diagnosis is important for the treatment and for the prognosis of mother and child as some pregnancy dermatosis can be associated with fetal and maternal health risk.

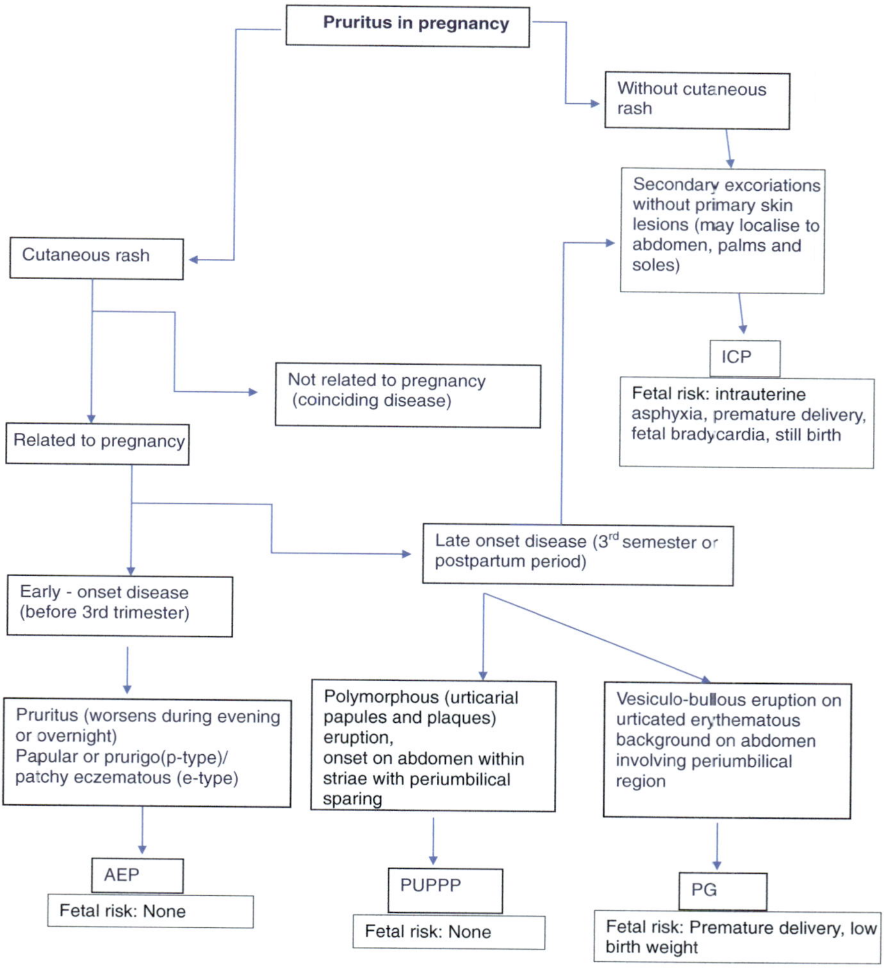

Flow Chart 19.1 Brief diagnostic approach for various specific dermatoses of pregnancy

References

1. Ambros-Rudolph CM, Mullegger RR, Vaughan-Jones SA, Kerl H, Black MM. The specific dermatoses of pregnancy revisited and reclassified: Results of a retrospective two-center study on 505 pregnant patients. Am Acad Dermatol. 2006;54:395–404.
2. Savervall C, Sand FL, Thomsen SF. Pemphigoid gestationis: current perspectives. Clin Cosmet Investig Dermatol. 2017;10:441–9.
3. Engineer L, Bhol K, Ahmed AR. Pemphigoid gestationis: a review. Am J Obstet Gynecol. 2000;183(2):483–91.

4. Hallaji Z, Mortazavi H, Ashtari S, Nikoo A, Abdollahi M, Nasimi M. Pemphigoid gestationis: Clinical and histologic features of twenty-three patients. Int J Womens Dermatol. 2016;3(2):86–90.
5. Kroumpouzos G, Cohen LM. Dermatoses of pregnancy. J Am Acad Dermatol. 2001;45(1):1–22.
6. Piechota J, Jelski W. Intrahepatic cholestasis in pregnancy: review of the literature. J Clin Med. 2020;9(5):1361.
7. Kang S, Amagai M, Bruckner AL, Enk AH, Margolis DJ, McMichael AJ, Orringer JS, editors. Fitzpatrick's Dermatology, 9e. McGraw Hill; 2019.
8. Roth MM, Cristodor P, Kroumpouzos G. Prurigo, pruritic folliculitis, and atopic eruption of pregnancy: Facts and controversies. Clin Dermatol. 2016;34(3):392–400.

Neoplastic Conditions in Pregnancy 20

Bhagyalaxmi Nayak, Sony Nanda, and S. K. Giri

Any new, uncontrolled growth of cells, not under any physiologic control is termed as neoplasia. Neoplasms are divided into benign and malignant. Benign neoplasms proliferate and divide, but do not invade the surrounding tissues, nor metastasize, whereas neoplasms that invade and/or metastasize are malignant.

Neoplasms both benign and malignant can occur during pregnancy. In this chapter, we plan to discuss some neoplasms (both benign and malignant) encountered during pregnancy.

The most common ovarian tumors encountered during pregnancy are functional cysts diagnosed incidentally during the first trimester ultrasound, which often regress spontaneously. The most frequent benign ovarian tumor diagnosed during pregnancy are dermoid cysts and cystadenomas.

Benign neoplasms are common and include leiomyomas, ovarian neoplasms, and endocervical polyps. Cancer in these organs may also complicate pregnancy, and of these, cervical neoplasia makes up the majority [1].

20.1 Benign Neoplasia

20.1.1 Cervix

20.1.1.1 Endocervical Polyp

Usually appears as elongated fleshy masses of different sizes arising from the endocervical canal and protruding through the external os. May present with bleeding per vaginum.

S. Nanda · S.K. Giri · B. Nayak (✉)
Department of Gynaecologic Oncology, AHPGIC, Cuttack, Orissa, India

R. Sharma, A. Kumar (eds.), *Systemic Disorders in Pregnancy*,
https://doi.org/10.1007/978-981-96-4876-4_20

Management

Asymptomatic lesions may be left alone. Symptomatic, bigger polyp needs removal and histopathological examination, as dysplasia is diagnosed in up to 0.5%, and malignant transformation in up to 0.1% [2, 3].

20.1.1.2 Epithelial Neoplasia

The incidence of abnormal cervical cytology during pregnancy is as high as that of nonpregnant women. Pregnancy provides an opportunity to screen an unscreened woman. Colposcopy and targeted biopsy may have to be performed on detection of cytological abnormality to rule out malignancy.

20.1.2 Uterus

20.1.2.1 Leiomyoma (Fig. 20.1)

The incidence of leiomyoma during pregnancy is about 2% [4, 5].

It does not require intervention unless complication(s) is encountered. Some myomas can undergo infarction, which is termed red degeneration with associated acute abdominal pain and low-grade fever. Analgesics and close observation usually take care of this condition and rarely myomectomy may be required. Twisted pedunculated myoma requires laparoscopic removal.

20.1.2.2 Endometrial Lesions

Very rare. Occasionally endometriosis can develop after cesarean or episiotomy.

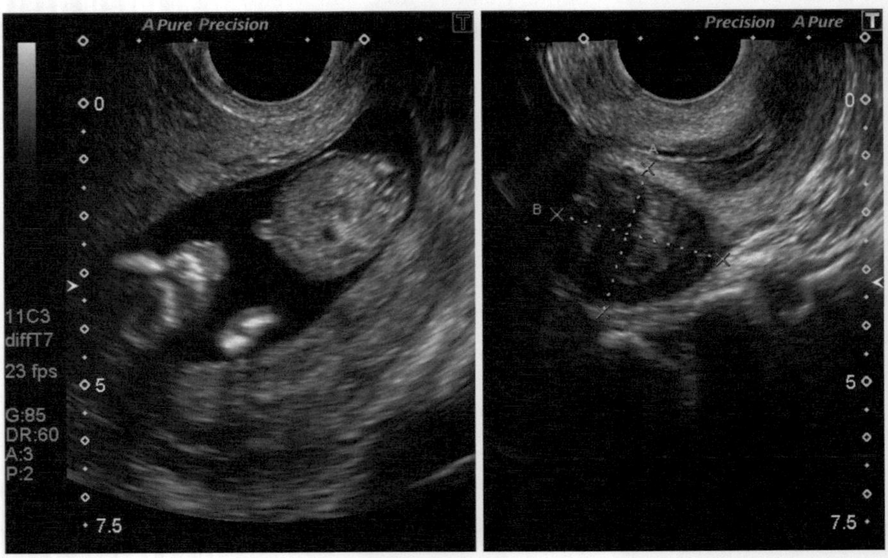

Fig. 20.1 Myoma with early pregnancy

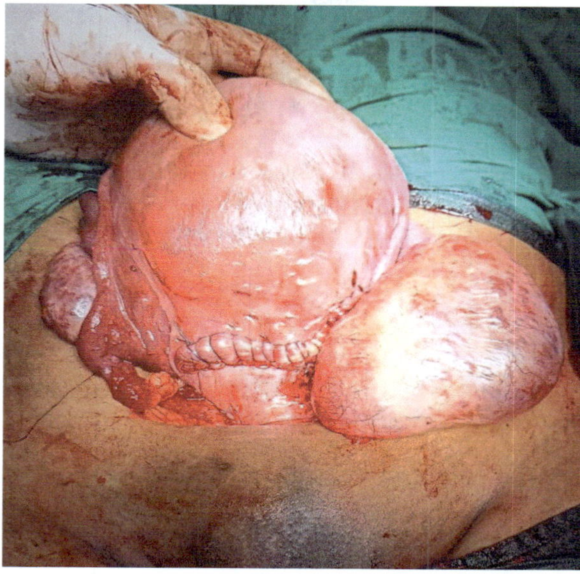

Fig. 20.2 Ovarian tumor at LSCS

20.1.3 Ovary (Fig. 20.2)

The common types of ovarian masses are corpus luteum cysts, endometriomas, benign cystadenomas, and mature cystic teratomas. Mostly they are asymptomatic, can present with acute or chronic abdominal pain due to torsion, rupture, or hemorrhage.

Proper evaluation to rule out malignancy by ultrasound or MRI is required. When torsion is diagnosed, a laparoscopic or laparotomy procedure should be performed, and either cystectomy or oophorectomy is required. There is a concern about pregnancy loss if an oophorectomy is done in early pregnancy, hence should be avoided. If mandatory, progestational support has to be ~~is~~ advocated.

Pregnancy Luteoma: A rare tumor, develops from the effect of various pregnancy hormones on ovarian stroma. The size varies from microscopic to >20 cm. The features confuse with that of granulosa cell tumor, thecoma, Sertoli–Leydig cell tumor. Does not require treatment unless complicated with torsion, hemorrhage, torsion, etc.

20.2 Malignant Lesions

As pregnant women are young, malignant tumors and borderline ovarian tumors are relatively uncommon. Malignant tumors during pregnancies complicate up to 1 per 1000–2000 cases and their prevalence is increasing due to sociodemographic causes like delay in marriages and advanced maternal age at the time of starting a family [6–8].

Breast, cervix, ovary, thyroid, and hematologic malignancies are the most common malignancies during pregnancy [8, 9].

Lung and gastric cancers though less frequent are associated with a worse prognosis [10, 11].

Furthermore, noninvasive prenatal testing (NIPT), one of the newer screening techniques for fetal aneuploidies, may unintentionally aid in the detection of concealed cancers in expectant mothers by disclosing aberrant genome representation profiles such as somatic copy number variants [12, 13].

20.2.1 Diagnosis

Pregnancy by itself is not a risk factor for cancer [2, 7]. However, because some symptoms could be mistaken for the effects of the pregnancy itself, cancer diagnoses are frequently delayed [2, 3]. The pregnant uterus and breast alterations might make physical examination challenging. Additionally, the physician could be less inclined to order the necessary tests due to worries about the accuracy of laboratory results or the potential risks associated with radiologic testing.

Obstetricians face particular obstacles in management and treatment because they must deal with moral, psychological, and therapeutic issues [2]. Therefore, treatment planning has to be individualized with a multidisciplinary team (MDT) including a gynecological oncologist, radiologist, medical oncologist, and perinatologist since treatment decisions involve both the maternal and fetal outcomes [1]. A thorough examination, including palpation of breasts, lymphnodes, and examination of the cervix with pap tests, and possibly further investigations are essential in diagnosing.

20.2.1.1 Laboratory Testing

It should be kept in mind that pregnancy-induced elevation of tumor markers does occur leading to low sensitivity and specificity of the same during pregnancy. CA 15–3 used in breast cancer, CA 125 used in epithelial ovarian cancer, and squamous cell carcinoma (SCC) antigen can be elevated during normal pregnancy, whereas levels of Inhibin B, anti-Mullerian hormone (AMH), and lactate dehydrogenase (LDH) are not altered [14].

B-hCG, and alpha-fetoprotein used in germ cell tumors are physiologically elevated in pregnancy.

20.2.1.2 Imaging

When choosing the appropriate imaging methods, fetal safety, risk of metastases, and pregnancy-induced changes that might hamper interpretation of imaging must be kept in mind.

Radiation exposure greater than 100 mGy has been linked to pediatric malignancies and fetal anomalies [8]. Adequate abdominal shielding should be given if X-rays are required. Due to the breast tissue's density and physiological hypervascularity, mammography images are difficult to interpret during pregnancy [15].

Because of the unacceptable cumulative radiation and contrast dosages, computed tomography (CT scan) is best avoided during pregnancy. Due to the potential risk of radiation exposure to the fetus, the use of positron-emission tomography (PET) imaging during pregnancy is controversial [16].

Ultrasound is the most commonly employed diagnostic technique. It is noninvasive and useful for guided lymph node and breast biopsies.

It is safe to have magnetic resonance imaging (MRI) during any trimester of pregnancy. It is the preferred imaging method for staging and diagnosis. Contrast agents are better avoided [17].

Tissue histopathology offers a conclusive diagnosis of tumor type and grade. It is important to inform the pathologist that the patient is pregnant to prevent misdiagnosis due to pregnancy-related tissue alterations [18].

20.2.2 Specific Cancers

20.2.2.1 Breast Cancer

The most frequent cancer encountered during pregnancy and the postpartum period is breast cancer. Pregnancy-related alterations in the breast and diagnostic obstacles that cause these tumors to remain undiscovered until the first postpartum year may be the cause of the difficulties and delay in diagnosis. Pregnant women who get breast cancer typically have larger tumors, are node-positive, Stage II or III high-grade invasive ductal carcinomas, and are typically ER/PR/HER2/neu-negative.

It is best to get a diagnosis as early as possible. The best imaging modalities are mammography with shielding and ultrasonography. The recommended modality for confirmation is core needle biopsy [19].

Metastatic workup for breast cancer during pregnancy should include a chest X-ray, liver ultrasound, and a non-contrast skeletal MRI, preferably a diffusion-weighted imaging (DWI) MRI if available [20].

Treatment aims to achieve local control and prevent distant metastases; Pregnant patients are treated similarly to nonpregnant women. In the initial trimester, the preferred course of treatment is modified radical mastectomy with axillary staging. Radiation therapy can be administered after delivery and adjuvant chemotherapy can be given in the second trimester [21]. It is safe to perform breast-conserving surgery during the second and third trimesters.

In the second and third trimesters, adjuvant chemotherapy using anthracycline-based regimens, such as different combinations of doxorubicin, fluorouracil, and cyclophosphamide, might be initiated. There have been reports of oligohydramnios and anhydramnios with trastuzumab, hence it is contraindicated. Because of the increased risk of birth abnormalities, endocrine medications such as tamoxifen, aromatase inhibitors, and LHRH analogues should not be used while pregnant. It is advisable to counsel pregnancy termination if a woman becomes pregnant while taking tamoxifen [19].

There is no significant survival difference in treated breast cancer in pregnancy and nonpregnant states considering all prognostic factors [22, 23].

20.2.2.2 Cervical Cancer

In pregnant women, cervical cancer is commonly diagnosed at an early age and stage compared to nonpregnant women and mostly in the first and second trimesters [24].

The same FIGO 2018 staging applies to these patients. Staging is mainly clinical but MRI without contrast can be done in all trimesters with no or minimal risks. Comprehensive treatment of pregnancy complicated with cervical cancer depends upon the histopathological type, stage of disease, lymph node status, gestational age, and desire to continue pregnancy.

Management of Preinvasive Disease

Treatment can be deferred until 6–8 weeks after delivery in CIN 1 to CIN 3 [25]. However, to assess lesion size and disease progress, a colposcopy is performed in each trimester. Because of increased vascularity and genital edema, it is challenging to perform a colposcopy during pregnancy [26].

Management of Invasive Disease (Fig. 20.3)

(a) *Pregnancy Continuation Desired with GA Less than 22 Weeks*

Tumor size and lymph node involvement are the most important prognostic factors in patients with cervical cancer in pregnancy. MRI is not a reliable modality for the detection of nodal metastases.

Lymph node staging can be done by both laparotomy and laparoscopy. It is advisable to restrict laparoscopy up to 14 to 16 weeks of gestation and reserve laparotomy beyond 16 weeks up to 22 weeks, beyond which lymph node retrieval is inadequate. However, lymphadenectomy is not indicated in Stage- IAI without LVSI [18].

Sentinel lymph node biopsy is contraindicated during pregnancy using patent blue (risk of anaphylactic reaction) and technetium (high radiation dose) but indocyanine green is a reasonable alternative.

If LN Negative

Stage IA1 with LVSI- conization is adequate and relatively safe. The cone margin should not be too deep to damage the fetal membranes and preventive cerclage can be done to reduce the risk of premature birth [25].

Best performed between 12 and 20 weeks and keeping in mind the risk of hemorrhage and pregnancy complications. Excision of a coin-shaped specimen can prevent many complications [27].

Stage I A2-I B1 ($\leq$2 cm size)—Conization or simple trachelectomy (excision of the cervix 1 cm above the tumor border) can be done with the fetus in situ [28].

In stage 1B2, neoadjuvant chemotherapy (NACT) is followed by cesarean radical hysterectomy after fetal maturity is advocated.

The parametrial extension in such cases is seen in less than 1% of women. Radical trachelectomy during pregnancy was found to have too many patient and fetal complications and is therefore discouraged during pregnancy [18].

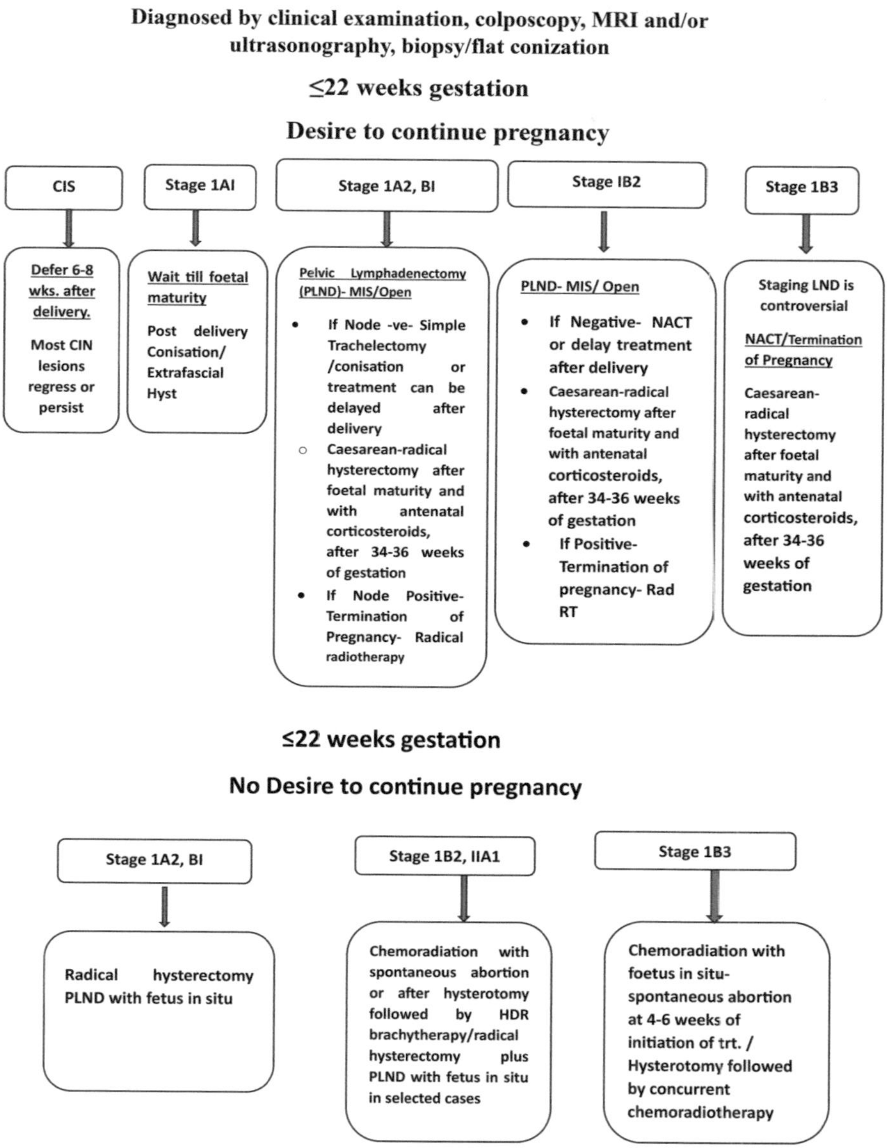

Fig. 20.3 Algorithm for management of cervical cancer in pregnancy

If LN Positive

In patients with lymph node metastases, termination of pregnancy is recommended and they should receive primary chemoradiation.

(b) *Pregnancy Continuation Desired with GA More than 22 Weeks*

In stages, IB: >2-cm tumors (IB2, IB3) neoadjuvant chemotherapy (NACT) is a good approach to halt the disease progression, though the efficacy is under clinical trial. Delayed treatment after delivery with regular follow-up can be started in cases with gestation beyond 22 weeks, though follow-up without treatment may compromise the prognosis [18].

In locally advanced cancer and advanced pregnancy NACT can also be given to prolong pregnancy duration until fetal maturity (35–36 weeks) when cesarean delivery followed by concurrent chemoradiation is recommended [29].

The most commonly used regimen in pregnancy is platinum-based, mainly cisplatin (50–100 mg/m^2) and paclitaxel (175 mg/m^2), every 3 weekly for six cycles or cisplatin alone. Due to the risk of spontaneous onset of labor after 35 weeks, it is better not to give the last dose after 34 weeks. It will also prevent fetal bone marrow suppression and accumulation of cytotoxic drugs in neonates. It is recommended to discontinue chemotherapy 3 weeks before delivery because of the risk of hematopoietic suppression in the mother and the newborn [30].

Optimal Timing and Route of Delivery

Due to the risks associated with preterm birth, it is reasonable to delay delivery until 37–39 weeks of gestation but premature delivery occurs in some patients because of tumor progression. The route of delivery is determined by the presence or absence of a tumor. In stages, IA1, IA2, and IB1, vaginal delivery is possible after conization or simple trachelectomy. In the presence of a tumor, a C-section is the preferred mode of delivery to prevent an episiotomy scar recurrence. In the case of locally advanced disease, transverse incisions during cesarean section should be avoided because of the risk of cutting through the tumor. Classical vertical incision avoids damaging the blood vessels of tumors and is preferred. Postoperatively placenta should be sent for histopathological examination to determine the presence of any metastasis. C-section can be combined with simple or radical trachelectomy, and simple or radical hysterectomy depending upon the stage of disease and further desire for fertility [21].

(c) *Pregnancy Non-Preserving Management*

When patients are unwilling to continue the pregnancy in early-stage disease, radical hysterectomy in an operable disease (IA2-IB2) with fetus in utero (during the first- or early-second trimester). Radical hysterectomy in the late second trimester also can be done after hysterotomy. It is quite a safe procedure with a good oncological outcome. Tissue edema makes dissection easier. Careful handling of engorged vessels is important to prevent unnecessary blood loss.

In IB3 and advanced disease higher stages, (stage IIB or higher or lymph node metastases), treatment is by chemoradiation in the first trimester with fetus in utero. Fetal death occurs and spontaneous abortion occurs within 4–6 weeks after the initiation of treatment. In the second trimester hysterotomy is performed to reduce obstetric complications before chemoradiotherapy [18].

20.2.2.3 Ovarian Cancer (Fig. 20.4)

Incidence of adnexal masses is found in the tune of 1 in 600 to 1 in 1500 pregnancies. Out of which about 1–3% are malignant and the rest are benign. Seventy percent of adnexal masses that are discovered during pregnancy dissolve by the second trimester, and the majority of them are functional cysts [31].

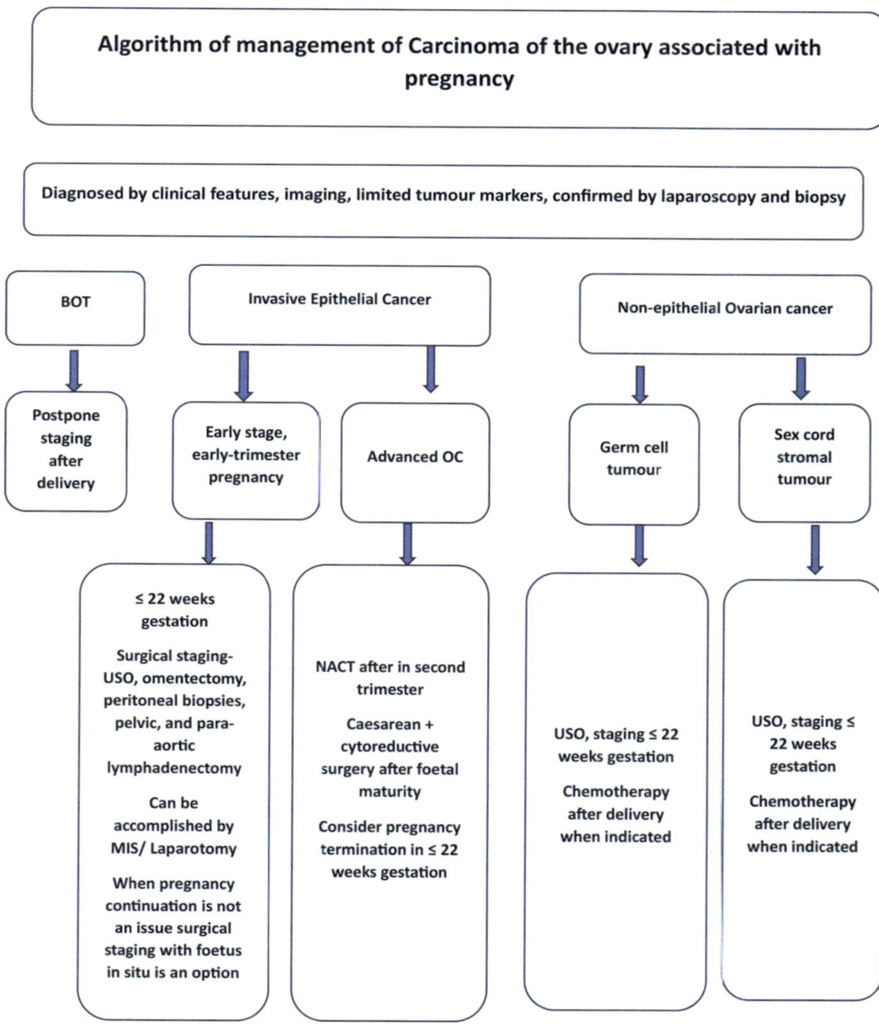

Fig. 20.4 Algorithm for management of carcinoma ovary with pregnancy

Germ cell tumor is the most commonly encountered, followed by sex cord-stromal tumors, borderline tumors, and epithelial cancers [31].

Most of the malignant tumors are detected at Stage I during routine ultrasonic screening. Abdominal combined with transvaginal ultrasound can detect the adnexal masses with reasonable accuracy. Employment of IOTA can differentiate benign, borderline, and malignant adnexal masses and treatment can be directed accordingly. However, MRI offers the most accurate diagnosis in assessing peritoneal disease extent and nodal involvement [32].

As CA 125, alpha-fetoprotein, and beta hCG are normally raised during pregnancy, they are not useful markers. However, as Inhibin B, anti-Müllerian hormone, HE4, CA 19–9, and lactate dehydrogenase are not raised during pregnancy, their estimation can be of use during pregnancy [25].

20.2.3 Management

20.2.3.1 Borderline Ovarian Tumor (BOT)

BOTs are managed as in nonpregnant patients. The treatment of choice is thorough surgical staging with peritoneal wash cytology, unilateral salpingo-oophorectomy, omentectomy, and peritoneal biopsies. As pelvic peritoneal assessment is difficult, and BOTs in pregnancy are more aggressive, restaging by laparoscopy may be planned after delivery [33].

20.2.3.2 Invasive Epithelial Ovarian Cancer (EOC)-

As mentioned earlier, they are detected in the early stage. In a situation when the patient is keen to continue the pregnancy and is in the early second trimester (around 22 weeks), surgical staging procedures including unilateral salpingo-oophorectomy, omentectomy, peritoneal biopsies, pelvic, and para-aortic lymphadenectomy can be undertaken if feasible without much handling of the gravid uterus [34].

This can be accomplished by both laparotomy and laparoscopy, keeping in mind that no spillage occurs during surgery. Adjuvant platinum-based chemotherapy can safely be administered in the second and third trimester. However, withholding of chemotherapy is required 3 weeks before expected delivery or after 35 weeks of gestation to avoid myelosuppression in neonates. Bevacizumab is not recommended during pregnancy. Vaginal delivery is an ideal route in such patients treated surgically. Breastfeeding is not advisable during therapy.

In the advanced stage of the disease in the first and second trimesters of pregnancy, and when the continuation of pregnancy is not an issue, primary surgical staging with fetus in situ followed by adjuvant chemotherapy is the treatment of choice. In the late second trimester and third trimesters or if the patient is keen on continuing pregnancy, NACT is recommended until fetal maturity is achieved. Cesarean delivery along with cytoreductive surgery is a feasible option, with similar oncological outcome as nonpregnant women [35].

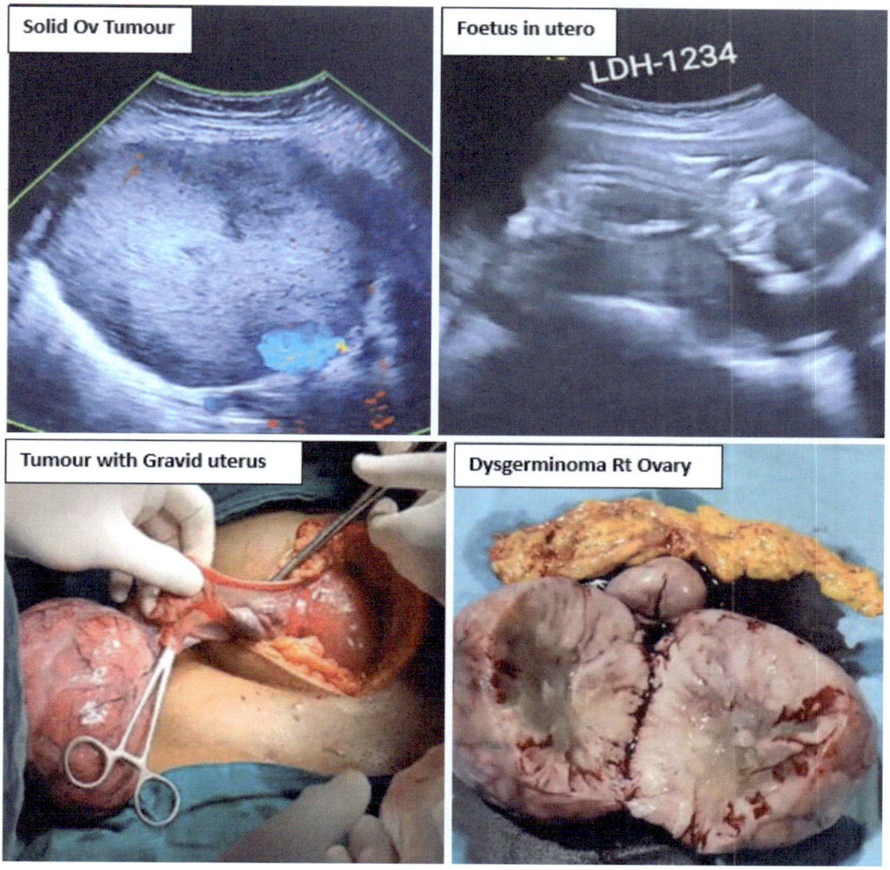

Fig. 20.5 Pregnancy with dysgerminoma ovary

20.2.3.3 Germ Cell and Sex Cord-Stromal Tumors (Fig. 20.5)

They are treated in the same way as in nonpregnant women in the early stages. In advanced stages, NACT with a BEP regimen is not recommended because of the probability of fetal growth restriction and high neonatal complication.

20.2.4 Vulval Cancer

Incidence is very low. The suspicious lesion should be biopsied. Once diagnosed, treatment is the same as for nonpregnant women. Radical local excision with unilateral or bilateral lymph node dissection or sentinel node procedure (SNLB) is followed. If lymph nodal involvement is detected after SNLB of lymphadenectomy, termination of early pregnancy and planned delivery in the late trimester to enable the application of inguinofemoral radiotherapy. A 6–8 weeks delay of radiotherapy is acceptable. If lymph node metastasis is detected preoperatively, termination of pregnancy is advised and concurrent chemoradiotherapy is advocated.

Delivery should be by cesarean section to avoid trauma to vulval lesions and surgical wounds [18].

20.2.5 Malignant Melanoma

Even though skin changes during pregnancy are common, a thorough evaluation of any suspected lesion is necessary [36].

Surgical excision combined with a lymphadenectomy should only be done as a last resort for treating early-stage melanoma. Due to the high risk of placental metastases, a thorough histologic examination of the placenta is necessary [37].

Novel targeted or immunotherapies as advocated in nonpregnant states, are not compatible with pregnancy and, hence not advocated.

20.2.6 Hematological Malignancies

Hodgkin lymphoma, with an incidence of 1 per 6000 births, is the most prevalent hematological malignancy in pregnancy, followed by leukemia (1 per 75,000–100,000 pregnancies) and non-Hodgkin lymphoma [38].

Treatment for lymphoma is the same as for women who are not pregnant, and pregnancy termination is advised if chemotherapy is required during the first trimester [39].

Regardless of gestational age, leukemia treatment must begin right away because waiting worsens the disease outcome [39].

20.2.7 Cancer Treatment and Pregnancy

20.2.7.1 Surgery

Surgery can be performed during pregnancy whenever indicated to diagnose, treat, and stage cancer. It should be individualized and an expert team of gynecologic oncologists, obstetricians, anesthesiologists, and pediatricians familiar with the management should be involved in the management. The optimal time for surgery is during the early second trimester to avoid spontaneous abortion. Because of the size of the uterus, surgery during the second trimester is technically less complex than during the third. The uterus should not be handled excessively. After the first trimester, oophorectomy can be performed safely on one or both sides. However, at any gestational age definitive surgery can be performed with a fetus in situ. Pelvic lymphadenectomy can be performed either by laparoscopy or laparotomy before 22 weeks, as it becomes difficult after this period of gestation. Because of the possibility of aspiration, regional anesthesia is favored over general anesthesia whenever feasible. During surgery, a lateral tilt could lessen the risk of aortocaval compression.

When delivery is planned, corticosteroids are used to improve lung maturity and premature labor should be avoided with tocolytics [18].

20.2.7.2 Radiotherapy

Planning radiotherapy for a pregnant patient is very important. Reducing both direct and indirect radiation exposure to the fetus is the responsibility of the physicist and radiation oncologist. Fetal dosages shouldn't go over 50–100 mGy [39].

Pelvic radiotherapy should be avoided when pregnancy continuation is a concern. Even with appropriate shielding, radiation leakage and scattering remain a problem. Because of the heavy materials employed, shielding the gravid uterus can be challenging, particularly in advanced pregnancy.

20.2.7.3 Chemotherapy

Most chemotherapeutic drugs can be used quite safely after the first trimester. Chemotherapeutic drugs vary greatly in their transplacental transport; for example, paclitaxel crosses the placenta at a low rate, anthracyclines cross the placenta at an intermediate rate, and carboplatin crosses the placenta at a high rate. Despite this, the growing baby appears to be unaffected by carboplatin given after 12–14 weeks of pregnancy [40].

The risk of congenital malformation is closely correlated with gestational age; before 12 weeks, anomalies of blood, ocular, and auditory systems are a possibility, and risk is reduced after complete organogenesis.

As myelosuppression is an effect of chemotherapy, the risk of maternal infection is increased.

The long-term effect of chemotherapy on children does not show any significant impact on general health, cognitive development, or cardiac function in comparison to the general population.

Breastfeeding should be avoided within 3 weeks from the last chemotherapy [41]. The placenta should be examined for evidence of metastasis [18].

20.2.7.4 Hormonal and Targeted Therapy

The available evidence is not in favor of the use of hormonal and targeted therapy during pregnancy hence not to be used [42].

20.2.7.5 Immunotherapy

Anti-PD1/PDL1 are not safe in pregnancy.

20.3 Conclusion

Medical experts, patients, and families may find it challenging to manage cancer during pregnancy. Pregnancies complicated by a cancer diagnosis should be overseen by a multidisciplinary team of doctors. The goal of treatment and diagnosis for pregnant cancer patients should be the same as that of nonpregnant women, with no detrimental impact on the long-term prognosis or development of the fetus. Surgery is a possible choice even in cases of gynecological cancer, and it is ideally performed during the second trimester.

From the time organogenesis is complete until 3 weeks before delivery, the majority of chemotherapy medications can be administered without risk. The time after delivery should be set aside for radiation treatment. Preventing iatrogenic preterm delivery is advisable because it is the most important factor that decides the long-term outcome.

Key Points

1. Though rare both benign and malignant neoplasms are encountered during pregnancy.
2. Clinical examination, ultrasound, and MRI are useful for detecting neoplasms.
3. A multidisciplinary team consisting of obstetricians, gynecologic oncologists, medical oncologists, neonatologists, and counselors to be involved to deliver the best.
4. Management should be individualized.
5. Surgery when indicated should be deferred till the second trimester.
6. When there is a need for chemotherapy, it can also be offered in the second trimester, when organogenesis is complete.
7. Chemotherapy regimens should be judiciously chosen.
8. Cesarean delivery is preferred in invasive cervical cancer and treated vulval cancer.
9. Radical oophorectomy and staging surgery along with cesarean delivery in operable cancer ovary is undertaken after fetal maturity. This can also be done after NACT.
10. Neonates should be handled by an expert neonatologist.
11. Avoid breastfeeding at least 3 weeks from the last chemotherapy.

References

1. Neoplastic Disorders. In. Williams Obst 25th Edn. 2018 Edn. F. Gary Cunningham, Kenneth J. Leveno, Steven L. Bloom, Jodi S. Dashe, Barbara L. Hoffman, Brian M. Casey, Catherine Y. Spong. Publisher McGraw Hill Education.
2. Esim Buyukbayrak E, Karageyim Karsidag AY, Kars B, et al. Cervical polyps: evaluation of routine removal and need for accompanying D&C. Arch Gynecol Obstet. 2011;283(3):581.
3. Long ME, Dwarica DS, Kastner TM, et al. Comparison of dysplastic and benign endocervical polyps. J Low Genit Tract Dis. 2013;17(2):142.
4. Qidwai II, Caughey AB, Jacoby AF. Obstetric outcomes in women with sonographically identified uterine leiomyomata. Obstet Gynecol. 2006;107:376.
5. Stout MJ, Odibo AO, Graseck AS, et al. Leiomyomas at routine second-trimester ultrasound examination and adverse obstetric outcomes. Obstet Gynecol. 2010;116(5):1056.
6. Eibye S, Kjaer SK, Mellemkjaer L. Incidence of pregnancy-associated cancer in Denmark, 1977–2006. Obstet Gynecol. 2013;122:608–17.

7. Lee YY, Roberts CL, Dobbins T, et al. Incidence and outcomes of pregnancy-associated cancer in Australia, 1994–2008: a population-based linkage study. BJOG. 2012;119:1572–82.
8. Smith LH, Danielsen B, Allen ME, et al. Cancer associated with obstetric delivery results of linkage with the California cancer registry. Am J Obstet Gynecol. 2003;189:1128–35.
9. de Haan J, Verheecke M, Van Calsteren K, et al. Oncological management and obstetric and neonatal outcomes for women diagnosed with cancer during pregnancy: a 20-year international cohort study of 1170 patients. Lancet Oncol. 2018;19(3):337–46.
10. Azim HA Jr, Peccatori FA, Pavlidis N. Lung cancer in the pregnant woman: to treat or not to treat, that is the question. Lung Cancer. 2010;67:251–6.
11. Lee HJ, Lee IK, Kim JW, et al. Clinical characteristics of gastric cancer associated with pregnancy. Dig Surg. 2009;26:31–6.
12. Amant F, Verheecke M, Wlodarska I, et al. Presymptomatic identification of cancers in pregnant women during noninvasive prenatal testing. JAMA Oncol. 2015;1:814–9.
13. Lenaerts L, Vandenberghe P, Brison N, et al. Genomewide copy number alteration screening of circulating plasma DNA: potential for the detection of incipient tumors. Ann Oncol. 2019;30:85–95.
14. Han SN, Lotgerink A, Gziri MM, et al. Physiologic variations of serum tumor markers in gynecological malignancies during pregnancy: a systematic review. BMC Med. 2012;10:86.
15. Ayyappan AP, Kulkarni S, Crystal P. Pregnancy-associated breast cancer: Spectrum of imaging appearances. Br J Radiol. 2010;83:529–34.
16. Almuhaideb A, Papathanasiou N, Bomanji J. 18F-FDG PET/CT imaging in oncology. Ann Saudi Med. 2011;31:3–13.
17. Michielsen K, Vergote I, Op de Beeck K, et al. Whole-body MRI with diffusion-weighted sequence for staging of patients with suspected ovarian cancer: a clinical feasibility study in comparison to CT and FDG-PET/CT. Eur Radiol. 2014;24:889–901.
18. Amant F, Berveillere P, Boereal IA, Cardonick E, Fruscio R, et al. Gynecologic cancers in pregnancy: guidelines based on a third international consensus meeting. Ann Oncol. 2019;30:1601–12.
19. National Comprehensive Cancer Network. NCCN clinical practice guidelines in oncology (NCCN guidelines). Breast Cancer. 2017; https://www.nccn.org. Accessed 1 Feb 2018.
20. Han SN, Amant F, Michielsen K, et al. Feasibility of whole-body diffusion-weighted MRI for detection of primary tumour, nodal and distant metastases in women with cancer during pregnancy: a pilot study. Eur Radiol. 2017;28(5):1862–74.
21. Zagouri F, Dimitrakakis C, Marinopoulos S, Tsigginou A, Dimopoulos MA. Cancer in pregnancy: disentangling treatment modalities. ESMO Open. 2016;1:e000016.
22. Amant F, von Minckwitz G, Han SN, et al. Prognosis of women with primary breast cancer diagnosed during pregnancy: results from an international collaborative study. J Clin Oncol. 2013;31:2532–9.
23. Loibl S, Han SN, von Minckwitz G, et al. Treatment of breast cancer during pregnancy: an observational study. Lancet Oncol. 2012;13:887–96.
24. Van der Vange N, Weverling GJ, Ketting BW, Ankum WM, Samlal R, Lammes FB. The prognosis of cervical cancer associated with pregnancy: a matched cohort study. Obstet Gynecol. 1995;85(6):1022–6.
25. Botha MH, Rajaram S, Karunaratne K. Cancer in pregnancy. FIGO CANCER REPORT 2018. Int J Gynecol Obstet. 2018;143(Suppl. 2):137–42.
26. Hunter MI, Monk BJ, Tewari KS. Cervical neoplasia in pregnancy. Part 1: screening and management of preinvasive disease. Am J Obstet Gynecol. 2008;199:3–9.
27. Hunter MI, Monk BJ, Tewari KS. Cervical neoplasia in pregnancy. Part I: screening and management of preinvasive disease. Am J Obstet Gynecol. 2008;199:3.
28. Rob L, Skapa P, Robova H. Fertility-sparing surgery in patients with cervical cancer. Lancet Oncol. 2011;12:192–200.
29. Ricci C, Scambia G, De Vincenzo R. Locally advanced cervical cancer in pregnancy: overcoming the challenge. A case series and review of the literature. Int J Gynecol Cancer. 2016;26:1490–6.

30. La Russa M, Jeyarajah AR. Invasive cervical cancer in pregnancy. Best practice and research. Clin Obstet Gynaecol. 2016;33:44–57. https://doi.org/10.1016/j.bpobgyn.2015.10.002.
31. Leiserowitz GS, Xing G, Cress R, Brahmbhatt B, Dalrymple JL, Smith LH. Adnexal masses in pregnancy: how often are they malignant? Gynecol Oncol. 2006;101(2):315–21. https://doi.org/10.1016/j.ygyno.2005.10.022.
32. Thomassin-Naggara I, Fedida B, Sadowski E, et al. Complex US adnexal masses during pregnancy: is pelvic MR imaging accurate for characterization? Eur J Radiol. 2017;93:200–8.
33. Fauvet R, Brzakowski M, Morice P, et al. Borderline ovarian tumors diagnosed during pregnancy exhibit a high incidence of aggressive features: results of a French multicenter study. Ann Oncol. 2012;23:1481–7.
34. Amant F, Maggen C. Cancer in pregnancy. In: Berek & Hacker's Gynecologic Oncology. 7th ed. Philadelphia: Wolters Kluwer; 2021.
35. Fruscio R, de Haan J, Van Calsteren K, Verheecke M, Mhallem M, Amant F. Ovarian cancer in pregnancy. Best Pract Res Clin Obstet Gynaecol. 2017;41:108–17.
36. Alexander A, Samlowski WE, Grossman D, Bruggers CS, Harris RM, Zone JJ, Noyes RD, Bowen GM, Leachman SA. Metastatic melanoma in pregnancy: risk of transplacental metastases in the infant. J Clin Oncol. 2003;21(11):2179–86. https://doi.org/10.1200/JCO.2003.12.149.
37. O'Meara AT, Cress R, Xing G, Danielsen B, Smith LH. Malignant melanoma in pregnancy. A population-based evaluation. Cancer. 2005;103(6):1217–26. https://doi.org/10.1002/cncr.20925.
38. Brenner B, Avivi I, Lishner M. Haematological cancers in pregnancy. Lancet. 2012;379(9815):580–7. https://doi.org/10.1016/S0140-6736(11)61348-2.
39. Barzilai M, Avivi I, Amit O. Hematological malignancies during pregnancy. Mol Clin Oncol. 2019;10(1):3–9. https://doi.org/10.3892/mco.2018.1759.
40. Shaw P, Duncan A, Vouyouka A, Ozsvath K. Radiation exposure and pregnancy. J Vasc Surg. 2011;53(Suppl.1):28S–34S.
41. Stopenski S, Aslam A, Zhang X, Cardonick E. After chemotherapy treatment for maternal cancer during pregnancy, is breastfeeding possible? Breastfeed Med. 2017;12(2):91–7.
42. Lambertini M, PeccatoriFA AHA. Targeted agents for cancer treatment during pregnancy. Cancer Treat Rev. 2015;41:301–9.

21 Surgical Disorders in Pregnancy

Asayas Bosco

This chapter is to understand the various surgical disorders in pregnancy and the surgeon point of view. Pregnancy is not a contraindication to the standard practice of the surgical management. Pregnancy is a normal physiological condition. But during this physiological condition, surgical pathology can confound the physiological condition and lead to an unfavorable outcome.

Individually, surgery in nonpregnant women will have the risks associated to any individual at that age and her fitness for surgery. But pregnancy and the changes associated to it make the management a very challenging task from the obstetrics and the surgeon's point of view; because technically they are two patients with different physiological composition.

Diagnosing a surgical disorder, more so an abdominal condition, with pregnant uterus is very challenging to the clinical obstetrician and the whole surgical team to avoid wrong or delayed diagnosis. Hence, a multispecialty team approach involving the obstetrician, surgeon, anesthetist, pediatrician, and a nursing department is mandatory and a balancing act will give the best outcome of the pregnancy for the safety of the mother and the child.

The most common concern in the multispecialty team is that well-being of the child and the mother apart from the general risk involved in the without the surgical conditions.

We are left with a pregnant mother and a surgical problem, what should be the approach to avoid risk to mother and child and also do justice to the surgical standard care of the surgical disorders. If surgery has to be done, then how to time the surgery with the pregnancy status. And if conservative route is opted then what is the implication if the disease gets worse.

Most of the time confusion is between the surgical condition that can complicate pregnancy in terms of delayed diagnosis or suboptimal treatment for the fear of fetal

A. Bosco (✉)
Sri Lakshmi Narayana Institute of Medical Sciences, Pondicherry, India

R. Sharma, A. Kumar (eds.), *Systemic Disorders in Pregnancy*,
https://doi.org/10.1007/978-981-96-4876-4_21

loss, stillbirth, etc., can lead to the danger over diagnosis, hence a proper differential diagnosis is warranted.

The following conditions are at most concern from the surgeon point of view apart from a wide range of surgical diagnosis.

Sl. No	System involved	Disease condition
1.	Endocrine disorders	Diffuse hyperplastic goiter Multinodular goiter Graves' thyrotoxicosis Thyroid carcinomas Papillary (most common) Pheochromocytoma
2.	Breast disorders	Fibroadenomas Breast carcinoma Intraductal carcinoma
3.	Abdomen	Cholelithiasis Cholecystitis Appendicitis Pancreatitis Intestinal obstruction Trauma
4.	Hernias	Paraumbilical hernia Inguinal hernia
5.	Perianal disorders	Fissure in ano Hemorrhoids Fistula in ano

Note: The above list includes the common problems for which a surgical team is called; nevertheless other surgical conditions can also may be present like in any nonpregnant women

21.1 Thyroid Disorders

Thyroid disorders are very common and are a part and parcel of pregnancy. Risk of thyroid enlargement is present due the associated physiological stress of pregnancy and present as a diffuse goiter that needs no surgical intervention except investigation. Thyroid-related concerns are hypothyroidism, diffuse hyperplastic goiter, Graves' thyrotoxicosis, thyroid nodules, and malignancy.

It is a routine practice to have thyroid function done in all pregnancy. Hypothyroidism needs only thyroid hormone supplement. Thyrotoxicosis treatment with methimazole (MMI) 3–4% and propylthiouracil (PTU) 2–3% is associated with birth defects. The American Thyroid Association recommends stopping of PTU in the first trimester and change to MMI to avoid risk if liver cell failure in mother. Radioiodine is a contraindication in pregnancy.

A goiter present needs evaluation as the possibility of malignancy is always present. Basic investigation of neck ultrasound and fine needle aspiration cytology (FNAC) has no specific contraindication in any or the trimesters. But a proven malignancy can't wait for 9 months of pregnancy. This waiting period can lead to a lot of risk to the patient and to the fetus. There is clear evidence of adverse pregnancy outcomes in cases of untreated overt hypothyroidism and hyperthyroidism in pregnant women (Level III).

21.2 Pheochromocytoma

This condition can remain silent and present at any time of pregnancy and has a 50% maternal mortality if it remains undiagnosed [1, 2]. This disorder has to be considered in pregnancy when the patient presents with features of preeclampsia, and it comes as a hypertensive emergency.

If detected early, laparoscopic adrenalectomy is possible in the first and second trimester following an alpha blockers administration, still a risk of fetal loss is present. If identified in the third trimester, then elective lower segment cesarean section (LSCS) and adrenalectomy after 6 weeks in the postnatal period.

21.3 Breast Disorders in Pregnancy

Parity is a protective factor for development of breast carcinoma. About 0.3 to 1% of patients do have a simultaneous breast lump, which needs evaluation. As a dictum any lump in the breast is malignant unless proved otherwise. So a minimum of investigation has to be done.

Noninvasive investigation like ultrasound of the breast has no contraindication and can give basic clue to whether the lump is solid or cystic. A limitation to investigation is that mammography or CT scan cannot be done for the fear of radiation to fetus.

Invasive tests like FNAC of the lump is not a contraindication in any trimester but gives very good confirmation of whether it is benign or malignant.

If it is a benign breast lump, then there is no need for surgical intervention during the pregnancy period.

If it is a malignant disease, we need to assess the extent of the disease and the metastatic status, but limitations exist. So, further management still can be done as in a non-obstetric patient, but waiting till the term might carry the risk of metastasis rendering the impossibility of surgical cure for the patient.

The choice of treatment between surgery or chemotherapy, obviously chemotherapy is not the option while the mother is pregnant, we need to plan for surgical cure as a prime modality of treatment. Radiation option in pregnancy is not considered and hence a breast conservative surgery is not possible; therefore, a modified radical mastectomy has to be done with the axillary clearance.

21.4 Breast Abscess

Breast abscess 3–4% is seen more common in puerperal period. It starts as a localized uniductal infection and later grows to a full-blown mastitis involving the entire breast and presents as a tender, erythematous, indurated breast, and with pyrexia. Later a fluctuant mass (abscess),requires urgent drainage under the cover of antibiotics and irrespective of gestational age. This condition is caused mainly by the surface bacteria, namely, the gram positive *Staphylococcus aureus.*

This can be avoided if clinical examination of breast and areola is done at the first visit to the obstetrician. A cracked nipple is always predisposing, so proper care and local hygiene is the key to avoid the problem. Cracked nipples are also a risk factor for galactocele and lactational abscess.

Pregnancy cures a retracted nipple, so this is not a worry.

21.5 Abdominal Disorders and Pregnancy

In abdomen most of the things are complex when it comes to an emergency condition and needs a multidisciplinary team appoarch [3] for the best outcome. For simplification, the abdomen is divided into quadrants to localize a particular organ-specific diagnosis relevant to the quadrant but practical difficulties arise; as the pregnancy progresses, the gravid uterus occupies almost all the quadrants.

About 2% of pregnant women require a non-obstetric operation during pregnancy; the most common operation is appendectomy, followed by cholecystectomy [4].

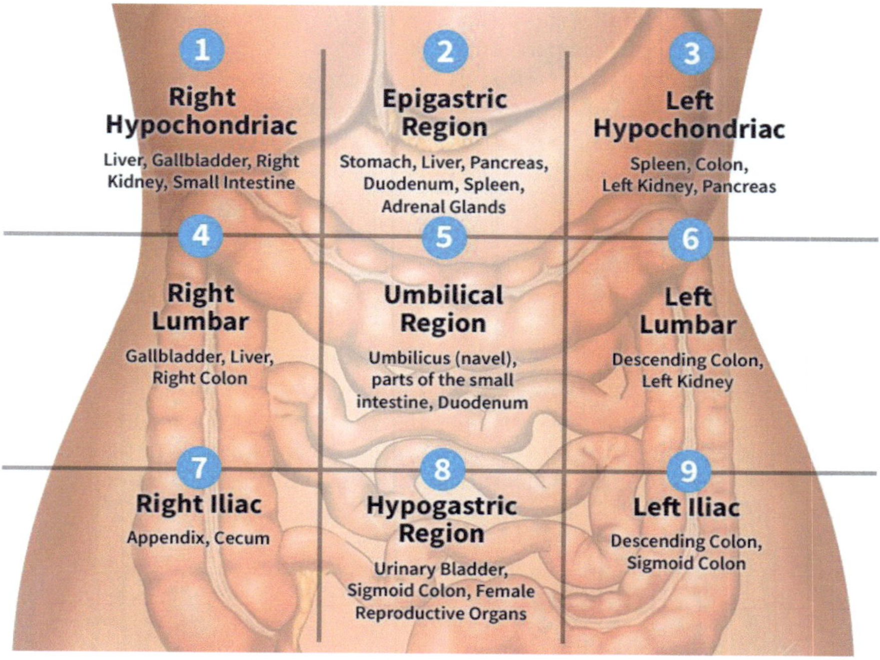

And the specific surgical diagnosis expected in a nonpregnant patient is as given below (Table 21.1).

The above table is a rough guide but as the pregnancy progresses the concept of quadrant specific diagnosis does not hold good for all the trimester. So, the team involved in patient care should keep it in mind that this can be applicable only say first trimester.

Another important dilemma is the role of minimally invasive surgery and pregnancy. As in any non-obstetrics abdomen, diagnosis laparoscopy is gold standard for certain disease like the cholecystectomy but consensus is present only for

Table 21.1 Quadrant-specific differential diagnosis

Right hypochondrium	*Epigastric*	*Left hypochondrium*
Gastroesophageal reflux Peptic ulcer disease Acute cholecystitis Biliary colic	Acute pancreatitis Acute appendicitis	Splenic trauma
Right lumbar	*Umbilical*	*Left lumbar*
Renal or ureteral colic Pyelonephritis Hydronephrosis of pregnancy	Paraumbilical hernia	Renal or ureteral colic Pyelonephritis Hydronephrosis of pregnancy
Right iliac	*Hypogastrium*	*Left iliac*
Acute appendicitis ureteral colic	Inflammatory bowel disease Irritable bowel syndrome	Inflammatory bowel disease Irritable bowel syndrome

selected group of conditions and patients. And important is the trocar placement with only minimal uterine manipulation.

Laparoscopy can be safely performed during any trimester of pregnancy when operation is indicated. And proper intraoperative fetal monitoring is necessary with a minimum pneumoperitoneum possible.

Society of American Gastrointestinal Endoscopic Surgeons recommends the following guidelines for laparoscopic surgery during pregnancy like a proper prior consent, and if possible delay the procedure after second trimester, with proper DVT prophylaxis intraoperatively like pneumatic compression.

For patients either operative or nonoperative treatment of biliary diseases other than acute cholecystitis in the third trimester, endoscopic retrograde cholangiopancreatography rather than common bile duct exploration for symptomatic choledocholithiasis, applying the same criteria for emergent surgical intervention in pregnant and non-pregnant IBD patients, utilizing an open rather than minimally invasive approach for pregnant patients requiring emergent surgical treatment of IBD, and managing pregnant patients with active IBD flares in a multidisciplinary team with IBD expertise [5] ensure best results.

21.6 Acute Appendicitis

Acute appendicitis also poses a diagnostic dilemma with an Incidence of 1:1500–2000 pregnancies and a fetal loss of 3–5% [6]. A diagnosis over clinical suspicion in pregnancy and planning surgery is not recommended in any trimester unless hard evidence is there for appendicitis. The solution to this condition despite inconclusive ultrasonography is an MRI that has a sensitivity of 91.8% and a specificity of 97.9% for appendicitis diagnosis in pregnancy. A complicated appendicitis like perforation has a very high maternal mortality rate. Surgical management is recommended [6].

21.7 Blunt Abdomen Trauma

This is mainly caused by road traffic accidents and domestic violence. Primarily there is no difference in the management except the investigation like serial CT of abdomen indicated cannot be done due the radiation risk to fetus [7].

Blunt abdomen injury in pregnancy can cause abruption of placenta, preterm labor/delivery in addition to uterine rupture and pelvic injuries like a pelvic fracture. Hence effective institution protocol is mandatory for a special situation like this. And nowadays management is purely based on the hemodynamic stability of the patient and most of the treatment plan is toward conservative line [8] and can be managed with multiple transfusion and resuscitation methods, which itself is sufficient in 90% of solid organ injuries with hemoperitoneum. The remaining needs an explorative laparotomy, which has a high rate of miscarriages, which is the last resort of management, and risk has to be taken to prevent maternal mortality at any trimester.

21.8 Pancreatitis

Acute pancreatitis has an incidence of 3 in 10,000 pregnancies. The risk factor being symptomatic gall stone disease present untreated before pregnancy and the other cause is the hyperlipidemia [9]. The severity of the disease can be scored by various scoring systems but by and large RANSON's criteria is followed in assessing the severity of the disease. For better diagnosis, CT with contrast is required but pregnancy is the contraindication for the CT and the contrast, hence has to be managed with ultrasound or MRI scan. Acute pancreatitis range from just a mild disease to a very severe disease causing multiorgan failure to acute respiratory distress syndrome (ARDS) and has very high mortality rate.

21.9 Burns

Burns during pregnancy is very difficult to manage. Minor burns are not an issue but major burns have to be treated as any other burns, the percentage of burns have to be calculated and Parkland formula for fluid management and same thing nothing much fluid replacement and other things so that also needs to be taken into account the problems if there is extensive burns the assessment of mothers fundal height to fetal monitoring all this becomes a very complicated issue especially if the burns are over the abdomen. Fluids management to choice of higher antibiotic is all limited. So a restricted way of treatment balancing the fluids and the antibiotics along with monitoring of fetus is essential.

21.10 Perianal Disorder

The problems are most common in the third trimester and very distressing to the other pregnancy-related problems of the gravid uterus. Upright posture and staying in a sitting or a standing posture for long hours with an already existing perianal problem makes it worse in the third trimester.

21.11 Fissure in Ano

Fissure in ano is caused purely by constipation, created by the gravid uterus and improper dietary habits. In pregnancy, fissures are seen in unusual position and often multiple. About 80% of the fissure in ano is a self-limiting problem and can be treated with high fiber diet and laxatives in moderate dose to relieve constipation,

Local creams can also be used. Fissure in ano rarely requires lateral sphincterotomy.

21.12 Hemorrhoids

Hemorrhoids are present in about 60% of the pregnant mothers. The grade of haemorriods progress as the trimester progresses as the compression of the gravid uterus on the rectal venous system and cause a physiological engorgement. So in third trimester a worse grade of hemorrhoids is present. Just palliative management of avoiding sitting and standing for longer duration should be avoided. Sitz bath and topical antihemorrhoidal cream application is recommended. And surgery is indicated if there is profuse bleeding with clots. A hemorrhoidectomy with the necessary fetal monitor can be done in the third trimester. Most hemorrhoids can be managed conservatively [10] with lifestyle modifications.

21.13 Perianal Abscess

Perianal abscesses are caused by infection of the perianal glands and ascending infection, and septicemia is a common feature in pregnancy. This condition requires surgery, irrespective of the trimester [11]. And surgery is done under the cover of antibiotics with preferably a spinal anesthesia. Crohn's disease is to be considered in multiple fistulation with abscess.

References

1. Singh S, Sandhu S. Thyroid disease and pregnancy. Treasure Island: StatPearls Publishing; 2024.
2. Roderick J. Clifton-Bligh, the diagnosis and management of pheochromocytoma and paraganglioma during pregnancy. Rev Endocr Metab Disord. 2023;24(1):49–56.
3. Vujic J, et al. Non-obstetric surgery during pregnancy—an eleven-year retrospective analysis. BMC Pregnancy Childbirth. 2019;19:382.
4. Nan X, et al. Laparoscopic cholecystectomy in pregnancy: a seven-year retrospective study from an Australian tertiary center. Cureus. 2023;15(12)
5. Kumar SS, et al. SAGES guidelines for the use of laparoscopy during pregnancy. Surg Endosc. 2024;38:2947–63.
6. Smolkin C, Kiridly A, Pryor A. Appendicitis during pregnancy: Best surgical practices and clinical management. Open Access Surg. 2023;2023(16):95–103.
7. Murphy NJ, Jeffrey D. Quinlan, Trauma in pregnancy: assessment, management, and prevention. Am Fam Physician. 2014;90(10):717–24.
8. Greco PS, Day LJ, Pearlman MD. Guidance for evaluation and Management of Blunt Abdominal Trauma in pregnancy. Obstet Gynecol. 2019 Dec;134(6):1343–57.
9. Madro A. Pancreatitis in pregnancy—comprehensive review. Int J Environ Res Public Health. 2022;19:16179.

10. Poskus T, et al. Preventing hemorrhoids during pregnancy: a multicenter, randomized clinical trial. BMC Pregnancy Childbirth. 2022;22:374.
11. Bužinskiene D, Sabonyte-Balšaitiene Ž, Poškus T. Perianal diseases in pregnancy and after childbirth: frequency, risk factors, impact on women's quality of life and treatment methods. Front Surg. 2022;9:788823.

MIX
Papier aus verantwortungsvollen Quellen
Paper from responsible sources
FSC® C105338

If you have any concerns about our products,
you can contact us on
ProductSafety@springernature.com

In case Publisher is established outside the EU,
the EU authorized representative is:
Springer Nature Customer Service Center GmbH
Europaplatz 3, 69115 Heidelberg, Germany

Printed by Libri Plureos GmbH
in Hamburg, Germany